Y0-BCL-384

Florida Hospital College of
Health Sciences Library
800 Lake Estelle Drive
Orlando, FL 32803

2013
DF
In print
classic

CHILDBIRTH

*Changing Ideas and Practices in Britain and
America 1600 to the Present*

Series Editor
PHILIP K. WILSON
Truman State University

Assistant Editors
ANN DALLY
*Wellcome Institute for the History of
Medicine (London)*

CHARLES R. KING
Medical College of Ohio

Florida Hospital College of
Health Sciences Library
800 Lake Estelle Drive
Orlando, FL 32803

A GARLAND SERIES

Series Contents

VOLUME

3

METHODS AND FOLKLORE

Edited with introductions by

PHILIP K. WILSON

Truman State University

W Q
160
.W 752
1996
v. 3

19942

GARLAND PUBLISHING, Inc.
New York & London
1996

Florida Hospital College of
Health Sciences Library
800 Lake Estelle Drive

Introductions copyright © 1996 Philip K. Wilson
All rights reserved

Library of Congress Cataloging-in-Publication Data

Childbirth : changing ideas and practices in Britain and America
    1600 to the present / edited with introductions by Philip K.
    Wilson.
        p.   cm.
    Includes bibliographical references.
    Contents: v. 1. Midwifery theory and practice — v. 2. The
medicalization of obstetrics: personnel, practice, and instruments — v. 3. Methods and folklore — v. 4. Reproductive science, genetics, and birth control — v. 5. Diseases of pregnancy
and childbirth.
    ISBN 0-8153-2230-5 (v. 1 : alk. paper). — ISBN 0–8153–
2231–3 (v. 2 : alk. paper). — ISBN 0–8153–2232–1 (v. 3 : alk.
paper). — ISBN 0–8153–2233–X (v. 4. : alk. paper). — ISBN 0–
8153-2234–8 (v. 5 : alk. paper)
    1. Childbirth—United States—History.   2. Childbirth—Great
Britain—History.   3. Obstetrics—United States—History.   4. Obstetrics—Great Britain—History.   I. Wilson, Philip K., 1961–.
    [DNLM: 1. Obstetrics—trends.   2. Midwifery—trends.
3. Pregnancy Complications.   4. Reproduction Techniques.
5. Genetic Counseling.   6. Contraception. WQ 100C5356   1996]

RG518.U5C47   1995
618.4'0973—dc20
DNLM/DLC
for Library of Congress   96–794
                                                                   CIP

Printed on acid-free, 250-year-life paper
Manufactured in the United States of America

CONTENTS

ALTERNATIVE METHODS OF CHILDBIRTH

Painless Childbirth

Cesarean Sections

LIST OF ILLUSTRATIONS

SERIES INTRODUCTION

Since "most women are interested in the process of giving birth and all men have been born," it would appear, claimed Johns Hopkins University obstetrician Alan Guttmacher, that the topic of childbirth would above all other topics have "universal appeal." Birth is also one of the most individual moments in each of our lives, but although we all share the experience of being delivered, the processes of delivery have been diverse. The social gathering around the childbed common in earlier times has, for many, been replaced by a more isolated hospital bed. Maternal fears of the pain and peril of procreation have, or so prevalent historiography would have us believe, intensified with the intervention of male midwives and obstetricians bringing along new "tools" of the trade. Markedly divergent beliefs about assisting in labor have created polarized factions of attendants. Some have followed wisdom similar to what Britain's Percivall Willughby first espoused in 1640:

> Let midwives observe the ways and proceedings of nature for the production of her fruit on trees, or the ripening of walnuts or almonds, from their first knotting to the opening of the husks and falling of the nut . . . . These signatures may teach midwives patience, and persuade them to let nature alone perform her work.

Opposing factions adhered to claims similar to that of the early nineteenth-century Philadelphia midwifery professor, Thomas Denman, that belief in:

> labour, being a natural act, . . . not requiring the interference of art for either its promotion or its accomplishment . . . has, from its influence, retarded, more perhaps than any other circumstance, the progress of improvement in this most important branch of medical science.

Other comparisons among midwifery writings suggest that although expectant women may no longer avoid the same "longings and cravings" of pregnancy as did their eighteenth-century forebears, contemporary concern about exposing pregnant women and their fetuses to nicotine, alcohol, known teratogenic agents, and unwarranted stress evokes similar warnings. Indeed, as the works included in this collection illustrate, many similar concerns have been shared by expectant mothers and their labor attendants for centuries.

Although there is a substantial literature on childbirth, it typically lacks the full medical, historical, and social contextualization that these volumes provide to readers. This series attempts to fill the gap in many institutions' libraries by bringing together key articles illuminating a number of issues from different perspectives that have long concerned the expectant mother and the attendants of her delivery regarding the health of the newborn infant. Primary and secondary sources have been culled from British and American publications that focus on childbirth practices over the past three hundred years. Some represent "classic" works within the medical literature that have contributed towards a more complete understanding of pertinent topics. The series draws from historical, sociological, anthropological, and feminist literature in an attempt to present a wider range of scholarly perspectives on various issues surrounding childbirth.

Childbirth: Changing Ideas and Practices is intended to provide readers with key primary sources and exemplary historiographical approaches through which they can more fully appreciate a variety of themes in British and American childbirth, midwifery, and obstetrics. For example, general historical texts commonly claim that childbed (puerperal) fever, a disease that has claimed hundreds of thousands of maternal lives, provoked much fear throughout most of British and American history. In addition to supplying readers with historians' interpretations, *Childbirth: Changing Ideas and Practices* also provides discussions of the causes and consequences of particular cases of childbed fever taken directly from the medical literature of the nineteenth and twentieth centuries, thereby enabling a better understanding of how problematic this disorder initially was to several key individuals who, after first increasing its incidence, ultimately devised specific methods of its prevention.

The articles in this series are designed to serve as a resource for students and teachers in fields including history, women's studies, human biology, sociology, and anthropology. They will also meet the socio-historical educational needs of pre-medical and nursing students and aid pre-professional, allied health, and midwifery instructors in their lesson preparations. Beyond the content of many collections on the history of childbirth, readers frequently need access to the primary sources in order to develop their own interpretive accounts. This five-volume series expands the readily accessible knowledge base as it represents both actual experiences and socio-historical interpretations on select developments within the history of British and American childbirth, midwifery, and obstetrics.

Given the vast and expanding literature on childbirth, it is virtually impossible anymore for any single source to provide a complete coverage of such a broad topic. Selecting precisely what articles to include has been, at times, a painstaking process. We have purposefully excluded works on abortion as many of these articles have recently been reprinted elsewhere. Additionally, we have only touched upon midwifery/obstetrical education, the legal issues surrounding childbirth, marriage, sex, and the family, and genetic engineering since numerous contemporary works in print thoroughly discuss these themes. Seminal articles that are currently available in other edited collections as well as general review articles were, with a few exceptions, not considered for reprinting in this series. There are several areas, including eclampsia, the development and role of the placenta, pregnancy tests throughout history, and Native American childbirth practices, for which suitable articles are wanting. Related topics such as gynecology and gynecological diseases, pediatrics, neonatology, postnatal care and teratology, though of considerable concern to many pregnant women and health care providers, appear beyond the scope of our focus and the interest of our generalist readers. Space did not allow for me to cover childbirth from the viewpoint of what have historically been considered alternative or complementary healing professions such as herbalism, homeopathy, or osteopathy, even though thousands of healthy children have been delivered by practitioners in these professions. The exorbitant permission charges that some journals charge for reprinting their articles has prohibited us from including many important articles. Finally, we have opted not to reprint biographical articles as the typical lengthy accounts of individuals would have precluded addressing more general relevant issues.

Series Acknowledgments

I am grateful to the many individuals who offered their assistance, suggestions, and support throughout the gestation of this project. Foremost, I wish to thank my co-editors, Dr. Charles R. King and Dr. Ann Dally, both highly valued "team players" in what truly became an international collaborative creation. Their medical expertise and historiographical suggestions strengthened the content of this series. Laura Runge, my undergraduate research student and Ronald E. McNair Post-Baccalaureate Achievement Program Scholar, provided exemplary editorial assistance throughout the growth of this project. In addition, she introduced Melissa Blagg-Holcomb to our team, a truly exceptional undergraduate scholar, without whom this project would not have been completed in such a timely manner. Melissa's professional interest in nurse midwifery expanded the scope of the literature we reviewed. Our research would have been impossible without the assistance of many librarians, archivists, and other members of the research staff. In particular, I wish to thank Lyndsay Lardner (The Wellcome Institute, London), Susan Case (Clendening Medical History Library, Kansas City), and Janice Wilson (Hawaii Medical Library, Honolulu; Sterling Medical Library, New Haven, and Pickler Memorial Library, Kirksville) for their exemplary library assistance. The unfailing efforts of Sheila Swafford, in Pickler Library's Reference Department, to secure necessary material are deeply appreciated. The editors also wish to thank Jane Carver, Prof. Mark Davis, Prof. Robbie Davis-Floyd, Nancy Dellapenna, Clare Dunne, Prof. Paul Finkelman, Andy Foley, Dr. Denis Gibbs, Ferenc Gyorgyey, Gwendolyn Habel, Jack Holcomb, Charlene Jagger, Maggie Jones, Carol Lockhart, Barb Magers, Andrew Melvyn, Jean Sidwell, Prof. John Harley Warner, Prof. Dorothy C. Wertz and the staffs of the Library of the Royal Society of Medicine (London), the National Library of Medicine (Bethesda), Pickler Memorial Library (Kirksville) and Rider Drug and Camera (Kirksville) for their assistance in preparing certain parts of this series. Leo Balk of Garland Publishing, Inc., proved to be a stable sounding board during the conception stage of *Childbirth*, a role that Carole Puccino has deftly carried on throughout the later progressions of this work. I also wish to thank my colleagues at the University of Hawaii-Manoa, Yale University, and Northeast Missouri State University (soon to be Truman State University) for their support and critical commentary on this project. Northeast Missouri State University provided a Summer Faculty Research Grant which allowed for the timely completion of this project. Finally, I remain indebted to my wife, Janice, for providing astute critique, able reference library assistance, and continual support and encouragement.

Philip K. Wilson

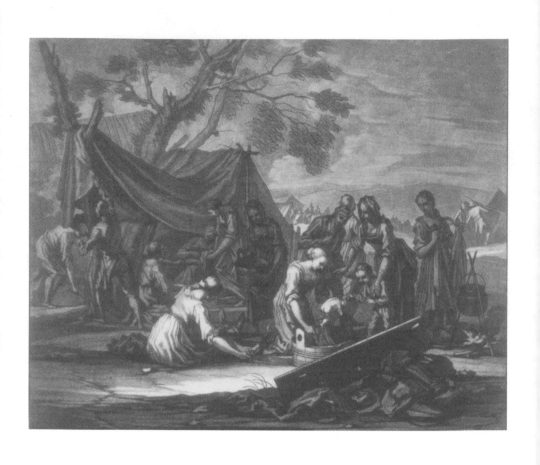

INTRODUCTION

Before the application of medical science to the study of pregnancy and childbirth, common wisdom about childbearing was intertwined with folklore, superstition, and old wives' tales. The folklore of pregnancy typically concerns predicting outcomes: knowing or controlling the sex of the baby, predicting the difficulty of the delivery, and prognosticating the health of mother and child. Two common examples of this folklore are that a pregnant woman should never reach up over her head to avoid tangling the umbilical cord, and a sharp object under the birthing bed would make for a faster delivery.

Similar knowledge about proper behavior still abounds. People still predict the sex of the baby by whether the mother carries high or low, wide or out front. The pregnant woman rubs olive oil or commercial creams on her belly to prevent stretch marks. There are still innumerable regional and individual variations of what to do and what not to do in order to avoid the tragedies of death and deformity, such as waiting until the fetus is thought to be viable before preparing a nursery or avoiding images of children with visible birth defects.

Even if a pregnant woman does not believe that viewing horrific images can make an impression upon the infant she carries, she may, herself, be deeply affected by photographs of potential pathological outcomes of pregnancy. Many obstetrical texts are filled with such nightmare-inducing images. Who wouldn't take comfort in doing all the right things, being extra careful, when her fantasies of the perfect baby are haunted by monsters? No fairy tale changeling would look more horrific than the long-dead, grossly misshapen infants in many clinical texts and teratological treatises.

There are precious few stories or images in either popular or clinical literature of severely deformed infants—to some, the worst imaginable outcome of pregnancy—that emphasize the baby, the life, and the family rather than the clinical aspects of the deformity. In *Spiritual Midwifery,* midwife Ina May Gaskin tells the story of Ira, a child born at home with anencephaly, or a marked developmental deformity of the brain and lack of a cranial covering.[1] He was taken to the hospital, but reclaimed by his parents after they learned that he was being given no food or drink in anticipation of his inevitable death. Ira's mother made little hats to cover his exposed brain and fed him from an eye dropper. A photo in the book shows him in his hat, held in a friend's arms. In some ways, he resembles the textbook image of anencephaly: bulging eyes, broad trunk, long arms. The midwife and family found themselves correcting Dr. Williams, the family physician: "When he talked about these babies he would use the medical term, 'anencephalic monster,' and we'd say, 'No, a baby, not a monster, a *baby*,' and that you should treat them like babies."[2]

The word "monster" has largely fallen out of vogue within medicine, after centuries of use. In the past, as Dudley Wilson described,

> the monster—whether or not seen as sign or portent—was definitely regarded as being outside human society, where human society is equated with normality. . . . When the New World begins to be discovered in the sixteenth century, its inhabitants are seen as aspects of humanity so unusual as to be put into the monster class.[3]

In the nineteenth century, natural scientists, medical men and teratologists began to more closely examine "monsters," but with very few exceptions, they did not approach them as patients. As Robert Bogdan has lucidly argued,

> Science and medicine had not gained control over human deviation. People with physical and mental anomalies were still in the public domain—curiosities. Later, in the twentieth century, however, as the power of professions increased, people with physical and mental anomalies came under the purview of professionals. Many were secluded from the public. Their conditions were to be treated, and possibly cured, behind closed doors. They were to be pitied and, from a eugenics perspective, feared. They needed to be locked away for the protection of society. This trend was followed by the growth of organized charities, the rise of professional fundraising, and the invention of the poster child, with "pity" used as the dominant mode of presenting human differences.[4]

Modern perceptions of cause and effect during fetal development are quite different than in the days of Blondel and Turner's debate about the "monstrous" imagination, described in an article in this volume by Wilson. Superstition has been replaced with the findings of clinical research. Monsters are not caused by the mother's imagination; neural tube defects are caused in part by insufficiencies in the mother's diet and in part by genetic factors. Medical management of pregnancy and childbirth is based on clinical evidence rather than hindsight and anecdote—or so we tend to assume.

Barbara Katz Rothman, in her introduction to *In Labor: Women and Power in the Birthplace,* describes the social location of medical knowledge:

> The obstetrical perspective on pregnancy and birth is held to be not just one way of looking at it, but to be the truth, the facts, science: other societies may have beliefs about pregnancy, but we believe our medicine has the *facts*. But obstetrical knowledge, like all knowledge, comes from *somewhere*: it has a social, historical, and political context. Medicine does not exist as 'pure,' free of culture or free of ideology.[5]

Although some aspects of obstetrical practice are, indeed, the results of research supported by repeated study, some of it really is folklore validated by medical tradition more than anything else.

A growing awareness of the socially constructed nature of obstetric practice has opened the field up to the criticism of consumers and scholars, as well as clinicians. Some childbearing women and their families have started rejecting as medical folklore many aspects of obstetric practice long held to be grounded in science. Social and clinical researchers have reevaluated nearly every aspect of childbearing, examining the objective merit of standard practices.

One vivid example of this reevaluation is seen in the VBAC (vaginal birth after cesarean) movement which holds that, contrary to medical tradition, a woman who has been delivered by cesarean section may subsequently have a vaginal delivery that is at least as safe as having another cesarean. The principle of "once a cesarean, always a cesarean" was established within obstetrics at a time when the procedure was first being transformed from a commonly lethal, last, desperate measure into an established surgical intervention with reasonably positive outcomes. The scar from the "classical" incision technique then in use tended to rupture unpredictably in subsequent pregnancies, threatening the lives of both mother and infant. Repeat cesareans prevented maternal and fetal mortality.[6]

However, the classical incision was eventually replaced by the lower segment transverse incision. This variation leaves a scar much less likely to rupture, and less likely to cause adverse effects for mother or infant if it does rupture; but the perception remained among obstetricians that repeat cesareans were a necessary and life-saving intervention. Although several studies support the assertion that a repeat cesarean poses a greater risk of maternal and fetal morbidity and mortality than does VBAC with the lower segment transverse incision, and most cesareans are now performed using this technique, repeat cesareans are still common practice.[7]

The current broad range of childbirth practices reflects attempts by groups and individuals to impose definitions on the biological universals of reproduction. Natural childbirth advocates see a healthy process where obstetricians see risk, in the same way that Ina May Gaskin saw a spiritual being where Dr. Williams saw a monster. Each individual responds to the situation out of his or her own experience and training.

Another widespread example of the attempted imposition of beliefs permeates the writings of Grantly Dick-Read, Fernand Lamaze, and Frederick Leboyer on "painless childbirth." "Lamaze" and other techniques consciously create a definition of the situation via training for the expectant family, intended to facilitate less medicated births. According to Lamaze, "Painless childbirth is a fact." There is no "miracle, . . . illusion or subterfuge" to the method Lamaze promotes. Rather, he steadfastly argues that any woman can *learn* how to give birth, "in the same way that she learns how to swim, or write or read; and she does so without pain."[8]

Recent research supports the idea that there is room for multiple interpretations of childbirth. Knowing the historical context of the development of existing views allows further evaluation of them on their own terms, rather than by the folklore of one tradition. Markedly divergent beliefs about the extent of assisting in labor and childbirth have created polarized factions of attendants. Some have followed the wisdom of letting nature perform the work while others have insisted that withholding all possible assistance only retards the progress towards improving the obstetrical art. The first section of this volume, "Alternative Methods of Childbirth," examines eighteenth- through twentieth-century attempts to relieve maternal pain during childbirth as well as the religious opposition to the use of anesthesia. Additional articles present case descriptions and biosocial concerns of cesarean sections. Various methods of natural childbirth are examined from the viewpoint of relieving pain, changing birthing positions, and moving birth from home to hospital then home again. The second section examines the "Oral Traditions and Folklore of Pregnancy and Childbirth," including an account of pregnancy and childbirth among "primitive people," beliefs about the formation of "monsters," and a medical dispute over the power of the maternal imagination.

Philip K. Wilson

NOTES

1. Ina May Gaskin, *Spiritual Midwifery* (Summertown, Tenn.: The Book Publishing Company, 3rd edition, 1990), 455–56.
2. Gaskin, *Spiritual Midwifery,* 456.
3. Dudley Wilson, *Signs and Portents: Monstrous Births from the Middle Ages to the Enlightenment* (London: Routledge, 1993), 4.
4. Robert Bogdan, *Freak Show. Presenting Human Oddities for Amusement and Profit* (Chicago: University of Chicago Press, 1988), 277–78.
5. Barbara Katz Rothman, *In Labor: Women and Power in the Birthplace* (New York: Norton, 1982), 33.
6. N. Cohen and L. Estner, *Silent Knife: Cesarean Preventions and Vaginal Birth After Cesarean* (South Hadley, Mass.: Bergin and Garvey, 1983).
7. Jeffrey P. Phelan and Steven L. Clark, eds., *Cesarean Delivery* (New York: Elsevier, 1988).
8. Fernand Lamaze, *Painless Childbirth: Psychoprophylactic Method* (New York: Pocket Books, 1965), 167, 16.

FURTHER READING

Adams, Alice E. *Reproducing the Womb: Images of Childbirth in Science, Feminist Theory, and Literature.* Ithaca and London: Cornell University Press, 1994.

Apple, Rima D., ed. *Women, Health, and Medicine in America: A Historical Handbook.* New York and London: Garland Publishing, Inc., 1990.

Arney, William Ray and Jane Neill. "The Location of Pain in Childbirth: Natural Childbirth and the Transformation of Obstetrics." *Sociology of Health and Illness* 4 (1982): 1–24.

Bailey, Flora L. "Suggested Techniques for Inducing Navaho Women to Accept Hospitalization During Childbirth and for Implementing Health Education." *American Journal of Public Health* 38 (1948):1418–23.

Bradley, Robert A. *Husband-Coached Childbirth.* New York: Harper and Row, 1965.

Campbell, Marie. *Folks Do Get Born.* New York: Garland Publishing, Inc., 1985. Originally published: New York: Reinhart and Co., 1946.

Chertok, L. *Psychosomatic Methods in Painless Childbirth: History, Theory and Practice.* New York: Pergamon Press, 1959.

Cohen, N. and L. Estner. *Silent Knife: Cesarean Preventions and Vaginal Birth After Cesarean.* South Hadley, Mass.: Bergin and Garvey, 1983.

Cohen, Nancy Wainer. *Open Season: A Survival Guide for Natural Childbirth and VBAC in the 90s.* Westport, Conn.: Greenwood Publishing Group, 1991.

Cosslett, Tess. *Writing Childbirth: Modern Discourses of Motherhood.* Manchester, England: Manchester University Press, 1994.

Davis-Floyd, Robbie E. "The Technological Model of Birth." *Journal of American Folklore* (Oct./Dec. 1987): 479–95.

DeVries, Raymond G. "The Alternative Birth Center: Option or Co-optation?" *Women and Health* 5 (1980): 47–60.

Dick-Read, Grantly. *Childbirth without Fear.* London: Heinemann, 1942.

Dougherty, Molly C. "Southern Lay Midwives as Ritual Specialists." in *Women in Ritual and Symbolic Roles,* edited by Judith Hoch-Smith and Anita Spring, 151–64. New York: Plenum Press, 1978.

Dundes, L. "The Evolution of the Maternal Birthing Position." *American Journal of Public Health* 77 (May 1987): 636–41.

Eakins, Pamela, ed. *The American Way of Birth.* Philadelphia: Temple University Press, 1986.

Eakins, Pamela. "The Rise of the Free Standing Birth Center: Principles and Practice." *Women and Health* 9 (1984): 49–64.

Engelmann, G.J. *Labor Among Primitive Peoples.* St. Louis: J. H. Chambers & Co., 1883.

Forbes, Thomas R. "Chalcedony and Childbirth: Precious and Semi-Precious Stones as Obstetrical Amulets." *Yale Journal of Biology and Medicine* 35 (April 1963):390–401.

Goldfarb, Connie Serouya. "The Folklore of Pregnancy." *Psychological Reports* 62 (1988): 891–900.

Haire, Doris. *The Cultural Warping of Childbirth.* Hillside, N.J.:

International Childbirth Education Association, 1972.

Henriksen, E. "Pregnancy Tests of the Past and Present." *Western Journal of Surgery, Obstetrics and Gynecology* 49 (1941):567–75.

Kay, Margarita Artschwager. *Anthropology of Human Birth*. Philadelphia: F.A. Davis Company, 1982.

Lamaze, Fernand. *Painless Childbirth*. trans. by L.R. Celestin. Chicago: Henry Regnery, 1970.

Leboyer, Frederick. *Birth Without Violence*. London: Fontana, 1977.

Martin, Emily. *The Woman in the Body: A Cultural Analysis of Reproduction*. Boston: Beacon Press, 1987.

Michaelson, Karen L., et al. *Childbirth in America: Anthropological Perspectives*. Massachusetts: Bergin and Garvey, Inc., 1988.

Nash, Anedith and Jeffrey E. Nash. "Conflicting Interpretations of Childbirth: The Medical and Natural Perspectives." *Urban Life* 7 (1979): 493–511.

National Institutes of Child Health and Human Development. *Cesarean Childbirth* (NIH Final Report). Bethesda, MD: NIH, 1981.

O'Connor, Bonnie B. "The Home Birth Movement in the United States." *Journal of Medicine and Philosophy* 18 (1993): 147–74.

Park, Katharine and Lorraine J. Daston. "Unnatural Conceptions: The Study of Monsters in Sixteenth and Seventeenth-Century France and England." *Past and Present* 92 (1981): 20–54.

Phelan, Jeffrey P. and Steven L. Clark, eds. *Cesarean Delivery*. New York: Elsevier, 1988.

Poppers, P. J. "The History and Development of Obstetric Anesthesia." *Anaesthesia: Essays on Its History*, edited by Joseph Ruprecht, et al., 133–40. New York: Springer-Verlag, 1985.

Porter, Roy. "The Secrets of Generation Display'd: *Aristotle's Masterpiece* in Eighteenth-Century England." *Eighteenth-Century Life* 9, n.s. 3 (May 1985): 1–21.

Rothman, Barbara Katz. *In Labor: Women and Power in the Birthplace*. New York: W. W. Norton & Co., 1991.

Sakala, Carol. "Medically Unnecessary Cesarean Section Births: Introduction to a Symposium." *Social Science & Medicine* 37, no. 10 (1993) 1177–98.

Sandelowski, Margarete. *Pain, Pleasure, and American Childbirth: From the Twilight Sleep to the Read Method, 1914–1960*. London and Westport, Conn: Greenwood Press, 1984.

Schutte, Anne Jacobson. "'Such Monstrous Births': A Neglected Aspect of the Antinomian Controversy." *Renaissance Quarterly* 38 (1985):85–106.

Sullivan, Deborah A., and Rose Weitz. *Labor Pains: Modern Midwives and Home Birth*. Yale University Press, 1989.

Stewart, David and Lee Stewart, eds. *Safe Alternatives in Childbirth*.

Chapel Hill, NC: NAPSAC, 1976.

Tew, Marjorie. *Safer Childbirth? A Critical History of Maternity Care*. London: Chapman and Hall, 2nd ed., 1995.

Todd, Dennis. *"Imagining Monsters: Miscreations of the Self in Eighteenth-Century England."* Chicago: University of Chicago Press, 1995.

Wertz, Richard W. and Dorothy C. Wertz. *Lying-In: A History of Childbirth in America*. New York and London: Macmillan, 1977.

Wilson, James G. and Josef Warkany. "The History of Organized Teratology in North America." *Teratology* 31 (1985): 285–96.

Young, J. H. *Caesarean Section: The History and Development of the Operation from Earliest Times*. London: H. K. Lewis & Co., Ltd., 1944.

Alternative Methods of Childbirth

Painless Childbirth
Cesarean Sections
20th-Century Natural Childbirth

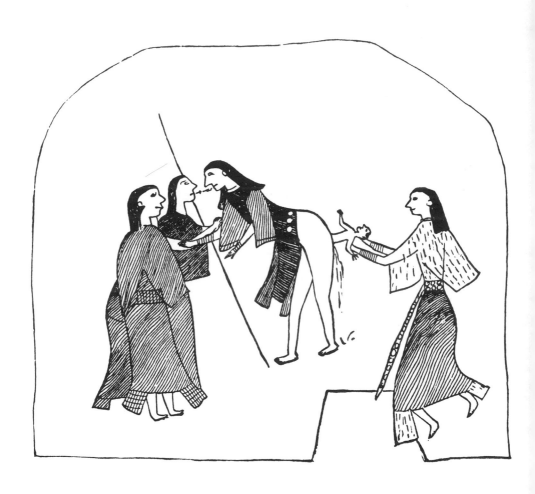

Painless Childbirth

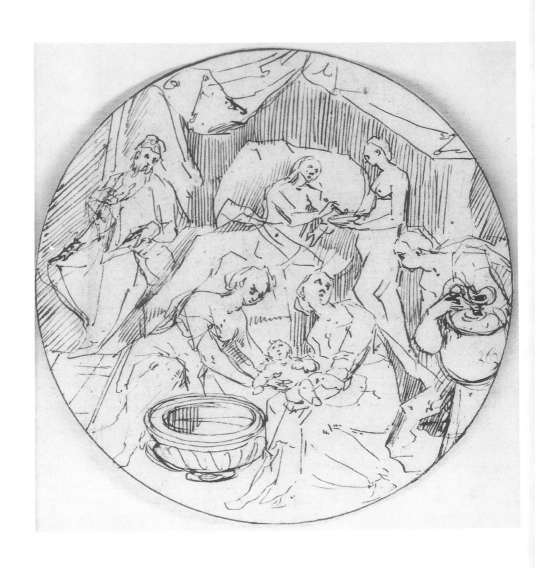

An Eighteenth Century Method of Pain Relief in Obstetrics

In 1803, Benjamin Rush, who unquestionably was the outstanding figure in American medicine at the time, wrote that in 1795 "he was led to suppose that blood-letting might be effectual in lessening the violence of the disease and pains of parturition." In his writings Rush always considered pregnancy and labor as diseases, although in his lectures he treated them under physiology. He attributed the ease with which Turkish women delivered their children to their use of sweet oil in the last months of pregnancy. Climate in the Brazils, in Calabria, in Sicily, and in several of the West Indian Islands exerts a similar influence, he said. The scanty diet of the Indian women enables them to resume their work after an unaided labor of a few hours. He noted that labor in the last stages of chronic diseases is short and comparatively easy, and both Rush and Dewees regarded pain as evidence of disease. For pain relief he advocated (i) bloodletting (30 ounces) in the beginning of labor, (ii) purgation, (iii) a low diet for ten to fourteen days before the patient is confined. In all fairness it should be said that he did not recommend bloodletting in all cases. Where there had been great previous inanition and where there were marks of languor and feeble action of the

5

system the remedies should be of an opposite nature, *i.e.,* supportive. He mentioned that Dr. Dewees had used bloodletting for the relief of pains of parturition when he was in practice in Abington, Pennsylvania.

William Potts Dewees (1768–1841) was the earliest great American obstetrician. His *Compendious System of Midwifery,* first published in 1824, went through twelve editions and kept abreast of the times. Thoms, in his *Chapters on American Obstetrics,* is surprised at "the small amount of real progress that has been made in obstetrical science since his time."

Dewees was graduated and received an M.B. from the University of Pennsylvania in 1789. He began practising in the village of Abington, just outside of Philadelphia, and it was there in September 1789 that he first noticed the beneficial effect of bleeding on the course of difficult labor. The patient had a history of very hard labors, many of her babies having to be delivered with the crotchet. He was very apprehensive about the outcome of the present pregnancy. To make matters worse she had a severe hemorrhage from the lungs at the onset of labor, but to everyone's astonishment the patient had a quick, easy labor. Dewees reasoned "it could be from no other cause than relaxation, produced by exercise and alarming haemorrhagy. I quickly resolved to take advantage of this kind hint, by endeavoring to imitate this good example." His subsequent experiences in Abington confirmed his reasoning and when in 1793 he returned to Philadelphia to practise and to get his M.D. degree, he chose this subject as his graduation thesis. It was dedicated to William Shippen, M.D., Professor of Anatomy; Benjamin Rush, M.D., Professor of the Institutes of Practice of Physic, etc.; Caspar Wistar, M.D., Adjunct Professor of Anatomy; James Woodhouse, M.D., Professor of Chemistry; Benjamin Smith Barton, M.D., Professor of Materia Medica; and Philip Syng Physick, M.D., Professor of Surgery in the University of Pennsylvania. The publication of this thesis gained for him so great a reputation that he became a candidate for the newly created chair of midwifery which was established at the University of Pennsylvania in 1810. In 1819 he reprinted an enlarged, 156-page edition of his thesis.

This subject was also used as a graduation thesis by Peter Miller in 1804, which would seem to be enough proof that the method had met with favor in Philadelphia or at least in the University of Pennsylvania. Fittingly enough, Peter Miller's thesis was dedicated to Philip Syng Physick, for the "Father of American Surgery" was a great believer in the relaxing effect of copious bloodletting. Miller cited the case of an irreducible dislocation of the shoulder that Physick easily and painlessly reduced after a free venesection.

What, if any, was the basis of the faith of these early Philadelphians in bloodletting as a means of relieving the pains of parturition? In the beginning of the nineteenth century Philadelphians were no longer pioneers. The women, while not subjected to the hardships of the frontier, were not exposed to the enervating influences of running water, indoor toilets, telephones, and household electricity. Dr. John Redman, under whom Dewees "read medicine," and who was considered the most skilful obstetrician of his time, saw only complicated cases. William Shippen (1736–1808) was the first in Philadelphia to have an obstetric practice, and he had time to be the Professor of Anatomy at the University of Pennsylvania in addition. So far as is known, he was not concerned about the pains of parturition. It is more than likely the average patient took labor as a matter of course and did not consider it particularly painful.

It was only in the presence of dystocia that medical attention was invoked. When the dystocia was due to bony deformity or malposition, some destructive operation was usually resorted to. (Be it remembered the first successful Cæsarean section in the United States was in 1793.) When the dystocia was uterine, the doctor was helpless. The long, tedious cases, especially if there was a constriction ring present, were particularly painful. The patient in such instances feels severe pain but makes no progress. Dewees recognized two general classes of dystocia — that due to bony deformity and that due to faulty behavior of the soft parts. He was concerned in his essay only with the latter. He regarded pain as an evidence of "disease" and in his efforts to solve the cause of the pain he studied the various forms of uterine contractions. He concluded that contraction of the circular fibres, such as hour-glass contraction, caused no pain, but when such contraction was present, the action of the longitudinal fibres necessary to overcome this obstruction caused severe pain. He enumerated several means of relieving the diffiulty. Morphine was not without its drawbacks. Warm baths had been tried, but bloodletting was the remedy *par excellence*. He related the first case (cited above) that directed his attention to this remedy and many other cases, all quite dramatic.

In Case XXIII, Dewees actually demonstrated a constriction ring.

1798, Dec. 18th. I was called to Mrs. Z——, in labour with her third child; she had been in labour eight and forty hours; waters discharged, thirty-six; the uterus well dilated; pains severe, but no advancement of the labour; during the pain the child's head, which was well situated, would be forced down, but as soon as it ceased it would again be retracted; this had been the case for many hours before I saw her. In order to ascertain the cause of this delay, I introduced my hand into the uterus, and presently found the cause of the child not advancing; a circle, as it were, of the uterus had closed between the shoulders of the child and the head, which prevented their passing. I bled her to fainting; pains soon came on, and she was quickly delivered.

Cases of this kind have frequently occurred to me; but in some cases I have been obliged to turn, after the bleeding, (which before was impossible) and in one or two others I have been obliged to use the forceps. These cases resemble each other so much in almost every respect, that I do not think it necessary to detail but one.

In his 1819 edition Dewees says: "We can, with a confidence that should only be produced by experience, recommend this operation, not only as a safe, but a certain remedy for all the objects we have just contemplated: and feel the more

7

security in doing this, since it met the approbation of the late venerable and ex-perienced professor of anatomy and midwifery, Dr. Shippen; who declared with a candour which did him honour, he could have spared much pain and misery to many of his patients had he used the lancet more freely in tedious and painful cases from rigidity."

In conclusion, he says he had never seen puerperal fever, milk abscess, or the swelled leg, take place in any patient who had suffered large or repeated bleed-ings during their labor; "it seems to ward off every blow aimed at the puerperal state."

There remains the problem of explaining why the remedy that was so ex-tensively used and which evidently had merit disappeared so completely from the obstetrician's armamentarium. Venesection was the prime remedy for in-flammation both in medicine and surgery. Benjamin Rush used it routinely in the great yellow fever epidemic, and maintained that he cured patients who would have died otherwise. Others were just as strongly of the opinion that he had done harm. The discussion grew acrimonious and ended in a famous lawsuit which settled nothing except that Cobbett, Rush's opponent, and editor of *Rush Light,* had to leave the State. The next generation, under the leadership of Louis and his statistical method, settled such controversies in a more scientific method. The verdict in regard to venesection was adverse. The reaction against bloodletting was so intense that the procedure disappeared completely even in such fields as congestive heart failure and eclampsia, where there was no doubt as to its effi-ciency. It was almost a hundred years before venesection began to be used again. Now it is used in some cases of congestive heart failure and certain cases of eclampsia. Substitution transfusions for erythroblastosis might be considered a modern adaptation of the oldfashioned bloodletting. Quite recently bloodletting for surgical hemostasis has been advocated by Donald Hale. Before the pro-fession had recovered from the marked and universal reaction against venesection, anesthesia had been discovered and obstetricians became engrossed in ether controversies, chloroform controversies, twilight sleep, etc.

Summary

A method of pain relief, when the pain was due to irregular or spasmodic uterine contraction, was extensively used in Philadelphia at the end of the eight-eenth and the beginning of the nineteenth century. It was advocated by two of the outstanding physicians of the country and served as a graduation thesis in at least two instances. An explanation as to why an apparently worthwhile method of treatment was abandoned is suggested.

It is interesting that Dewees in the beginning of the nineteenth century and Grantly Dick Read in our own times should have emphasized the importance of relaxation in comfortable childbirth and it is also interesting that Dewees should have chosen the quicker and more certain means of causing relaxation.

REFERENCES

RUSH, B. *Medical Repository*, 1803, 6, 26.

DEWEES, W. P. *The means of lessening pain and facilitating certain cases of difficult parturition*. Philadeiphia, 1806, p. 95.

DEWEES, W. P. *Ibid.*, Philadelphia, 1819. p. 156.

MILLER, PETER. An essay on the means of lessening pains of parturition. Philadelphia, 1804.

Richmond, Virginia   M. PIERCE RUCKER

ORIGINAL COMMUNICATION.

Notes on the Employment of the Inhalation of Sulphuric Ether in the Practice of Midwifery. By J. Y. SIMPSON, M.D., Professor of Midwifery in the University of Edinburgh.

ABUNDANT evidence has of late been adduced, and is daily accumulating, in proof of the inhalation of sulphuric ether being capable, in the generality of individuals, of producing a more or less perfect degree of insensibility to the pains of the most severe surgical operations. But whilst this agent has been used extensively, and by numerous hands, in the practice of surgery, I am not aware that any one has hitherto ventured to test its applicability to the practice of midwifery. I am induced, therefore, to hope that the few following hurried and imperfect notes, relative to its employment in obstetric cases, may not at the present time prove uninteresting to the profession.

Within the last month I have had opportunities of using the inhalation of ether in the operation of turning, in cases of the employment of the long and of the short forceps, as well as in several instances in which the labour was of a natural type, and consequently required no special form of artificial aid.

The first case in which I employed the ether vapour, occurred on the 19th of January. Some details of the result have been already published in the last number of this Journal (see p. 639). The pelvis of the mother was greatly contracted in its conjugate diameter from the projection forwards and downwards of the promontory of the sacrum; the lumbar portion of the spine was distorted; and she walked very lamely. The present was her second confinement. Her first labour had been long and difficult; she began to suffer on a Monday, and after a protracted trial of the long forceps, was at last delivered by craniotomy late on the subsequent Thursday night. Even after the cranium had been fully broken down, a considerable time and much traction had been required to drag the diminished and mutilated head of the infant through the contracted brim of the pelvis; and she was long in recovering. Contrary to the urgent advice of her medical attendant, Mr Figg, he was not made aware of her present or second pregnancy till she had arrived at nearly the end of the ninth month. It was thus too late to have recourse to the induction of premature labour, which had been strongly pressed upon her as the only means of saving her child, should she again fall in the family way. The pains of her second labour commenced in the forenoon of the 19th. I saw her with Mr Figg at five o'clock in the afternoon, and again at seven. The os uteri was pretty well dilated, the liquor amnii not evacuated, the presenting head very high, mobile, and difficult to touch; and a pulsating loop of the umbilical cord was felt floating below it in the unruptured bag of membranes. From five to nine o'clock the pains seemed only to push the circle of the os uteri further downwards, without increasing its dilatation, or making the head in any degree enter into the pelvic brim. Assisted by Dr Zeigler, Dr Keith, and Mr Figg, I shortly after nine o'clock made the patient inhale the ether vapour. As she afterwards informed us, she almost immediately came under the anodyne influence of the ether. But in consequence of doubts upon this point, its use was continued for nearly twenty minutes before I proceeded to turn the infant (as I had previously predetermined to do). A knee was easily seized, and the child's extremities and trunk readily drawn down ; but extreme exertion was required in order to extract the head. At length it passed the contracted brim with the anterior part of its right parietal bone deeply indented by pressure against the projecting promontory of the sacrum, and the whole cranium flattened and compressed laterally. The infant gasped several times, but full respiration could not be established. The transvere or biparietal measurement of its head, at the site of the indentation, was, in its compressed state, not more than $2\frac{1}{2}$ inches. Hence we judged the conjugate diameter of the pelvic brim not to exceed this. The infant was large, and rather above the usual size. It weighed 8 lbs. On afterwards examining the head and removing the scalp, no fracture could be found at the seat of the indentation. The thin parietal bone had merely bent inwards.

On questioning the patient after her delivery, she declared that she was quite unconscious of pain during the whole period of the turning and extracting of the infant, or indeed from the first minute or two after she first commenced to breathe the ether. The inhalation was discontinued towards the latter part of the process, and her first recollections on awaking were " hearing," but not " feeling," the head of the infant " jerk " from her (to use her own expressions), and subsequently she became more roused by the noise caused by the preparation of a bath for the child. She quickly regained full consciousness, and talked with gratitude and wonderment of her delivery, and her insensibility to the pains of it. Next day I found her very well in all respects. I looked in upon her on the 24th (the fifth day after delivery), and was astonished to find her up and dressed, and she informed me that on the previous day she had walked out of her room to visit her mother. Mr Figg informs me that her further convalescence has been interruptedly good and rapid.

I have previously alluded to two cases of delivery by the forceps, in which the patients were under the action of ether at the time of the operation. The woman in the first of these cases was brought into the Royal Maternity Hospital, in strong labour, early on the morning of the 3d February. It was her second confinement. At her first accouchement (seven years before), she had been delivered by instruments, in Ireland, and had been informed by the attendant practitioner, that artificial delivery would be similarly required at her future labours. I saw her between ten and eleven o'clock A.M. The os uteri was well dilated, the membranes ruptured, and the pains extremely strong and frequent; but the large head of the child seemed not to enter fully into the brim, and was little affected by the powerful uterine contractions under which the patient was suffering. By three o'clock her pulse had risen to above 125 beats a minute, and it appeared to the medical officers present, that it would be improper to allow the ineffectual and exhausting efforts of the patient to be longer continued. She was then, at my request, brought under the influence of ether. Dr Moir, with great skill, applied the long forceps upon the head of the child. He subsequently was obliged to use strong traction during the pains that followed, and becoming temporarily fatigued with his efforts, I supplied his place. After the head fully passed the brim, the forceps were laid aside, and one or two uterine contractions finished the delivery. The child was large and strong, and cried vigorously soon after it was expelled. During the whole of this severe operation the patient appeared quiet and passive. The cries of her child speedily roused her from her etherized state, and she subsequently assured Dr Moir that she had felt comparatively little or no pain during the whole operation and delivery.

On the evening of the 12th February, I saw another forceps case with my friend, Dr Graham Weir. The patient was advanced in life, and it was her first confinement. The waters had escaped early, and the anterior lip of the uterus had subsequently become forced down in a very swelled and œdematous state before the head of the infant. After this obstruction was overcome, the child's head speedily descended upon the floor of the pelvis; but it was there impeded in its further progress by the narrow transverse diameter of the outlet. Under the compression of the converging tuberosities of the ischia, the bones of the fœtal cranium soon began to overlap; but at last, no further progress being made, the patient becoming exhausted by a continuous labour of about twenty-four hours, and the soft parts being evidently well relaxed and prepared, Dr Weir applied the short forceps, and extracted a living infant. For a considerable time before this operation was adopted, I exhibited the vapour of ether to the patient; under it she speedily became quite narcotized. Its action was kept up, and the pains appeared to be so strong as almost to warrant the idea that nature would yet be sufficient; but ultimately, instrumental delivery was, as I have already stated, had recourse to. The mother did not fully recover from her state of etherization for ten or fifteen minutes after delivery, and then stated that she was quite unaware of anything that had been done, and of what had occurred.

As far as they go, the preceding cases point out one important result. In all of them, the uterine contractions continued as regular in their recurrence and duration after the state of etherization had been induced, as before the inhalation was begun.—The emotion of fear has appeared to me to suspend, in one or two nervous patients, the recurrence of the first pains, after the apparatus was adjusted and its employment commenced; but this effect speedily passed off; and as yet I have seen no instance in which the pains were sensibly diminished in intensity or frequency after the ether had fairly begun to act.—Indeed, in some cases they have appeared to me to have become increased as the consciousness of the patient was diminished. This has more particularly occurred with one or two patients, who breathed ether, combined with tincture of ergot, or containing a solution of its oil. A woman was brought into the Maternity Hospital on the 28th February, after being in labour for 30 or 40 hours. It was her second child. Subsequently to her entering the hospital, at seven P.M., scarcely any decided uterine contraction could be said to take place. The os uteri was well opened, but the head was still high in the pelvis; and when I saw her at four A.M. of the following morning, nine hours after her entrance into the hospital, little or no advance whatever had been made, and the case was becoming an anxious one. She was then made to inhale equal parts of sulphuric ether and tincture of ergot. In the course of a few minutes a series of extremely powerful uterine contractions supervened, and the child was born within a quarter of an hour of the commencement of inhalation. The mother subsequently declared that she recollected nothing at all of her delivery, except the removal of the after-birth. In this case, was the re-excitement of strong pains the result of the action of the sulphuric ether, or of the ergot, or of both? Or was it a simple but very strange coincidence? More facts than I yet possess are necessary to decide such a question; but I have seen some cases which lead me to believe that other therapeutic agents besides those I have named may be readily introduced into the system by means of pulmonary inhalation.[1]

A more extensive and careful series of investigations than I have yet been able to institute, may perhaps show that in some constitutions, and under some circumstances or *degrees* of intensity, the process of etherization may possibly interfere with the uterine contractility, particularly in the earlier stages of the labour. At the same time, various analogies would lead us to expect that, as I have hitherto found, the action of the uterus would go on uninterruptedly, when the psychical influence of the mind and purely cerebral functions was suspended, as in the more complete states of etherization. At all events, if we may judge from the analogous

---

[1] Dr Richard Pearson, who, in 1795, was, I believe, the first person that recommended the inhalation of sulphuric ether as a therapeutic agent (see his Account of the Nature and Properties of different kinds of Airs, p. 24) suggested also the use of it impregnated with opium, squill, cicuta, &c.; and he speaks of the effect of " an emetic given in this manner." He employed the simple sulphuric ether vapour in some cases of phthisis, asthma, hooping cough, croup, and catarrh, recommending it to be inhaled, after being rectified and washed, from a cup, through an inverted funnel, or, with children, by " wetting a handkerchief with it, and holding it near the nose and mouth." See Fort Simmons' Medical Facts and Observations, vol. vii. p. 96. In the 13th volume of the Dictionnaire des Sciences Medicales (1816) p. 385, Nysten has described a particular apparatus, like some of our modern forms, for the inhalation of sulphuric ether. See also vol. xvii. p. 134. Vaporizable substances, when introduced into the system in this manner, probably pass undigested and unchanged into the circulation, and " seem (observes Wagner) to make their way into the blood through the unbroken vascular membrane [of the bronchial cells] with the *same* certainty and ease as when they are injected *directly* into the veins " (Elements of Physiology, 1842, p. 443.) Will this not explain both the rapidity and intensity of their action when thus used?

experiments of Vollkmann, Bidder, Kölliker, and others, upon the simple contractions and rhythmic actions of the heart, intestines, &c., the motory nervous powers of the uterus belong to the ganglionic and to the spinal systems, and are not in any necessary dependence upon the brain or mind. Indeed, Ollivier and Nasse have published cases of perfect paraplegia, notwithstanding which the act of parturition in the human female proceeded regularly in its course, and without conscious pain. In the one case (Ollivier's), the cord was compressed and destroyed from the first to the fourth dorsal vertebra by a collection of acephalo cysts;[1] and, in the other instance (Nasse's), complete paralysis had followed a fracture of the third and fourth cervical vertebræ.[2]   Of course such lesions necessarily prevented the brain exerting any influence upon the uterus, or its contractions.

Long ago, in discussing this subject, Haller adduced the authority of Harvey, Smellie, Lamotte, &c., to prove that uterine contractions and labour may go on with the mother, " ignara, stupida et sopita, et immobili, et apoplectica, et epileptica, et convulsionibus agitata,[3] et ad summum debili."[4]   Deneux mentions a fact still more in point, because in it the analogy with the operation of ether is still stronger, or indeed identical. " A woman," says he,[5] " was brought to the Hotel Dieu at Amiens in a comatose state, in consequence of her taking spirituous liquors since the commencement of labour. She was delivered in the natural manner in this state; the sleep continued for some time after delivery. The woman, on awaking, much surprised at finding her delivery completed, congratulated herself on having made so happy a discovery, and declared she would make use of it if she had again occasion."[6]

In obstetric as in surgical practice, the degree of insensibility produced by etherization, and its accompanying phenomena, differ much in different instances. In some, a state of total apathy and

---

[1] Traité de la Moelle Epiniere, p. 784.
[2] Untersuchungen zur Physiologie, &c. — Dr Cheyne reports a case of fatal hemorrhagic apoplexy and hemiplegia, in which, without any apparent pains, "the uterus (observes Dr Kellie) appears, as an involuntary muscle, to have acted in the most perfect manner in expelling the fœtus and secundines," the day before death. The child was born alive. Cases of Apoplexy and Lethargy, p. 91 and 161.
[3] " During the continuance of puerperal convulsions, uterine action is *not* suspended, although no signs of pain are manifested by the woman, if she remain comatose." Dr F. Ramsbotham's Obstetric Medicine (1844) p. 455.
[4] Elementa Physiologiæ, tom. viii. p. 420.
[5] Receuil Periodique de la Societé de Medicine, April 1818.
[6] The celebrated case of the Countess de St Geran is sufficiently remarkable in relation to the present subject. See full and long details of it in Gayot's Causes Celebres, tom. i. p. 142 to 266.   After the Countess had been nine hours in labour with her first child, the midwife in attendance exhibited to her a potion (*breuvage*), which rendered her insensible till the following morning. When the Countess then awoke to consciousness, she found herself bathed in blood, the abdominal tumour fallen, and all the signs of recent delivery present; but the child born during her state of insensibility had been removed, and its existence was even denied to her. It was years afterwards proved, to the satisfaction of the French law courts, that the Countess had been delivered of a male child during an induced lethargic condition, and that the infant had been surreptitiously conveyed away to a distance, and brought up as the son of a poor man. The child's claims were, after much litigation, fully acknowledged, he was restored to his parents, and ultimately succeeded to his father's title. What Nepenthean " breuvage" could possibly produce the alleged effect?

insensibility seems to be produced; others move about and complain more or less loudly during the uterine contractions, though afterwards, when restored to their state of common consciousness, they have no recollection of any suffering whatever, or, indeed, of any thing that had occurred during the inhalation and action of the ether; others again, remain quite aware and conscious of what is going on around them, and watch the recurrence of the uterine contractions, but feel indifferent to their effects, and not in any degree distressed by their presence; and in another class again, the attendant suffering is merely more or less diminished and obtunded, without being perfectly cancelled and annulled.

On the evening of the 13th inst, in two cases that rapidly followed each other, I witnessed, in the above respect, two very different conditions induced by the use of the ether. The patients (who each had borne several children previously) were both placed under the influence of it just as the os uteri became fully opened, and in neither did the full expulsion of the infant through the pelvic passages require above twelve or fifteen minutes. My first patient (the wife of a clergyman) subsequently stated, that she knew all that was said and done about her, was aware of the pains being present, but felt no distress from any of them till the supervention of the last strong contraction which drove the head out of the vulva, and the feeling then seemed to partake of the character of strong pressure, rather than of actual pain. Subsequently she told me, she could only look back with regret to the apparently unnecessary suffering she had endured in the birth of her former infants. The second patient, a lady of a timid temperament, and very apprehensive about the result of her present confinement, was induced with difficulty to inhale the ether vapour; but it speedily affected her when once she did begin. In two or three minutes she pushed the apparatus from her mouth, talked excitedly to a female relative present, but was immediately induced to recommence the inhalation; and subsequently, according to her own statement, " wakened out of a dream, and unexpectedly found her child born." Like many others, she thought hours instead of minutes had elapsed, from the commencement of the inhalation to the period of the complete restoration of consciousness. Making apparently an effort of memory, she afterwards inquired if she had not once awakened out of her dreamy state, and spoken some nonsense to her friend.

A careful collection of cautious and accurate observations will no doubt be required, before the inhalation of sulphuric ether is adopted to any great extent in the practice of midwifery. It will be necessary to ascertain its precise effects, both upon the action of the uterus, and of the assistant abdominal muscles; its influence, if any, upon the child; whether it gives a tendency to hemorrhage or other complications; the contra-indications peculiar to its use; the most certain modes of exhibiting it; the length of time it may be employed, &c.[1] In no case have I observed any harm whatever

---

[1] I have, during labour, kept patients under its influence for upwards of half an hour. In exhibiting it, the first, or exhilarating stage of its effects should be passed

to either mother or infant, follow upon its employment. And, on the other hand, I have the strongest assurance and conviction, that I have already seen no small amount of maternal suffering and agony saved by its application. The cases I have detailed sufficiently show its value and safety in cases of operative midwifery. And here, as in surgery, its utility is certainly not confined to the mere suspension and abrogation of conscious pain, great as, by itself, such a boon would doubtlessly be. But in modifying and obliterating the state of conscious pain, the nervous *shock* otherwise liable to be produced by such pain, particularly whenever it is extreme, and intensely waited for and endured, is saved to the constitution ; and thus an escape gained from many evil consequences that are too apt to follow in its train.[1] Granting that experience will yet be able to prove its safety and efficacy in modifying and annulling the pains of labour, will (I have repeatedly heard the question asked) the state of etherization ever come to be generally employed with the simple object of assuaging the pains of *natural* parturition ? Or (as the problem has not unfrequently been put to me) would we be " justified" in using it for such a purpose ? In conclusion, let us consider this point for a moment.

Custom and prejudice, and, perhaps, the idea of its inevitable necessity, make both the profession and our patients look upon the amount and intensity of pain encountered in common cases of natural labour, as far less worthy of consideration than in reality it is. Viewed apart, and in an isolated light, the degree of actual pain usually endured during common labour is as great, if not greater, than that attendant upon most surgical operations. I allude particularly to the excessive pain and anguish, which in nine out of ten cases accompany the passage of the child's head through the outlet of the pelvis and external parts. Speaking of common or natural labour in its last stages, Dr Merriman observes, the pulse gradually " increases in quickness and force ; the skin grows hot ; the face becomes intensely red ; drops of sweat stand upon the forehead ; and a perspiration, sometimes profuse, breaks out all over the body ; frequently violent tremblings accompany the last pain, and at the moment that the head passes into the world, *the extremity of suffering seems to be beyond endurance.*"[2]

---

through as rapidly as possible, and the patient never allowed to be excited or irritated by the nurse or others. I have heard its use strenuously denounced on the ground that its effects, though good, are still of an intoxicating character. But on the same ground, the use of opium, &c. &c., in medicine, to relieve pain, and procure sleep, should be equally reprobated and discarded.

[1] On what division or divisions of the nervous system does the nervous shock operate—the cerebral, spinal, or ganglionic? If on the former, it should be kept in abeyance by due etherization. I once saw Dr Robertson amputate, at the shoulder joint, an arm sadly shattered an hour or so before by a railway injury. The man received the injury, during the operation, and for several hours afterwards, when he was in a state of insensibility from deep intoxication; and at last wakened up, not knowing what had happened. His recovery was rapid and uninterrupted. Would it have been so if his nervous system had been sufficiently alive to the double shock of the operation and injury ? Out of eighteen cases of primary amputation, mentioned in Dr Peacock's Report, and performed during four years in the Edinburgh Hospital. this man and another patient were the only two that survived.

[2] Synopsis of Parturition, p. 15.

Or, take the picture of the suffering of the mother in the last stage of natural labour, as pourtrayed by the most faithful of living observers—Professor Naegele of Heidelberg—"The pains (he observes) of this stage are still more severe, painful, and enduring; return after a short interval, and take a far greater effect upon the patient, than those of the previous stage. Their severity increases so much the more from the additional suffering arising from the continually increasing distention of the external parts. They convulse the whole frame, and have hence been called the *dolores conquassantes*. The bearing down becomes more continued, and there is not unfrequently vomiting. The patient quivers and trembles all over. Her face is flushed, and with the rest of the body, is bathed in perspiration. Her looks are staring and wild; the features alter so much that they can scarcely be recognised. Her impatience rises to its maximum with loud crying and wailing, and frequently expressions which, even with sensible, high principled women, border close upon insanity. Everything denotes the violent manner in which both body and mind are affected."[1]

I have stated that the question which I have been repeatedly asked is this—will we ever be "justified" in using the vapour of ether to assuage the pains of natural labour ?   Now, if experience betimes goes fully to prove to us the safety with which ether may, under proper precautions and management, be employed in the course of parturition, then, looking to the facts of the case, and considering the actual amount of pain usually endured (as shown in the above descriptions of Merriman, Naegele, and others),[2] I believe that the question will require to be quite changed in its character. For, instead of determining in relation to it whether we shall be "justified" in using this agent under the circumstances named, it will become, on the other hand, necessary to determine whether on any grounds, moral or medical, a professional man could deem himself "justified" in withholding, and *not* using any such safe means (as we at present pre-suppose this to be), provided he had the power by it of assuaging the agonies of the last stage of natural labour, and thus counteracting what Velpeau describes as "those piercing cries, that agitation so lively, those excessive efforts, those inexpressible agonies, and those pains apparently intolerable,"[3] which accompany the termination of natural parturition in the human mother.

EDINBURGH, FEBRUARY 1847.

---

[1] Lehrbuch der Geburtshülfe, p. 104. See British and Foreign Medical Review, vol. xix. p. 64.

[2] Dr Rigby in his System of Midwifery, p. 103, observes, " This is the moment of greatest pain, and the patient is quite wild and frantic with suffering; it approaches to a species of insanity," &c.

[3] Traité des Accouchemens, vol. i. p. 449. " Ces cris perçans, cette agitation si vive, ces efforts excessifs, ces angoisses inexprimables, ces douleurs qui parassaient intolerables," &c.

W. S. PLAYFAIR, M. D., F. R. C. P.,

CHAPTER IV.

ANÆSTHESIA IN LABOR.

A FEW words may be said as to the use of anæsthetics during labor—a practice which has become so universal that no argument is required to establish its being a perfectly legitimate means of assuaging the sufferings of childbirth. Indeed, the tendency in the present day is in the opposite direction, and a common error is the administration of chloroform to an extent which materially interferes with the uterine contractions and predisposes to subsequent post-partum hemorrhage.

Agents Employed.—Practically speaking, the only agent hitherto employed in this country is chloroform, although the bichloride of methylene and ether have been occasionally tried. Of late years, chloral has been extensively used by some, and, as I believe it to be an agent of very great value, I shall first indicate the circumstances under which it may be employed.

Chloral.—The peculiar value of chloral in labor is that it may be safely administered at a time when chloroform cannot be generally employed. The latter, while it annuls suffering, very frequently tends in a marked degree to diminish uterine action. This is a familiar observation to all who have employed it much during labor, as the diminution of the force and intensity of the pains, and the consequent retardation of the labor, often oblige us to suspend its inhalation, at least temporarily. Indeed, this very property of annulling uterine action is one of its most valuable qualities in obstetrics, as in certain cases of turning. For such purposes it is necessary to give it to the surgical extent, which we endeavor to avoid when it is used simply to lessen the suffering of ordinary labor. Still, it is not always easy to limit its action in this way, and thus it very frequently does more than we wish. Such diminution in the intensity of uterine contraction is comparatively of less consequence in the propulsive stage, and it is generally more than counterbalanced by the relief it affords. In the first stage it is otherwise, and, practically speaking, chloroform is generally not admissible until the head is in the pelvic cavity.

Chloral is especially the Anæsthetic of the First Stage.—Chloral, on the other hand, has no such relaxing effects on uterine contraction. It cannot, it is true, compete with chloroform in its power of relieving pain, but it produces a drowsy state in which the pain is not felt nearly so acutely as before. It is therefore in the first stage of labor, while the pains are cutting and grinding, and during the dilatation of the cervix, that it finds its most useful application. It is especially valuable in those cases, so frequently met with in the upper classes, in which the pains produce intolerably acute suffering, but with little effect on the progress of the labor. In them the os is often thin and rigid and the pains very frequent and acute, but little or no dilatation is effected. When the patient

19

is brought under the influence of chloral, however, the pains become less frequent but stronger, nervous excitement is calmed, and the dilatation of the cervix often proceeds rapidly and satisfactorily. Indeed, I know of nothing which answers so well in cases of rigid, undilatable cervix, and I believe its administration to be far more effective, under such circumstances, than any of the remedies usually employed.

Object and Mode of Administration.—The object is to produce a somnolent condition which shall be protracted as long as possible. For this purpose 15 grains of chloral may be administered every twenty minutes until three doses are given. This generally suffices to produce the desired effect. The patient becomes very drowsy, dozes between the pains, and wakes up as each contraction commences. It may be necessary to give a fourth dose at a longer interval, say an hour after the third dose, to keep up and prolong the soporific action; but this is seldom necessary, and I have rarely given more than a drachm of chloral during the entire progress of labor. Another advantage of this treatment is that, while it does not interfere with the use of chloroform in the second stage, it renders it necessary to give less than otherwise would be called for, and thus its action can be more easily kept within bounds. On the whole, therefore, I am inclined to consider chloral a very valuable aid in the management of labor, and believe that it is destined to be much more extensively used than is at present the case. So far as my experience has yet gone, I have not met with any symptoms which have led me to think that it has produced bad effects; and I have known many patients sleep quietly through labor, without expressing any excessive suffering or asking for chloroform, who under ordinary circumstances would have been most urgently calling for relief. It occasionally happens that the patient cannot retain the chloral from its tendency to produce sickness; it may then be readily given per rectum in the form of enema.

Chloroform.—Generally speaking, we do not think of giving chloroform until the os is fully dilated, the head descending, and the pains becoming propulsive. It has often, indeed, been administered earlier, for the purpose of aiding the dilatation of a rigid cervix; and there is no doubt that it often succeeds well when employed in this way, but I have already stated my belief that chloral answers this purpose better.

Only to be Given during the Pains.—There is one cardinal rule to be remembered in giving chloroform during the propulsive stage, and that is that it should be administered intermittently, and never continuously. When the pain comes on a few drops may be scattered over a Skinner's inhaler, which affords one of the best means of administering it in labor, or placed within the folds of a handkerchief twisted into the form of a cone. During the acme of the pain the patient inhales it freely, and at once experiences a sense of great relief; and as soon as the pain dies away the inhaler should be removed. In the interval between the pains the effect of the drug passes off, so that the higher degree of anæsthesia should never be produced. Indeed, when properly given consciousness should not be entirely abolished, and the patient, between the pains, should be able to speak and understand what is said to her. This intermittent administration constitutes the peculiar safety of chloroform administered in labor; and it is a fortunate circumstance that, as yet, there is, I believe, no case on record of death during the inhalation of chloroform for obstetric purposes.[1] This is obviously due to the effect of each inhalation passing off before a fresh dose is administered.

The effect on the pains should be carefully watched. If they become very materially lessened in force and frequency, it may be necessary to stop the inhalation for a short time, commencing again when the pains get stronger; which effect may be often completely and easily prevented by mixing the chloroform with about one-third of absolute alcohol, which, originally recommended, I believe, by Dr. Sansom, increases the stimulating effects of chloroform, and thus diminishes its tendency to produce undue relaxation. The amount administered must vary, of course, with the peculiarities of each individual case and the effect produced, but it need never be large. As the head distends the perineum and the pains get very strong and forcing, it may be given more freely, and to the extent of inducing even complete insensibility just before the child is born.

Ether as a Substitute for Chloroform.—In cases in which chloroform has lessened the force of the pains ether may be given instead with great advantage. It certainly often acts well when chloroform is inadmissible on account of its effects on the pains, and, so far as my experience goes, it has not the property of relaxing the uterus, but, on the contrary, has sometimes seemed to me distinctly to intensify the pains. Of late I have used a mixture of one part of absolute alcohol, two of chloroform, and three of ether. This is less disagreeable than ether, and has not the over-relaxing effects of chloroform.

Precautions.—Bearing in mind the tendency of chloroform to produce uterine relaxation, more than ordinary precautions should always be taken against post-partum hemorrhage in all cases in which it has been freely administered.

In cases of operative midwifery it is often given to the extent of producing complete anæsthesia. In all such cases it should be administered, when possible, by another medical man, and not by the operator, because the giving of chloroform to the surgical degree requires the undivided attention of the administrator, and no man can do this and operate at the same time. I once learnt an important lesson on this point. I had occasion to apply the forceps in the case of a lady who insisted on having chloroform. When commencing the operation I noticed some suspicious appearances about the patient, who was a large stout woman with a feeble circulation. I therefore stopped, allowed her to regain consciousness, and delivered her without anæsthesia, much to her own annoyance. Just one month after labor she went to a dentist to have a tooth extracted, and took chloroform, during the inhalation of which she died. This impressed on my mind the lesson that no man can do two things at the same time. The partial unconsciousness of incomplete anæsthesia, in which the patient is restless and tossing about, renders the application of forceps, as well as all other operations, very difficult.

[1 In the *Transactions of the American Gynæcological Society* for the year 1877 are five cases of chloroform-poisoning occurring in obstetrical cases, reported by Dr. W. T. Lusk of New York. In three, restoration was effected by artificial respiration, but in two death resulted absolutely.—ED.]

Therefore, unless the patient can be completely and fully anæsthetized, it is better to operate without chloroform being given at all.

[In the United States the dangers attending the use of chloroform in obstetric practice have, in large measure, banished it from the lying-in chamber. Some obstetricians in our chief cities still resort to it with little hesitation, believing that by great carefulness in its administration, and by the substitution of ether in exceptional cases, all danger may be avoided. Others have a very great fear of it, and universally trust to the safer anæsthetic. It is an error to suppose that the parturient state robs chloroform of much of its danger, the apparent immunity being due to its intermittent and incomplete administration; complete anæsthesia being but a fraction less dangerous than in surgical operations upon women who are not pregnant. Dr. Lusk, already quoted, after a large experience with the use of chloroform, says: " *Patients in labor do not enjoy any absolute immunity from the pernicious effects of chloroform.*"[1] It is much to be regretted that this more pleasant anæsthetic is so much more dangerous than ether as an inhalant; but in consideration of the difference of risk, that of their relative effects upon the nose and trachea is scarcely to be considered. Chloroform acts upon the respiratory centres just as ether does; and this is an element of danger in each, but is capable of being counteracted by artificial respiration. But, beyond this, chloroform is far more dangerous, in acting upon the motor ganglia of the heart and producing sudden death. According to the experiments of Vulpian upon animals, not more than one case of cardiac failure in forty can be restored by artificial respiration. He affirms that there is danger at the commencement, during the course, and at the close of chloroformization, and even some hours or days subsequent to it. Nélaton made the important discovery that the cerebral anæmia produced by chloroform, with its accompanying death-like condition, might be remedied by long perseverance in artificial respiration with the patient turned head downward.

Anæsthesia in labor is much less popular, both with obstetricians and patients in this country, than it was soon after its introduction. Improvements in the purity of sulphuric ether have made the narcosis more reliable, but the general effect upon patients varies very decidedly, being all that can be desired in some, and just the reverse in others. Some of the undesirable effects I have witnessed are intoxication, with cessation of labor, hysterical excitement, nightmare, and post-partum inertia and hemorrhage. I have also witnessed the most delightful results from ether that could be desired. In a small, delicate multipara, whose mother died of phthisis, and to whom I had been obliged to administer stimulants in the first and much of the second stage of labor, the use of ether had the effect to revolutionize her condition. Her pulse became strong ; her expulsive power increased ; she had no suffering : her placenta was expelled without accompanying blood ; and there was no subsequent uterine relaxation. But such cases are, unfortunately, exceptional.—Ed.]

[[1] *Opus cit.*]

A TREATISE

ON

ETHERIZATION IN CHILDBIRTH.

ILLUSTRATED BY

FIVE HUNDRED AND EIGHTY-ONE CASES.

BY WALTER CHANNING, M.D.

PROFESSOR OF MIDWIFERY AND MEDICAL JURISPRUDENCE IN THE UNIVERSITY
AT CAMBRIDGE.

PLAN AND OBJECTS OF THE WORK.

In May, 1847, I published a pamphlet, containing a few cases of labor in which I had employed sulphuric ether with entire success. In July of the same year, a second edition of the same pamphlet, somewhat enlarged, appeared. Cases have gradually accumulated in my practice, in which etherization has been employed. They have been of the different classes of labor, and in sufficient variety and number too, to authorize a cautious generalization. It occurred to me, that these cases might be published, and possibly be of some service as guides, or authority, towards the farther employment of etherization. They were recorded as soon after the labor was over as circumstances allowed. I often wrote the case out immediately upon my return home from it, and the hour is sometimes mentioned. After some thought, it was determined to print the cases just as they were first put down. A different course might have improved their strictly literary character; but it could hardly have happened otherwise than that the freshness, if not the truth, of the impression made by the case, would have been affected by any new labor upon them.

23

In the meantime, etherization was in use here, and in different parts of the country, in midwifery practice. We were hearing of results through journals and newspapers. They existed alone. The thought occurred to me, that, with very little personal trouble, I might collect from various sources, facts in regard to etherization which would, in a much surer manner, make my work useful, than would any thing of my own which it might contain. A circular letter was prepared, and addressed to many physicians in Boston and vicinity, containing questions which embraced some of the most important points regarding the use of ether and chloroform.

My great, I had almost said my sole, object in this circular, — in short, in my whole efforts, — was to ascertain here at home, in the birthplace of etherization, what had been the precise results of many experiments, made by many physicians, of the employment of the remedy of pain. My object was to learn if this use of it had been *safe*, — safe both to *mother* and to *child ;* and thus, as far as such results might reach, to contribute something towards settling the most important point concerning its further use, namely, that of its *safety*.

This matter of safety is especially dwelt upon, because much that is related to it, if not all else, has very little in it requiring present discussion or argument. I consider other questions as, in an important sense, settled, and therefore not demanding special attention. Thus we know that *pain* may be abolished by etherization. We know that voluntary or *animal power* is very much, if not wholly, suspended during this state. We know that *organic power* remains. Nay, more, we know that it is often increased, that of the womb for instance; and in the exceptional cases, in which uterine contraction is diminished, or in which it entirely ceases, we know that this is temporary, and that no danger to either mother or child has hence ensued. We know, finally, that during and in consequence of etherization, circumstances highly favorable to safe as well as to easy labor arise. Among these may be enumerated the increase of secretions in the organs immediately concerned in labor, and a more perfect relaxation or dilatability than existed before its use. Dubois first made this last observation, and my latest experience of etherization confirms his early and important statement.

It was, then, to the question of safety, in our experience of etherization here, that my attention was directed in the questions in the circular. But do not for a moment, reader, consider this as a very simple or a single question. It has regard, indeed, to a single fact, — the well-being of mother and child. But to show that, in its uses here, etherization has been safe in midwifery practice, is to declare a most important fact. Safety in this matter involves whatever exists or is done in etherization, as a condition towards this great end. These conditions are few, and cannot be too often repeated. They are, 1st, Purity in the article used. 2d, Such an instrument as will allow the freest escape of the expired or *exhaled* air, and the due admixture of atmospheric air with the *inhaled*. A hollow sponge for ether answers every purpose; for its structure is such as to ensure these conditions. 3d, When *etherization* is produced, inhalation is to cease. This state is declared by the relaxed condition of the limbs, the inability to raise the eyelids at command, and cessation of complaint. The books are full of other conditions, and in these the diversity of individual observations and views is sufficiently declared. Suffice it to say concerning the mode of exhibiting ether-vapors, that, of the two methods recommended in midwifery, the one by Professor Simpson, which directs so much to be used, and after such a manner, as shall in the shortest time produce the fullest effects, — and the other recommended by observers here in the same practice, which seeks its object by a less quantity, and that moderately administered, — I think, of these the latter is decidedly to be preferred.

I am very glad to find, that my old friend and class-mate, Professor Mussey, of Cincinnati, takes the same view of the matter, and even extends its application to surgery.

With regard to contra-indications to etherization which are founded in other conditions, whether of co-existing functional or structural disease, — whether of heart, head, or lungs, — I have no experience or observation to offer. I have met with none. I believe I am borne out by fact, when I say, that, in the examinations which have been made of those who have died after etherization, it has not happened, in more than a single case, that any disease existed in any of the organs referred to, whereby to explain the death. The exception occurred lately in New York, and will be referred to more particularly hereafter. And farther it will hereafter be shown, by cases of known and grave structural disease, in which etherization has been employed as a remedy amongst us, that great relief has been afforded by it, and no suspicion, much less proof, furnished, that any untoward results have been produced or death accelerated by it. A case of confirmed phthisis is this moment under my care, in which chloroform has been very excessively and imprudently employed, and from which no other apparent troubles than nausea and vomiting have followed. These ceased when inhalation was omitted. Of contra-indications to etherization arising in diseases and lesions above alluded to, I have no experience to offer.

The object of the circular was to learn what had been the whole result of etherization, so far as it has been employed in midwifery amongst ourselves; and this in order especially to ascertain whether those who had used it had done well or ill, had lived or had died, — the question of *safety*.

The circular was addressed to many physicians. From some I learned that they had never employed etherization in midwifery; from others, that their experience furnished nothing new. From one came the religious objection. One friend thus writes, and his short letter is a " whole history : " —

" Dear Doctor,
" I have used the ether in labor a considerable number of times, and with obvious benefit; but my observations have not been made with sufficient precision to be made the basis of statistical results.
" Yours, most truly,
" February 10." " ENOCH HALE.

I give this letter with great pleasure. It contains, as far as the writer's experience goes, a very important answer to the great question of the circular, namely, of the entire safety of etherization. It says that its author has employed ether " a considerable number of times, and with obvious benefit." The character, the intellectual habits, the deep interest in all questions of science, and the caution of the writer in stating results, give to this short testimony of my friend, in favor of ether, great value.

From some, to whom I took the liberty to address the circular, I have received no answer. Thinking that in some of these instances my communication had miscarried, I sent another; and this, because I had learned that the physicians so addressed had valuable information to impart. I regret that I sent my circular in these cases. I acknowledge I had no other right to do so than that which some interest in good science bestows. If I exceeded such privilege in the instances referred to, I here make my best apology, and promise to offend in like manner no more.

From a great many came answers, in more or less detail, to the questions proposed ; and, more than this, letters often accompanied them, giving at some length important cases and deliberate opinions. At first it was my purpose to publish, along with my own cases, tabular views of what I had been so very kindly and liberally favored with, together with the accompanying letters, and here rest the case. It was an after-thought to devote some pages to a few of the topics which my subject so directly involves. That subject forms one of the most important epochs in medical history. Was it not due to it to say something of its history, of what it is in itself, of what it has done, and what appears to be its destiny?

It will be perceived that from some of my friends the communication of facts is small, sometimes not exceeding a single case. But that single case, is it without its interest? I answer no. It has its place in what has been done with ether, and deserves a distinct record in its literature. In its entire success, it teaches that it does not stand alone because of a want of confidence in the *safety* and whole benefit of etherization, and so gives positive support to these facts in our history. From some I learn that they have used, and mean to use, ether or chloroform, only when desired by the patient. No one can question the propriety of this course; but in thus dividing the responsibleness, or laying its weight principally on the patient, I do not know of any one physician who has pursued this course because of his want of confidence in the perfect safety of etherization. Had he felt a doubt, had he had the smallest scruple concerning this its entire safety, would he have done that, or thought for a moment of doing it, which a sick and a most suffering woman asked for, nay demanded, but which to his mind involved the smallest danger? The whole question resolves into *safety* alone. It has nothing to do with men's notions of the value or the pleasure of pain. We dismiss this latter from the matter at once as wholly irrelevant. We know of *painless* labor, of labor wholly without *pain ;* and in too many instances, not now to refer to them, in which the patient was unconscious of delivery, or knew nothing more of it in regard to suffering than of an ordinary defecation, which for the most part is pleasurable rather than painful, and who did not pay the penalty of death for the involuntary violation or temporary suspension of a natural law.

Let the reader, then, look at the true point at issue; and, above all, let him not be misled in his judgments by ignorance, by prejudice, or more especially by *a priori* reasoning.

Since receiving answers to the circular, I have, upon every opportunity, talked to my brethren of what has happened concerning etherization in their practice since they commenced it. I am told by all, that not an untoward occurrence has attended or followed its later use. From one, I learned that, since the newspaper accounts of alarm-- ing and even fatal cases in surgical operations, patients and their friends have sometimes held back from etherization in midwifery, and that he waits for it to be asked for. The influence is natural upon patient and physician. And it is both natural and wise to act accordingly. It, however, makes nothing against the use of the remedy of pain in childbirth, in which it is known never to have done harm, if an untoward result come of its use in some two or more cases of surgical practice, and in some diseases which are almost invariably fatal, as tetanus and hydrophobia.

The reader may look in this volume for the enunciation of principles concerning etherization which have come out of its facts, and which establish its place in practical medi- cine. I have examined the journals and papers in which these facts are scattered with a profusion which the impor- tance of the subject certainly authorizes, and with a variety in reasoning or opinion which attaches to few other subjects, but which its novelty and extreme interest fully explain. We are told that every thing has two sides, and the one chosen depends on the point of sight. Etherization would seem to have as many sides as there are observers, and doc- trines concerning it seem only limited by the number of observers. There is Dubois, with his faith and his fears so well nigh balanced, that one feels that he has been so taken with all sides of the matter, that he hardly seems to have looked thoroughly at any. And there is Simpson of Edinburgh, with his hosts of cases, the living witnesses of the safety of etherization, full of faith and of zeal. Mr. Travers says a man may die as well five days after etherization as twenty-four hours; and that he has known a limb, five days after death, smell of ether, the stump having become gangrenous. And this case has by some been elevated into a principle, that ether makes stumps gangrenous, and kills people in five days or twenty-four hours. How was it with Mr. Wells, of the English navy, who gives *one hundred and six* operations, in which he used ether-vapor? " No serious effects followed in any case." Not a case of gangrene occurred in a single stump of hundreds of amputations collected by Simpson, and not one after a single surgical operation in our own Hospital. Tetanus has been cured by ether, or recovery has followed its use. But it has not cured all. M. Roux has failed; and a writer says concerning this case, that " any such trials (namely, in cases of hydrophobia and tetanus) will assuredly end in disappointment; these diseases being *diseases of motion, not of sensation.*" The physiology may be true, but the fact is diverse. Patients do grow still, when etherized, both in hydrophobia and in tetanus. Spasms are controlled, nay, entirely overcome, by it. Positive *rest* ensues. We *infer* the abolition of *sensibility*. We *know* that *mobility* is abolished in etherization. Midwifery is full of teaching on this point. Muscles of voluntary motion become powerless. The limbs to which they are attached fall as dead, when raised and left to themselves; and, even when consciousness returns, this want of power sometimes remains. Ask a person in this condition of first waking after ether or chloroform, to raise the head to drink, or if he says he will do this, after handing him the vessel, witness his absolute, sure failure, and the question of the physiological action of ether, in this regard, is settled.

Mr. B. Cooper thinks much of the benefits of pain, which he calls a " *premonitory condition ;* no doubt fitting parts, the subject of lesions, to *reparatory action.*" He farther speaks of vessels losing the power of retraction, and so hemorrhage from small vessels follows. How wholly unlike this is the experience of other surgeons! How different are the results in midwifery! I mean established results, not such as come of mere conjecture, and which are offered as such.

M. Flourens shows the progress of etherization in regard to the nervous centres from the hemispheres to the medulla oblongata, with the inferential caution, that we must not let it reach the last. This knowledge is derived from countless experiments upon all sorts of animals, — men among the rest. The latter, I believe, have all survived, and so did not complete in themselves the experiment. But the poor lower orders have suffered terribly. Vivisections have been done without number and without mercy. It would seem, that ether had come to destroy life, not to save it. I have read the reports over and over, and doubt not for a moment that many animals have suffered, and many more have been killed, in the toil. But the end is not yet. Who is ready to determine, or have determined for him, a wholly practical question, by results of experiments on animals, which, in their whole history and proof, have no possible relation to the case of a suffering human being? It were easy to extend this narrative of effort and of result, of individual and multiplied fact, and of resulting individual opinion, concerning etherization abroad. But I refrain. A moment for home. How has it been with the etherization question here? The question has various answers. Men have tried etherization; and they who have done this most, whether in surgery or midwifery, have most advocated it. Men have not tried it at all; and it would seem, from the tone of their avowal, that they do not mean to try it. These show it little favor. There are whole communities in which nothing has been done with etherization in midwifery, and very little in surgery. Here, in

2

Boston, it has been tried in both. There has been no rush about it, however. The cautiousness in our sectional phrenological development, if M. Flourens will allow the allusion, has prevented a rush. Etherization in midwifery has been employed here now for a year; and, with some industry, my collections of cases do not much exceed five hundred. I have no doubt that many more exist; but, of the certain, I know of those only of which I give reports. The number is not large. But just add them to the hundreds and thousands which are furnished abroad, and they perform a distinguished part in a most important history. They, with all the rest, show that there has not been a case in which, during etherization in labor, any untoward circumstance has occurred. I cannot point to a single established case of disaster, during this state, for an exception even to the rule.

I had written thus far when I lighted upon two letters which much interested me, and from which I will make some extracts. The first is from Professor Simpson, of Edinburgh, to Professor Meigs, of Philadelphia. The extracts will occupy some space; but this matters little, if they will at all aid our inquiries.

Professor Simpson's letter is dated Edinburgh, January 23, 1848. He says: —

" The statements which I have already made, may show you to what an extent the chloroform is used in this country ; and our chemists tell me that the demand for it steadily increases with them.

" In *surgery*, its use is quite general for operations, painful diagnosis, &c. My friend, Dr. Andrew Wood, has just been telling me of a beautiful application of it. A boy fell from a height, and severely injured his thigh. It was so painful that he shrieked when Dr. Wood tried to handle the limb ; and would not allow of a proper examination. Dr. Wood immediately chloroformed him — at once ascertained that the femur was fractured — kept him anæsthetic till he sent for his splints — and did not allow his patient to awake till his limb was all properly set, bandaged, and adjusted.

" In *medicine*, its effects are being extensively tried as an anodyne, an anæsthetic, a diffusible stimulant, &c. Its anti-spasmodic powers in colic, asthma, &c. are everywhere recognized.

" In *midwifery*, most or all of my brethren in Edinburgh employ it constantly. The ladies themselves insist in not being doomed to suffer, when suffering is so totally unnecessary. In London, Dublin, &c. it every day gains converts to its obstetric employment; and I have no doubt that those who most bitterly oppose it now will be yet, in ten or twenty years hence, amazed at their own professional cruelty. They allow their medical prejudices to smother and over-rule the common dictates of their profession, and of humanity.

" No accidents have as yet happened under its use, though several hundred thousand must have already been under the influence of chloroform. Its use here has been a common amusement in drawing-room parties, for the last two or three months.

" I never now apply it with any thing but a silk handkerchief. In surgical cases and operations, the quantity given is not in general measured. We all judge more by the *effects* than the *quantity*. Generally, I believe, we pour two or three drachms on the handkerchief at once, and more in *a minute*, if no sufficient effect is produced, and we stop when sonorous respiration begins. Not unfrequently, spasms, rigidity, &c. come on; but they disappear as the effect increases, and none of us care for them any more than for hysteric symptoms; nor do they leave any bad effect. But the mere *appearance* of them is enough to terrify a beginner.

" I shall be glad to hear how the cause of anæsthesia gets on among you; and I remain, with great respect, very faithfully yours,

" J. Y. SIMPSON."

Professor Meigs, in reply, says: —

" I presume you will, ere this date, have received copies of Professor Warren's pamphlet on ' Etherization,' which may inform you very fully as to the use of the anæsthetic agent in the Massachusetts General Hospital and in Boston. That eminent gentleman is more reserved as to the obstetric employment of the agent; much more so, I understand, than either Dr. Channing, Dr. Homans, and other practitioners, who make use of it very commonly. In New York, as I learn, the surgical application of chloroform is common, while its obstetrical use has not as yet acquired a general vogue. . . . . . .

" As to its employment in midwifery here [in Philadelphia], notwithstanding a few cases have been mentioned and reported, I think it has not yet begun to find favor with accoucheurs. I have not exhibited it in any case; nor do I, at present, know of any intention in that way, entertained by the leading practitioners of obstetrical medicine and surgery, in this city. I have not yielded to several solicitations as to its exhibition addressed to me by my patients in labor. . . . .

" I freely admit — for I know it — that many thousands of persons are daily subjected to its power. Yet I feel that no law of succession of its action on the several distinct parts of the brain has been or can be hereafter ascertained, seeing that the succession is contingent. Many grave objections would perhaps vanish, could the law of the succession of influences on the parts of the brain be clearly made out, and its provisions ensured. There are, indubitably, certain cases in which the intellectual hemispheres are totally hebetized and deprived of power by it, while the co-ordinating lobes remain perfectly unaffected. In others the motor cords of the cerebro-spinal nerves are deprived of power, whilst the sensitive cords enjoy a full activity, and *vice versa*. . . .

" M. Flourens's experiments, and others, especially those by the younger Mr. Wakley, of the ' Lancet,' prove very conclusively that the aspiration of ether or chloroform, continued but a little longer than the period required for hebetizing the hemispheres, the cerebellum, the tubercula quadrigemina, and the cord, overthrows the medulla oblongata, and produces thereby sudden death. I fully believe, with M. Flourens, that the medulla oblongata is the *nœud vital ;* and that, though later brought under the power of chloroformization, it is always reducible under it. Hence I fear, that, in all cases of chloroformal anæsthesia, there remains but one irrevocable step more to the grave.

" I readily hear, before your voice can reach me across the Atlantic, the triumphant reply, that an hundred thousand have taken it *without accident !* I am a witness that it is attended with alarming accidents, however rarely. But should I exhibit the remedy for pain to a thousand patients in labor, merely to prevent the physiological pain, and for no other motive, and if I should in consequence destroy only one of them, I should feel disposed to clothe me in sackcloth, and cast ashes on my head for the remainder of my days. What sufficient motive have I to risk the life or the death of one in a thousand, in a questionable attempt to abrogate one of the general conditions of man? "

As Professor Meigs's letter is on chloroform, it did not appear to me perfectly clear that his remarks concerning it were meant to be extended to sulphuric and chloric ether. To learn how this was, I at once sent to Professor Meigs a copy of my circular in a letter, in which I took the liberty to ask him such questions as particularly interested me, concerning his trials and his views on the whole subject.

It will be seen, in my first extract from Professor Meigs's reply to Professor Simpson, that reference is made to a work by Professor Warren, of Boston, on "Etherization," which speaks of his reserve as to its employment in midwifery, and of the freer use made of it by Dr. Homans and Dr. Channing, of Boston. In my very first effort to obtain facts from my professional brethren respecting etherization in childbirth, and I believe before Professor Warren's book was published, I addressed a copy of my circular to him; feeling particularly anxious to obtain a precise statement both of facts and opinions concerning the employment of etherization, in this application of it, derived directly from his own observations of its effects in midwifery. I was the more desirous to obtain this information from this source, as Professor Warren was among the first to use etherization in important operations in surgery, of which midwifery is a department, and because of the weight of his opinions with the community in which he lives, and abroad. I have not received his reply; but my impression is, that his remarks were intended as a lesson of caution, and not as the results of actual experience.

From Professor Meigs, almost by return of mail, I received the following reply to my letter. It is written in a spirit of so much kindness, so much courtesy, — is expressive of an interest so deep in the important and the true, — of so hearty a love of science, that I cannot withhold this public expression of my thanks to its honored author. As a mere matter of taste, it may be questioned if somewhat of that which is especially personal to myself might not have been left out of the print. But I prefer to publish the letter just as it is, and to take the chances with my reader concerning other and purely inferential matters.

"Philadelphia, April 26, 1848.
"Dear Sir, — I feel much honored by your letter of the 21st instant, covering certain interrogatories relative to the use of anæsthetic agents

in midwifery; and I beg you to accept my sincere thanks for the attention.

"I believe I have read all the articles, within my reach, that have appeared upon the anæsthetic practice; and I misconceive of my own motives, if the hesitation which hitherto has prevented me from employing either chloroform or ether arises from any other than a conscientious scruple as to the administration of remedial agents, that I do not deem it indispensably necessary to employ. I have as yet met with no such case, and have therefore remained an interested observer of what my brethren have deemed it expedient, and certain of them indispensable, to do in the matter. I am therefore incapable of answering your interrogatories; being without any clinical experience in the case.

"Seeing that so many thousands of persons have taken, and do daily take, advantage of the insensibility produced by etherization, to avoid the pain of surgical operations, one might well charge me with being cautious overmuch in so long refraining from adopting the remedy in my own practice; but it seemed to me, that the motives set forth for my recusancy, in a published letter to Professor Simpson, ought to be of weight sufficient to determine my action in the premises. The results thus far attained, although they are doubtless beneficent in most cases, are nevertheless mixed up with elements of distrust, as to the permanency of present opinions and indications of practice, so considerable, that I am most anxious to have a candid exposition of the motive for or against it; comprising an amount of intelligence, drawn from different sources, sufficient to lead the body of the profession to clear views of duty upon the point.

"I hold myself in readiness to yield to conviction upon sufficient evidence of the necessity and propriety of etherization in midwifery; but I beg leave to say, that this is a case in which I should hardly yield my opinions to the force of statistical returns, because I have no doubt of some physiological and therefore needful and useful connection of the pain and the powers of parturition, the inconveniences of which are really less considerable than has by some been supposed. If I am not here in error, I submit that no statistics ought to have a real power to convince. There are a few of my brethren here who have exhibited chloroform or ether in their obstetric cases. The instances are not numerous. Dr. Hodge and Dr. Huston, who enjoy a large share of the public confidence as obstetricians, tell me they have not yet resorted to the anæsthesia, nor do they at present feel inclined to do so. Perhaps, sir, when the volume you are preparing for the press shall have appeared, and we shall have become masters of the results obtained and collected by you, we may all give our adhesion to the recommendation. I shall take great pleasure in studying your work with care, as soon as I can get it from the booksellers.

" I have to-day received Ed. Wm. Murphy's pamphlet, which he was so good as to send me by the ' Acadia.' Dr. Murphy gives us accounts of *seven* cases, five of which were under his own observation. I cannot say, that any influence has been produced upon my mind, to change my purpose, by reading Dr. Murphy's cases and observations. In the seventh case particularly, I do not perceive any good fruits of the administration. The success was extraordinary, but can by no means be attributed to the chloroform.

" It is obviously, my dear sir, so much more agreeable to say yes than to say no to any honorable invitation, and it is so clear that you have many distinguished names to sustain the practice now common in Boston, that I could almost feel ashamed not to be on your side also; but if, after reading your forthcoming work, I shall find all my objections swept away by the power of truth, I shall hasten to confess my conversion, and my obligation to you. It is certain, that those who establish great practical truths, that are efficient in meliorating man's condition, are deserving of all honor and commendation.

" The motives that govern me thus far are connected with, or rather dependent upon, my views of the nature and offices of different parts of the brain. If you will do me the favor to look over Mons. Flourens's pamphlet, a copy of which I beg you to accept, you will perhaps see the course of my reasoning against etherization in obstetricy.

" We both seek the truth. I hope that you may find and establish it. In the meantime, I rest, with the greatest respect and esteem, your most obliged and very faithful servant,   " CH. D. MEIGS."

" Professor Channing."

It will be perceived, that the objection of Professor Meigs is wholly and purely physiological Etherization being given, this objection demands for its removal the law of succession of its action on the several portions of the brain, from the hemispheres to the medulla oblongata, should it happen to reach so far; while it is at the same time obvious, that no such law as this can be ascertained. It is hence an impossible objection, and the true question is whether it should for a moment influence practice. We know not what is the succession of events from the slightest impression made by ether or chloroform on the hemispheres, or upon any intervening point between them and the medulla oblongata. We know not, and cannot know, where safety ends, and danger begins, by any known action of the agent,

or by any law of its action. Examinations after death from
etherization show every variety of results, from the slightest, or none at all, to the greatest. The heart is found in
every condition of emptiness and fulness, and the blood is
quite as remarkable for the varieties of lesion it presents.
So is it with the lungs; and, in short, so is it everywhere.
Then we have the results of vivisections, after etherization induced in animals expressly to produce death, that
its lesions may be made manifest. Now, vivisections are
accompanied by direct effects, which at once prevent all
true reasoning from them to the medicinal uses of etherization. The transcendental physiology of Flourens, of
Preisser and Melays, and the equally visionary teachings
of Snow, have really no pertinence to such an issue. They
explain nothing, and should not for a moment be allowed
to touch the questions involved in etherization.

I have directed as much, if not more, attention to the
state of the respiration and of the circulation, than to any
other facts in the history of etherization. These functions
have always seemed to me to demand the most attention.
They depend on the integrity of the medulla oblongata for
their regularity, and for their very continuance. Thus I
have counted the pulse and the breathings before etherization. Then, while it was getting established, and during
its most perfect state, I have known them to remain
wholly undisturbed in the midst and pressure of the total
abolition of consciousness and sensibility. The patient
has been in a state of entire and perfect repose. It has
been the completed work of a second. There has been
no time for succession in action, or it has been too small
to be measured, or the series of events noted. I have
known labor to advance in this state of things and to terminate, and not a limb or a muscle to move, or the face to
betray the slightest token of suffering. In another part of
this volume, I have related a case in which volition and
muscular power partially remained, or was regained during

deep etherization. The woman was evidently wearied with her position on the left side, and in the most methodical manner possible turned herself over to the right, and composed her limbs after such a manner as to secure to herself a most comfortable sleep; and sleep she did through the whole of the remainder of the labor. These cases have been perfectly safe.

I have said, that the law of succession of the action of etherization cannot be learned; and I will state some facts which show how impossible the attempt to learn this would, and must continue to be. This condition occurs in many, many instances in so short a time after inhalation as to make observation of any succession in events impossible. I have known it to take place completely after two full inspirations, so that not the least notice was taken of any thing said or done. I spoke of the state of the breathing of the pulse, and the subject will come up under other heads again. Let me here say, in addition to what was remarked of their general natural state, that sometimes we find the reverse. They are sometimes more rapid, sometimes slower, than natural. Sometimes the breathing is perfectly noiseless; at others it is a heavy, stertorous snoring. Professor Simpson speaks of this as occurring more frequently in his practice, than has been met with in the cases which have fallen under my own observation.

Not only has the physiological objection to the use of chloroform and ether prevented Professor Meigs employing them in midwifery practice, — and will continue to do so, since it is pretty clear that this objection cannot be obviated, — but it will be perceived, that this same objection has with the professor also destroyed the authority of statistics; a science which, in matters of fact, has been of the greatest practical regard and benefit. It makes no sort of odds, that a thousand or a million cases, duly reported and authenticated, have been most successfully and happily treated by etherization. The possibility, not the *proba-*

3

bility, — for this is denied in the very statement of the number who have safely used it, — the *possibility* of one case proving fatal *afterwards* (not in consequence of etherization, for this cannot be determined) would seem to be regarded as a valid objection by my highly respected correspondent to his ever employing it. At least, notwithstanding the thousands of cases in which etherization has been most successfully used by others, Professor Meigs, in amount, says he has not met with one in which he has thought this agency necessary, or in which it would have been usefully employed. The position of this distinguished professor, and the collateral support which that position, and especially his opinions in midwifery, get from the adhesion of Professors Hodge and Huston to the same, makes it a duty, in the discussion of our subject, to consider all the grounds of his not having employed the remedy of pain in labor. I do not understand, that his associates in doctrine and in practice, in this regard, have, any more than himself, employed ether or chloroform in childbirth. If they have not, is not the whole reasoning against their use strictly *a priori* in its whole nature? It is not only indifferent to, but wholly irrespective of facts, which are alike the sources and the basis of all inductive science. Its supporters do not ask, " What has occurred? — what has etherization done in childbirth? — how safe has it been to mother and child?" They ask what it *ought*, what it *should* do, upon certain physiological principles; and which show that, as far as we can see, it ought to be, or that it is very likely to be, fatal whenever used. The friends of etherization look to the simple fact, — to what actually has happened in childbirth, after using ether or chloroform. They can learn what this truly is, both from their own observation and from that of others. They know that these remedies of pain have been widely used, and with a success which attaches to no other known remedy in practical medicine. They look to the facts. They collect these;

and, when the time for philosophizing has come, they will with great pleasure use physiology, and all other collateral aid, in their important generalizations. While thus waiting, however, they do not reject the teachings of physiology. But in the very imperfect condition of this noble science, and more especially that department of it which concerns the nervous system, they are willing to take the guidance of simple fact, of daily observation, in the conviction that, if wisely followed, it will never lead them astray. It is simply and wholly in view of the great importance of our subject, that another opinion of Professor Meigs will now be referred to. It is a passage in his letter to Professor Simpson, and contains what seems to Professor Meigs a conclusive objection to the use of etherization in childbirth. We have already made the quotation, but repeat it for special remark : —

" I readily hear, before your voice can reach me across the Atlantic, the triumphant reply, that an hundred thousand have taken it *without accident !* I am a witness that it is attended with alarming accidents, however rarely. But should I exhibit the remedy for pain to a thousand patients in labor, merely to prevent the physiological pain, and for no other motive, and if I should in consequence destroy only one of them, I should feel disposed to clothe me in sackcloth, and cast ashes on my head for the remainder of my days. What sufficient motive have I to risk the life or the death of one in a thousand, in a questionable attempt to abrogate one of the general conditions of man ? "

The " alarming accidents " are not stated to have happened in midwifery practice, and probably were not observed in childbirth in which etherization was employed. This opinion is partly derived from the statement of Professor Meigs, that he has never used this agency in labor, and partly from what is stated immediately after concerning the employment of chloroform for the pain of disease, and of surgical operations to which no objection is made. It will be perceived, that the objection to etherization is still a physiological one ; for the *pain* of labor is obviously, from the whole language and reasoning of Professor Meigs, a *functional* pain. Now, here we join issue, and state what will be met with elsewhere in this volume, that the *functional* department of labor is the *contraction* of the womb, the dilatation of its mouth, vagina, and external organs, which are no more necessarily painful than are those which carry forward, and expel the contents of the rectum or bladder. There is no pain in the pure functional actions of the uterus. Pain is the consequence of *resistance* to the contractions of the womb, which the moving body, the fœtus, encounters in its progress to birth. Pain in labor is the result, first, of the imperfect harmony of functional dilatability of the mouth of the womb, with the contractions of the organ; secondly, of a like state of the vagina; and, thirdly and specially, of a like condition of the perineum and external organs. It is in these contingencies, not natural elements of labor, that the whole *pain* of labor has its cause. The pressure of the unyielding head on the sacrum also takes its share in the production of the resistance which makes up the whole pain of labor. I do not refer to morbid conditions of the passages, such as excessive sensibility and others, with which all practitioners of midwifery are so well acquainted. I merely refer to functional conditions or disturbances, which are ordinarily met with, and which give rise to the agony of childbirth. Now, this state is one which demands relief. It does not necessarily belong to labor, since painless, or nearly painless, cases of labor are too common to allow of such a statement for a moment. It is to relieve the unnecessary suffering which results from those conditions referred to, that etherization is employed. And it gives the demanded relief, by increasing dilatability, diminishing or suspending sensibility, preventing exhaustion, increasing the secretions, taking away the disturbing action of the will; and thus produces results which strike the observer of the first case in which he witnesses it, as if a miracle had been performed in his presence.

A husband sat at the bedside of his wife, and witnessed her sufferings during labor for some hours. Soon after my arrival, and no contra-indications to etherization being present, she inhaled sulphuric ether-vapor. She very soon experienced its most happy effects, and expressed the positive pleasure which had replaced so much agony. The effect upon her husband was such, of this sudden and entire change in her whole state, that he became faint, left the room, and did not return to it till after the child was born.

Let it, then, be distinctly borne in mind, that etherization is not used to suspend *uterine contractions* (which it most rarely does), but to prevent *pain ;* and, in this way, to make labor safe and happy to both mother and child, and to secure a successful convalescence. The cases that follow will abundantly show how true and how general is this alleged effect of etherization, — the rapid recovery which follows its use. Perhaps no effect has been so frequently alluded to by patients as this. They may be unconscious of what happened during etherization, and are insensible to pain; but the after condition is matter of distinct consciousness, and is always referred to with entire satisfaction.

Professor Meigs speaks of the depth of the sorrow he should endure, should he destroy one in a thousand cases, by using etherization in labor. Whence would come that sorrow? Not on account of wrong-doing, certainly. For what better argument could he or anybody else have for employing the remedy of pain in the thousandth case, than the preceding nine hundred and ninety-nine perfectly successful ones? Would it not at once occur to such experience as this, that the untoward result was in no sense the product of professional delinquency in the employment of a remedy, but that it was a result not to be looked for or anticipated, — which stands as the solitary exception to the universal rule, for such would such an exception make it, — which has hence no relation to practice, — and the

very existence and whole history of which begins and ends
with the fact itself?   Add to this the fact, that in not a single
instance of the thousands of recorded cases of childbirth,
has there been a single untoward result met with during
etherization; and what farther argument do we want to
support the position, that this agency in painful labor is
not only most reasonably demanded by the sufferer, but
that it is the solemn duty of the profession to afford to such
suffering its certain relief?

Do not for a single moment let the question be regarded
as an impertinence; for it has a most important bearing on
the subject.   It is this.   What becomes of the other physiological objection already noticed; namely, that etherization may quite unexpectedly reach the medulla oblongata,
and so suddenly destroy life?   I ask, what becomes of this
objection, in view of the open recommendation of this agent
in medical and surgical contingencies by the opponents of
its use in childbirth?   Certainly the risk is as great in
these, as in the childbirth employment of the same agent.
Nay, experience has shown it to be much greater; for fatal
results have come of it, as I shall show by and by, in surgical operations, while etherization has never touched the
medulla oblongata in any childbearing woman.

I do not mean to support my position regarding etherization in childbirth, by referring to the uncertainties of
therapeutics in practical medicine.   It may not, however,
be out of place to observe, that, often in the gravest diseases, the correctness of the treatment is a matter of inference from its results, rather than of *a priori* reasoning, or
mere experiment in other like cases.   And yet who would
or should question the propriety, the wisdom of that course
which has its determination in such reasoning or in such
experiment?   Sydenham, in his noble writings on epidemics, especially new ones; and Gooch, in his admirable paper
on puerperal fever, have settled the laws of practice in
most important diseases, and, in their wise cautions in the

44

use of powerful means, have proved that their confidence in their remedies and in themselves has not been misplaced, but has made the ages long to come their grateful debtors.

I have not confined myself to etherization in childbirth. I have devoted some pages to its employment in surgery and general medicine. I have done this for illustration, and especially for its bearings on labor, both in regard to its agency, and in explanation, and as argument for its safety in this practice. This part of the inquiry seems to me exceedingly pertinent to the whole object in my undertaking, and is surely one of the deepest interest. It forms a most important portion of the teachings of the remedy of pain, and shows how wide is the domain of human suffering which it covers and controls.

Another subject, — the untoward results of etherization. Cases have been collected from home and abroad, in which these results have been alarming, and even fatal. Where original sources of information concerning these cases could be reached, they have been referred to, and the answers to inquiries are recorded. Thus I have published from authentic sources important facts concerning the Cincinnati case; others from Dr. Bartlett, of New Bedford, of a case in which chloroform was inhaled for amusement; from Dr. Flint, of Roxbury; from Professor Parker, of New York; and an important correction of a newspaper report of a case of crushed thigh, in which amputation was done during insensibility from chloroform. The correction is by Dr. S. D. Townsend, one of the surgeons of the Massachusetts General Hospital.

The numbers which the cases bear belong to an arrangement for a special object. They have been retained, as answering the purpose quite as well as would initials of names, and without the objection which might have attached to their use.

The word *etherization* has been used as a generic term,

45

and to express that condition which follows the use of ethers of whatever kind. I have, for the most part, designated the particular agent employed for its induction; and, where this has not been done, no necessity existed for doing it.

The first seven cases in the series were published in a pamphlet referred to in the beginning of this section. They are reprinted without alteration, because of the personal interest with which they are regarded, and because of their immediate relation to, and direct agency in, what I have since done concerning etherization.

It has not been easy, in the composition of this work, to avoid occasional repetition of thought, doctrine, or fact. Reports of cases, and statements of opinion, have been constantly reaching me while writing; and I was not willing to withhold either, though at times it has not been always easy to give them the best place. But the repetitions referred to have not been without design. They sometimes present important truths in different aspects. Sometimes, in their wider application, they involve new and useful practical suggestions. Sometimes they are used for illustration.

As to arrangement, very little attempt has been made to render this exact. Subjects follow each other in sufficient order, however, to indicate somewhat their mutual dependence, while each section is complete in regard to the subject discussed.

In offering this work to my profession, I have only to say that it was undertaken, and is finished, in the hope of adding something to useful medical literature. It has occupied more time than I supposed would have been necessary for its completion. It has been written in the uncertain leisure of a professional life, which makes a daily and like demand on physical and intellectual power. It treats of a noble subject, — the *remedy of pain*. After ages of suffering, and of frequently and long intermitted pursuit of such a remedy, one has been discovered. It remains with the profession to say whether it shall take its place among the permanent and most important agents in the treatment of disease, and in abolishing pain; or whether it shall pass away with the unimportant and undeserving, until another and a truer age shall revive and give it a wider sphere of usefulness and a surer perpetuity.

I have stated my views fully and freely. They are believed to have a legitimate basis in numerous and well-established facts. These facts have been reported, not to sustain a vague opinion, or to give importance and currency to a poor and an unsafe hypothesis. It is no part of the purpose of the following treatise to teach, or to leave it to be inferred, that untoward results have not followed, or will not again follow, etherization. But I can and do say, that I have not met with an untoward result in any case of midwifery in which etherization has been induced, which, by any violence or ingenuity of explication, can be ascribed to this state as its cause. I have met with no record of such.

Sincerely do I hope, that what of earnestness may be discovered in the pages which follow, or in those which have preceded, will be ascribed to interest alone in the truth ; and that I shall be saved from any thing approaching the charge of a partizanship, of which neither my subject nor my self-respect need, or I trust would allow, the indulgence.   W. C.

178, TREMONT-STREET, BOSTON,
June, 1848.

ANGLO–AMERICAN REACTION TO OBSTETRICAL ANESTHESIA

JOHN DUFFY

In view of the breadth of the subject, no attempt will be made here to deal with the early history of anesthetics nor to become involved in the tangled web of claimants to the honor of having first introduced this revolutionary technique into medical practice. It is well to note, however, that in 1799 Sir Humphry Davy, in reporting on nitrous oxide, specifically cited instances of its analgesic effect and asserted that as it "appears capable of destroying physical pain, it may probably be used with advantage during surgical operations. . . ."[1] Although his suggestions fell on barren ground, less than fifty years later the advent of anesthesia through sulphuric ether and chloroform was immediately hailed as a medical triumph and found almost universal adoption.

As the history of every major break-through demonstrates, an invention or discovery can succeed only when advances in technology and changes in the cultural factors have created a favorable milieu. Although the evidence is scant, there is little doubt that throughout history man has sought to alleviate pain through drugs and herbs, or by means of sorcery. It was not until the advent of the nineteenth century, however, that men in the Western world seriously turned their attention to this problem. The story of obstetrical anesthesia closely parallels that of surgical anesthesia. For example, in 1591 when Eufame MacAlyane of Edinburgh sought relief from her childbirth pains, she was buried alive for the offense. If the method she used was no better than that prescribed by a Massachusetts colonist in 1677, her sacrifice was completely meaningless, since the latter prescription involved a lock of virgin's hair, twelve ant eggs, and various other items.[2]

By 1800 a scientific rationale had emerged and, although we may look askance at some of the results, more serious approaches were made toward the relief of pain. Influenced by Doctor Rush, no doubt, a young medical student at the University of Pennsylvania, in his dissertation, *An Essay on the Means of Lessening the Pains of Parturition*, proposed to induce

---

[1] Louis H. Bauer, ed., *Seventy-Five Years of Medical Progress 1878-1953* (Philadelphia: Lea & Febiger, 1954), pp. 15-16.

[2] Claude E. Heaton, "The history of anesthesia and analgesia in obstetrics," *J. Hist. Med. & Allied Sc.*, 1946, *1*: 567.

muscular relaxation by copious blood letting and thus to facilitate the parturition process. This same idea was set forth by William P. Dewees a couple of years later and can be found with some slight variations in a number of articles published in medical journals during the subsequent years.[3]

Quite obviously the pathway to modern medicine led to many blind alleys, a fact further illustrated by the emergence of phrenology and mesmerism. Even exploring blind alleys is not always unproductive, however, for negative findings frequently have value in themselves, and the sidelights they throw often indicate future pathways. In the case of mesmerism, which gained a measure of scientific standing in the late 1830's and the 1840's, some very real benefits were achieved in the relief of surgical and obstetrical pain. Although the English medical profession, led by Thomas Wakley, the irascible editor of *The Lancet,* stoutly opposed the use of mesmerism or hypnotism, its practitioners enjoyed varying degrees of success on the Continent and in the United States. The advent of chemical anesthesia in 1846, which provided a much simpler and much more certain method of relieving pain, relegated mesmerism to the role of an insignificant cult and dashed the hopes of its leading advocates. Nonetheless, the limited successes achieved by its practitioners and the ensuing heated controversies aroused in medical and lay publications alike helped pave the way for the immediate acceptance of sulphuric ether and chloroform.[4]

In view of the almost instant acceptance of surgical anesthesia following William T. G. Morton's demonstration on October 16, 1846, a surprisingly long delay occurred in the United States before ether, or Letheon as it was known, was applied in an obstetrical case, and this delay enabled Sir James Y. Simpson, a British obstetrician, to become the first to use chemical anesthesia for this purpose. Simpson administered ether on January 19, 1847, while the first recorded use of ether for obstetrics in the United States was made on April 14, 1847, by Nathan Colley Keep, a dentist. Almost at the same time as Doctor Keep, Walter Channing, professor of obstetrics at the Harvard Medical School, also began using ether in his practice and soon established himself as its leading American champion. Late in 1847, Simpson began searching for a better anesthetic agent, and on November 8 introduced chloroform into obstetrical practice.

[3] *Ibid.*
[4] A fine discussion of this topic can be found in George Rosen, " Mesmerism and surgery, a strange chapter in the history of anesthesia," *J. Hist. Med. & Allied Sc.,* 1946, *1* : 527-550.

Henceforth he became the staunchest advocate of obstetrical anesthesia and the leading exponent of chloroform.

While the introduction of anesthesia for surgical and obstetrical cases was hailed as a major triumph, strong opposition quickly developed, and the twentieth century was well advanced before the anesthetic question became largely academic. Although a few clergymen and theologians opposed obstetrical anesthesia on religious grounds, the attack from this front was never too serious despite a continued sniping for many years by some of the more fundamentalist clergymen. Surprisingly enough, the real threat to obstetrical anesthesia came from within the ranks of the medical profession itself. Few physicians openly supported the theological arguments against obstetrical anesthesia, but it is obvious that many were seeking in physiology a means for rationalizing their religious convictions. The opposition of a second group of doctors, the reactionaries, seems to have been based upon an instinctive resistance to anything new, while still another group was comprised of conservative physicians who were reluctant to endorse a radical innovation before it had been adequately tested.

The great debates which raged in the medical journals for a dozen or more years after 1847 make a separate story and all that can be done in a brief paper is to touch upon them. As early as March of 1847 Dr. W. Tyler Smith laid the basis for most of the subsequent medical arguments against obstetrical anesthesia in an article in *The Lancet* in which he asserted that, in addition to removing pain, the "inhalation of ether takes away from the parturient woman several other elements natural to her condition. . . ." Etherization, he wrote, affected the voluntary movements and in some instances caused a violent and irregular action "like the movements of ordinary intoxication." Furthermore, he said, pain was a preservative in labor, for when it became unbearable the patient cried out, "and her cry, by opening the glottis, takes away all expiratory pressure, and leaves the uterus acting alone." He conceded that the agonies of childbearing probably represented the most acute form of human suffering, but pointed out that this pain "sometimes acts as a stimulant, and as such is probably salutary rather than prejudicial." [5]

Over and above these purely physiological matters, he continued, were the emotional and moral considerations. In illustration he cited a number of instances in which erotic manifestations had occurred in women under

[5] W. Tyler Smith, "A lecture on the utility and safety of the inhalation of ether in obstetric practice," *Lancet*, 1847, *1*: 321-323.

the influence of anesthetics, and he suggested that it was possible that ether metamorphosed pain into pleasure. After declaring it well-known that eroticism was associated with parturition among lower animals, he noted that it was " reserved for the phenomena of etherization to show that, as regards sexual emotion, the human female may possibly exchange the pangs of travail for the sensations of coitus, and so approach to the level of brute creation." "If this be so," he continued, "women would scarcely part with pain, hard as their sufferings may be to bear; chastity of feeling, and, above all, emotional self-control, at a time when women are receiving such assistance as the accoucheur can render, are of far more importance than insensibility to pain." [6]

In the United States, Dr. C. D. Meigs of Philadelphia, one of the most prominent obstetricians of his day, led the attack against obstetrical anesthesia. He argued that the pains of childbirth were physiological and as such were an intimate part of the birth process. Pain was a "manifestation of the life force," and by avoiding it the mother risked both her health and her life. A well-known English obstetrician, Dr. Francis H. Ramsbotham, agreed in all essentials with Doctor Meigs but warned further that the lives of both mother and child were endangered by anesthesia. Moreover, he added, the process reduces a woman " to that condition which the law designates as ' *drunk and incapable.*' " [7]

Led by Simpson in England and Channing in America, a host of defenders laid aside their lancets and raised their pens in defense of anesthesia. In fact, as the battle swung decisively in favor of anesthesia, the views of its opponents can be learned largely by inference from the answers of its defendants. Suffice it to say, the arguments that pain was morally or physiologically essential to childbirth were demolished by 1860, and it is evident that henceforth the old guard conducted only a rearguard action.

Whatever may have been the reaction of doctors and clergymen, there was never any question of the patients' views on anesthesia, for parturient women seem to have been little concerned with abstract questions of morality, when an anesthetic agent was available. In the English-speaking world Queen Victoria's resort to chloroform in 1853 and 1857 gave obstetrical anesthesia the seal of complete respectability, but this royal approval merely confirmed what thousands of women had already

---

[6] *Ibid.*

[7] Francis M. Ramsbotham, *The Principles and Practice of Obstetric Medicine and Surgery, in Reference to the Process of Parturition* . . . (New American Edition, with notes and additions by William V. Keating, Philadelphia, 1857), p. 193.

accepted. In a paper read before the Massachusetts Medical Society in 1856 Dr. John G. Metcalf reported on his use of ether in some 223 obstetrical cases. Apropos of the reaction of his patients, Doctor Metcalf commented, " in every case, if I am called to a succeeding labor, the first question has invariably been, ' Have you brought the chloroform? ' " [8] Three years later, in Philadelphia, another American doctor stated that he had never found " a single instance where a patient would consent to its discontinuance after commencing its inhalations." " The universal cry," he concluded, " has been, ' give me more! ' " [9]

Although the main battle for obstetrical anesthesia had been won by 1860, the wide lag between medical developments and medical practice in the nineteenth century meant that the use of anesthesia was not nearly as universal as might have been expected. Relatively few doctors read medical journals, and many others opposed innovations in principle. Midwives, few of whom, at least in the United States, had any training, continued to attend the majority of normal deliveries. Thus it was that the question of the use of anesthesia in normal deliveries continued to be debated in lay and medical journals until the twentieth century. After 1860, however, the chief discussions in medical publications centered more on the relative values of the various anesthetic agents and on the methods for administering them. Until the development of satisfactory inhalation devices, ether was difficult to administer, and many doctors and patients objected to its odor. In fact, it was these characteristics of ether which led Sir James Simpson to his discovery of chloroform as an anesthetic agent.[10]

Although a number of anesthetic agents, including nitrous oxide, came into use, chloroform and ether dominated the field in the nineteenth century. Then, as now, the preference for one or another anesthetic was determined by the influence of medical schools, of individual personalities, or of other intangible factors. In Scotland and England, under the respective influences of Sir James Y. Simpson and Dr. John Snow, chloroform became the standard anesthetic in obstetrical cases. In the United States, practice varied somewhat, with the North stoutly adhering to ether and the Southern states clinging with equal determination to chloroform. The Northern faith in ether has been attributed in part to local pride,

[8] *College J. M. Sc.*, 1857, *2*: 78-80.

[9] D. W. Young, " Chloroform in parturition," *M. & S. Reporter*, 1859, *3*: 291.

[10] Sir James Y. Simpson, *Works*, vol. II: *Anaesthesia, Hospitalism, Hermaphroditism, and a Proposal to Stamp Out Small-Pox and Other Contagious Diseases*, Sir W. G. Simpson, ed. (Edinburgh, 1871), p. 27.

since Boston was the site of its first demonstration, and in part to the influence of the Harvard and University of Pennsylvania Medical Schools. In the South, New Orleans was the leading medical center, and the adoption of chloroform there undoubtedly contributed to its general use. It has been suggested that the warm climate of the Southern states inclined practitioners to the use of chloroform over the more volatile ether and, moreover, that possibly New Orleans was influenced by the French adoption of chloroform.[11] Whether or not these factors had any bearing, there is little question that chloroform won quick acceptance in New Orleans. A young interne in the city's Charity Hospital in 1849 reported on a series of eight obstetrical cases in which the patients had been anesthetized with chloroform. Chloroform, he commented, " is in constant use in the surgical and obstetrical practice of this hospital and is administered on a handkerchief held at a short distance from the mouth and nose so as to admit of a due mixture of atmospheric air with the vapor." [12] Ten years later the *New Orleans Medical News and Hospital Gazette* declared that ether was administered only for experimental purposes in the Charity Hospital, but that chloroform had been in almost daily use for medical, surgical, and obstetrical cases since 1848.[13]

The ease of administering chloroform soon made it the preferred anesthetic agent, but it was not long before evidence began to accumulate which showed its potential dangers. Although in 1848 the committee on obstetrics of the American Medical Association had strongly supported chloroform as the preferred anesthetic agent in obstetrics, by 1858 a Roxbury, Massachusetts, physician declared that chloroform has " proved to be a dangerous and often deadly agent." [14] At the same time the rising number of deaths in Great Britain was also causing serious second thoughts with respect to chloroform. John Snow, the world's first anesthetist, recognized the potential danger of chloroform and, by experimentation with animals, was able to establish the principle that a five per cent vapor was the maximum that could safely be inhaled. He knew, too, that ether was safer than chloroform, but, nonetheless, he continued to use chloroform because of its ease of administration. In his skillful

[11] Barbara M. Duncum, *The Development of Inhalation Anaesthesia with Special Reference to the Years 1846-1900* (London: Oxford Univ. Press, 1947), pp. 11-12.

[12] John T. McLean, "Anesthesia in midwifery with cases," *New Orleans M. & S. J.,* 1849, *6*: 418.

[13] "Chloroform in New Orleans," *New Orleans M. News & Hosp. Gaz.,* 1859, *6*: 312-313.

[14] B. E. Cotting, "Anaesthetics in midwifery," *Boston M. & S. J.,* 1858-1859, *59*: 369-370.

hands chloroform proved perfectly safe, but in the hands of careless and untrained individuals it was almost inevitable that deaths would occur.

By 1863 a total of 123 deaths were attributed directly to chloroform in Great Britain alone, and the Royal Medical College, urged on by *The Lancet* and other medical publications, appointed a committee to investigate the subject. This committee, which consulted with two of the leading anesthetists in England, issued a long report in 1864, conceding that chloroform was potentially dangerous and recommending that a search be made for a safer substitute. " Ether," the committee noted, " to a certain extent, fulfils these conditions, but its odour is disagreeable, it is slow in its operation, and gives rise to greater excitement than chloroform." For these reasons, the committee concluded, its use was impractical.[15] Within a few years a gradual improvement in inhalation devices simplified the administration of ether, and it, along with nitrous oxide, gained favor in England, where professional anesthetists were expected to give the patient and doctor some choice in the matter of anesthetic agents. John Snow's example helped to establish in Great Britain the concept that anesthesiology should be a field of its own. This fortunate state of affairs meant that although chloroform remained the prime anesthetic agent in nineteenth-century Great Britain, the creation of a group of relatively skilled anesthesiologists helped keep the number of deaths to a minimum.

In the United States in these years anesthetization was essentially a slapdash procedure. Usually chloroform was simply poured on a handkerchief or piece of cloth held over the face of the patient. A Texas physician reported in 1876 that, during a difficult labor lasting thirty hours, he had used seventeen ounces of chloroform, but he admitted that the imperfect administration of the anesthetic led to much wastage—a fact which may well account for the mother's survival![16] Ordinarily the anesthetic was given by the attending physicians, most of whom were convinced that chloroform was absolutely safe and could be sloshed on a towel or cloth with more or less impunity. Fortunately, as the nineteenth century drew to a close, inhalation devices were adopted in most of the better hospitals, but the average general practitioner still continued to use sponges, towels, handkerchiefs, or whatever else was available.

Since the obstetrical patient did not require a great degree of anesthetization, chloroform was relatively safe. Certainly most English and American physicians were convinced of this. Writing in a Cincinnati

[15] Duncum, *op. cit.*, pp. 179-180, 253-255.

[16] D. W. Brodnax, "The use of chloroform in puerperal convulsions," *Cincinnati M. News*, 1876, 9: 22-24.

medical journal in 1859 on the subject of anesthesia in parturition, Dr. Almon Gage referred to chloroform as " the highest known type " of anesthetic agent, and declared that its adaptability to labor was especially good.[17] In 1881, a textbook on anesthesia declared that chloroform was " the obstetrical anesthetic *par excellence*." [18] Six years later a New England physician, in extolling the virtues of chloroform, asserted that it involved no increase in the danger of postpartum hemorrhage and that it tended to hasten rather than retard labor. It was his opinion, furthermore, that heart disease was no " contra-indication to its use. . . ." [19] A Virginia physician summarized the general attitude towards the use of chloroform for maternity patients in an article in the *Journal of the American Medical Association* in the year 1895. He stated that during the past thirty-five years chloroform had been administered in literally millions of parturition cases, and yet there had been but few fatalities. This was particularly significant, he continued, in view of the manner in which chloroform was given in labor. " Often administered by ignorant nurses, husbands, by-standers, even by the patients themselves, and not infrequently, recklessly and injudicially by the attending physicians," he continued, " it is wonderful that evil results are so rare." He attributed this remarkable success to the " acquired force of the vasomotor system of the pregnant woman which enables her to resist the toxic action of chloroform to an extraordinary extent. . . ." [20]

The extensive use of chloroform in surgical cases in England may explain why the British increasingly became concerned with the growing number of deaths attributable to it. Yet here, too, obstetrical practice was considered in a class by itself, insofar as anesthesia was concerned. Addressing the Obstetrical Society of London in 1862, Dr. Thomas Skinner commented upon the growing opposition to chloroform appearing in the leading British and American medical journals. He blamed the increasing death toll on the lack of skill and experience of the operators and asserted: " There is a department of medicine which stands out in bold relief as a great and triumphant proof of the safety of chloroform as an anaesthetic, and of its superiority over ether in every respect: I allude to the obstetric department." Like some of his American counterparts, he

[17] Almon Gage, " Anaesthesia-chloroform in parturition," *College J. M. Sc.,* 1859, *4*: 482-484.

[18] *Cincinnati M. News,* 1881, *14*: 702-703.

[19] *Canada Lancet,* 1887, *20*: 24.

[20] Bedford Brown, " The therapeutic action of chloroform in parturition," *J. A. M. A.,* 1895, *25*: 354-358.

expressed the idea that pregnant women had a *"special tolerance* for chloroform." [21] *The Lancet,* which had been the first British medical magazine to take note of the deaths ensuing from chloroform, constantly urged caution in its use. For example, a brief note in an 1875 issue warned that a Strasbourg physician had shown that chloroform inhaled by the mother passed into the circulation of the foetus, and an editorial in 1889, which pointed out that many deaths among children had been attributed to chloroform, suggested that it was high time to reconsider its routine use in connection with young people.[22] The fears expressed in *The Lancet,* however, seem to have had little effect on English obstetrical practice. A textbook on midwifery published in London in 1887 declared that chloroform was suitable in any labor, normal or otherwise. Furthermore, the author declared: " No particular form of inhaler is necessary; a towel or a handkerchief molded in the form of a cone, answers every purpose." [23]

The Boston Medical and Surgical Journal, like its counterpart in England, *The Lancet,* did not share this felicitous view of chloroform and expressed a strong preference for ether. As one of the oldest and most respectable of American medical journals, it was widely read, but its influence on the chloroform issue seems to have been restricted to the relatively fertile grounds of New England and the Northeast. For example, a Doctor Cotting of Roxbury, Massachusetts, asserted in 1858 that ether was the only anesthetic which should be used in obstetrical cases.[24] Even Dr. Henry Lyman, whose book on anesthetics had described chloroform as the obstetrical anesthetic *par excellence,* conceded that for the graver operations of midwifery, ether was the preferred anesthetic.[25]

However the medical profession may have been divided on the issue, the evidence is clear that the general public welcomed anesthesia with open arms and with few reservations. Occasionally the doctors were accused of withholding relief, and even those doctors who had no objection to anesthesia *per se* but expressed legitimate doubts with respect to chloroform, on occasion found themselves under attack. *The Westminster Review* in England probably spoke for many laymen in 1859 when it expressed utter bewilderment at the wide diversity of views within the

---

[21] Thomas Skinner, " Anaesthesia in midwifery . . .," *Brit. M. J.,* 1862, *2*: 109.

[22] *London Lancet* (New York), 1875, *12*: 440; " Deaths under chloroform," *Lancet,* 1889, *2*: 802.

[23] Otto Spiegelberg, *A Text Book of Midwifery,* trans. from 2nd. German ed. by J. B. Hurry, 2 vols., (London, 1887-8), vol. I, pp. 266-269.

[24] Cotting, *loc. cit.,* p. 371.

[25] *Cincinnati M. News,* 1881, *14*: 702-703.

medical profession on the subject of obstetrical anesthesia. It pointed out that Doctor Channing of Boston advocated ether for every maternity case, that Professor Meigs of Philadelphia objected " to the use of anesthetics in labour under all circumstances," and that in Edinburgh, the birthplace of chloroform anesthesia, " scarcely a woman is ' confined' without drowning her pains in the Lethe of that fluid." With the doctors differing so widely, the author of the article commented, it is difficult for the public to decide. His tone, however, leaves little doubt that he considered the arguments against anesthesia to be specious. " The contest still rages fiercely," the author concluded, " and while these professional battles are being fought millions of Mothers are suffering agonies from which, according to the advocates of anesthesia, they might be surely and safely saved." [26] A few years later the same journal, evidently replying to the critics of anesthesia who argued that pain was essential to the birth process, concluded after reviewing the main points of argument that in all likelihood anesthesia tended to heighten, " instead of lower, the preventive efficacy of pain." [27]

Although the opposition to anesthesia on religious grounds proved no serious threat, individual ministers continued to inveigh against the practice throughout the nineteenth century, causing many devoutly religious women to hold grave misgivings. As late as 1888, the Reverend Henry Hayman denounced anesthesia on the grounds that pain is a " fountain of human affection." The birth pangs, he said, provided a physical basis for maternal love and helped to cement " more closely conjugal affection." [28] The need to reassure women with religious scruples is evident in an article appearing in *The Living Age* in 1898. With the magnificent aplomb and condescension of a nineteenth-century male addressing the delicate and childlike creatures of the opposite sex, the author expressed himself in the simple language reserved for such readers and personified the woman with religious qualms about anesthesia as " Devota." After carefully explaining to her that anesthesia was completely moral, he informed " Devota" that she had noble instincts but was not able to reason accurately. Having thus clarified the situation, he concluded his words of wisdom with the injunction: " And so let Devota take her chloroform and thank God for sending it." [29]

By the end of the nineteenth century the middle and upper classes, at

---

[26] " Chloroform and other anaesthetics," *Westminster Rev.*, 1859, *71*: 121-122.
[27] " The function of physical pain: anaesthetics," *Westminster Rev.*, 1871, *96*: 203.
[28] Henry Hayman, " The economy of pain," *Bibliotheca Sacra*, 1888, *45*: 7.
[29] William Barry, " The ethics of pain," *The Living Age*, 1898, *219*: 861-864.

least, had generally adopted anesthesia in maternity cases, and the author of an article in the *Atlantic Monthly* who proclaimed in 1896 that " childbirth has lost half of its terrors " was essentially correct.[80] It is still difficult to say, even during the early years of the twentieth century, what percentage of mothers were provided with an anesthetic agent. In 1914 the *Good Housekeeping Magazine* carried an article entitled, " When the stork arrives," which carefully explained the benefits to be derived from the use of anesthesia. The author assured his readers that " thanks to those supremest boons, chloroform and its twin sister, ether, it [was] no longer necessary in humane and competent hands, that a woman in labor should suffer agonizing pains." [81] Implicit in the article is the assumption that many mothers were still enduring the pains of childbirth. An article headed " Twilight Sleep in America," which was published in *McClure's Magazine,* April of 1915, carries this same implication. A prefatory editorial note stated that a previous story on twilight sleep, or the Freiburg method of painless childbirth, had brought hundreds of letters from women all over the country asking for further information. The article itself began by stating that from time immemorial each infant had entered the world " only at the cost of unimagined agony to its mother," but now " for the first time . . . there was at least a possibility that this suffering was to end." [82] In these same months the *Woman's Home Companion* was also discussing the topic of twilight sleep. In this journal, too, the editor mentioned the widespread interest aroused among its readers.[83] While many of them were interested in the Freiburg method primarily from the standpoint of wishing to participate in the birth process, the level of writing and the tone of the women's magazines indicate that many of their readers had had little experience with any sort of anesthetic.

One can readily understand the opposition of reactionary physicians to any innovation or the reluctance of conservative doctors to accept untried procedures. What is surprising, however, is the relatively large number of American physicians who even down to the end of the nineteenth century still either opposed obstetrical anesthesia totally or else used it only in difficult cases. A Dr. D. M. Barr, evidently appealing to this

[80] Edward Waldo Emerson, " A history of the gift of painless survery," *Atlantic Month.*, 1896, *78*: 679.

[81] Woods Hutchinson, " When the stork arrives," *Good Housekeeping Mag.*, 1914, *59*: 102-103.

[82] Constance Leupp and Burton J. Hendrick, " Twilight sleep in America," *McClure's Mag.*, 1915, *44*: 25.

[83] " Is the twilight sleep safe—for me?," *Woman's Home Companion,* 1915, *42*: 10.

group, began an address on anesthesia in labor in March of 1880 by stating: " I am here tonight to plead for ' Anaesthesia in Labor.' Not only in troublesome instrumental labor, but in all cases where the pains of travail fall upon women." [84] A year later in the same journal, Dr. D. M. Culver was quoted as saying: " I advise young physicians to use anaesthetics only in extreme cases—threatened convulsions or manual delivery —and let natural labors rest with nature's aid." [85] Dr. W. S. Ely conceded in the *New York Medical Journal* in 1886 that " the use of anaesthetics at some period in the progress of many obstetric cases was justifiable," thus leaving the impression that anesthesia should not be used in normal deliveries.[36] A year later, an Iowa physician proclaimed: " I do not use any anesthetic of any kind, especially in forceps cases. I want the patient to know what is going on." [37] Five years later, Dr. E. T. Rulison asked rhetorically: " Why are the great majority of our lying-in patients allowed to endure the travail of childbirth without the hand of science being extended to them in relief? " The answer, he said, lay in the tradition, " handed down by one old woman to another," which says it is " wicked to interfere with the laws of nature." [38] A Pennsylvania physician who stoutly espoused the cause of obstetrical anesthesia in 1893 was highly critical of some of his colleagues, who, he said, were too lazy to bother with anesthesia for their maternity patients and thus caused them to endure unnecessary suffering.[39] Quite obviously a large number of physicians, even fifty years after the introduction of anesthesia, were content to practice in the traditional manner. Moreover, the majority of babies were still being ushered into the world with the help of midwives, the majority of whom had virtually no formal training. For example, in Greater New York 48 per cent of the 80,735 births recorded by the Department of Health in 1901 were reported by midwives.[40] In rural areas, it seems logical to assume that midwives played an even greater role in maternity cases.

The gradual improvement in medical education and licensing standards which occurred during the second half of the nineteenth century, the upheaval created by the Flexner Report in 1909, and the improvements in

[84] D. M. Barr, " Anaesthesia in labor," *M. & S. Reporter*, 1880, *42*: 221.
[85] *Ibid.*, 1881, *44*: 279.
[36] *New York M. J.*, 1886, *44*: 25.
[37] A. D. Bundy, " Obstetrics in the country," *M. & S. Reporter*, 1887, *56*: 201.
[38] E. T. Rulison, " The use of chloroform in labor," *ibid.*, 1891, *65*: 851.
[39] John W. Groff, " One hundred cases of labor," *College and Clin. Rec.*, 1893, *14*: 301-302.
[40] Ralph Folks, " Obstetrics in the tenements," *Charities*, 1902, *9*: 429.

anesthesiology itself virtually guaranteed that by the outbreak of World War I some type of anesthesia was available for any parturient woman under a physician's care. The question of whether or not to use anesthesia in obstetrical cases was no longer seriously debated: henceforth the problem was essentially a medical one relating to the type of anesthetic agent or the technique of administration. There was no immediate relief for the thousands of women who still depended upon midwives, but the solution to this problem was at hand by virtue of the rapidly rising standard of living.

ANNALS OF SCIENCE, 40 (1983), 159–177

Religious Opposition to Obstetric Anaesthesia: a Myth?

A. D. FARR

Tullochvenus House, Lumphanan, Aberdeenshire AB3 4RN, Scotland

Received 24 September 1982

Summary

It has frequently been suggested that science and religion are innately in conflict. One example from the history of medicine is the introduction of anaesthesia into obstetrics in 1847, which is commonly said to have stimulated massive religious opposition. Historians have almost unanimously averred that such opposition arose from the belief that obstetric anaesthesia interfered with the primeval curse— 'In sorrow thou shalt bring forth children' (Genesis 3. 16). Despite considerable opposition to obstetric anaesthesia upon medical, physiological, and general moral grounds, evidence of genuine religious opposition in contemporary sources has proved to be virtually non-existent. On examination, this particular 'conflict' appears to be an artifact of historiography based upon a contemporary defence prepared against an attack which never materialized.

Contents

1. Introduction

Although there was only slight opposition to the introduction of anaesthesia into surgery in the 1840s, there was rather more resistance to its use in obstetrics, and only here is it said that religious arguments were adduced. The first operation in Britain using ether anaesthesia took place in Scotland on 19 December 1846.[1] Its use spread rapidly,[2] and ether was introduced in Edinburgh by her professor of midwifery, James

---

[1] W. Scott, 'Correspondence', *The Lancet*, 1872, ii, 585. This event has been investigated thoroughly by T. W. Baillie, 'The first European Trial of Anaesthetic Ether: the Dumfries Claim', *British Journal of Anaesthetics*, 37 (1965), 952. The nature of the operation performed is not recorded.
[2] J. Robinson, *A Treatise on the Inhalation of the Vapour of Ether for the prevention of pain in Surgical Operations* (London, 1847). This pamphlet collates a large number of ether operations. See also *The Lancet*, 1947, i, for a series of reports of operations performed in Britain under anaesthesia during the six months following its introduction. pp. 54, 77, 104, 132, 158, 184, 210, 237, 342, 367, 499, 549, 639, etc.

Young Simpson (1811–70), who was the first to apply it in obstetrics in January 1847. The need for some relief of pain during parturition was implicit even in a book written by Charles Meigs (subsequently one of the major medical opponents of obstetric anaesthesia), who said of the 'painful sensations' of a woman in labour that they were so great 'as to be absolutely indescribable and comparable to no other pain'.[3] This view was nowhere seriously rejected. The employment of general anaesthesia during labour involved more problems than in general surgery, it being necessary to determine its effects both upon the uterine contractions essential to delivery and upon the fetus, whose reaction to the anaesthetic may differ from that of the mother.

Simpson first employed ether in midwifery on 19 January 1847, soon following this case with two others and deducing that 'As far as they go the preceding cases point out one important result: in all of them, the uterine contractions continued as regular in their occurrence and duration after the state of anaesthesia had been induced, as before the inhalation was begun'.[4] Thus far Simpson was merely extending surgical anaesthesia, but on 13 February 1847 he employed ether in two cases in which no surgery or manipulations were indicated, the first patient subsequently telling Simpson 'she could only look back with regret to the apparently unnecessary suffering she had endured in the birth of her former infants'.[5]

Simpson posed the rhetorical question: 'will the state of etherization ever come to be generally employed with the simple object of assuaging the pains of natural parturition?'. After reviewing the extent of suffering due to labour pains he concluded that 'it will become...necessary to determine on any grounds, moral or medical, whether a professional man could deem himself "justified" in withholding, and not using any such safe means, as we at present presuppose this to be'.[6] Simpson's own practice was made clear some months later when he wrote of ether,

> that since for the first time directing the attention of the medical profession to its great use and importance in natural and morbid parturition, I have employed it, with few rare exceptions, in every case of labour that I have attended; and with the most delightful results. And I have no doubt whatever, that some years hence the practice will be general. Obstetricians may oppose it, but I believe our patients themselves will force the use of it upon the profession. I have never...once witnessed any disagreeable result follow to either mother or child; whilst I have now seen an immense amount of material pain and agony saved by its employment.[7]

[3] C. D. Meigs, *Obstetrics: the Science and the Art* (Philadelphia, 1849), p. 153.
[4] J. Y. Simpson, 'Notes on the Employment of the Inhalation of Sulphuric Ether in the Practice of Midwifery', *Monthly Journal of Medical Science*, 8 (1847), 721–8. Also reprinted as a pamphlet (Edinburgh. 1847).
[5] Ibid.
[6] Footnote 4. The two final paragraphs of the original paper were omitted from the reprinted pamphlet version of the paper.
[7] J. Y. Simpson, *Account of a New Anaesthetic Agent as a Substitute for Sulphuric Ether in Surgery and Midwifery* (Edinburgh, 1847). Reprinted by W. O. Priestley and H. R. Storer, editors, *Obstetric Memoirs and Contributions*, 2 vols (Edinburgh, 1885–6), II, pp. 722–32.

In the same paper he reported his discovery of 'a new anaesthetic agent, more efficient than sulphuric ether'—chloroform, which he had already employed in midwifery,[8] but he chided his colleagues outside Scotland:

> I am told that the London physicians, with two or three exceptions only, have never yet employed ether-inhalation in their midwifery practice. Three weeks ago, I was informed, in a letter from Professor Montgomery of Dublin, that he believed that in that city, up to that date, it had not been used in a single case of labour.[9]

Chloroform rapidly displaced ether in Britian until a number of fatalities led to further experiments resulting in the re-introduction of nitrous oxide.

Many twentieth-century commentators have alleged that part of the criticism of obstetric anaesthesia was on religious grounds, but examination of these allegations reveals little direct evidence of any such attack. The first hint (and it was no more) of religious criticism of anaesthesia came in 1847. Mr Parke, a Liverpool surgeon, visited Edinburgh during October and had several conversations with Simpson about anaesthesia, during which he learned with surprise that 'he advocated most strongly, its use, not as the *exception*, but as the *rule*, in midwifery cases—in cases of ordinary labour'.[10] It so happened that Parke, a member of the Liverpool Medical Institution, was asked by their secretary to provide a paper for a meeting on 25 November and he offered to read one 'On the Moral Propriety of Medical Men recommending the inhalation of Aether in other than Extraordinary Cases',[11] stating that 'it was on moral grounds alone I should treat it, and that by some it might be viewed as belonging to the Divine more than the Medical man'.[12]

Simpson heard of the impending paper and, in a post-script to a letter addressed to Mr Waldie of Liverpool on 14 November, indicated that he had a good idea of Parke's line of thought. The postscript is worth quoting *in toto*:

> By the bye, Imlach tells me Dr P. is to enlighten your medical society about the 'morality' of the practice [of obstetric anaesthesia.] I have a great itching to run up and pound him. *When* is the meeting? The true moral question is, 'Is a practitioner justified by *any* principles of humanity in not using it?' I believe every operation without it is just a piece of the most deliberate and cold-blooded *cruelty*. He will be at the primary curse, no doubt. But the word translated 'sorrow' is truly 'labour', 'toil'; and in the very next verse the very same word means this: Adam was to eat of the ground with 'sorrow'. This does not mean *physical* pain, and it was cursed to bear 'thorns and thistles', which we pull up without dreaming that it is a sin. God promises repeatedly to take off the two

---

[8] Ibid. This paper appeared, with some variations, in a number of places. The title quoted here was that used in *The Lancet*, 1847, ii, 549–50, dated 20 November. The original announcement was made on 10 November at a meeting of the Medico-Chirurgical Society of Edinburgh. Apart from several editions of the pamphlet (footnote 7 above), the report also appeared in the *London Medical Gazette*, new series 5 (1847), dated 22 November, and the *Medical Times*, 17 (1847–8), 90.
[9] Ibid. *The Lancet*, 550n.
[10] J. Parke, *Reasons for Not Using Chloroform Except in Cases of Extreme Necessity* (Liverpool, 1848), p. 5.
[11] The Institution's minute book gives the title of the paper as *On the Moral Propriety of Administering Aether in other than Extraordinary Cases*. The version quoted in the text is that given by Parke in his later pamphlet based upon the paper (footnote 10 above).
[12] Parke (footnote 10).

curses on women and on the ground, if the Israelites kept their covenant. See Deut, vii, 13, etc., etc. See also Isaiah xxviii. 23; extirpation of the 'thorns and thistles' of the first curse said to come from God. Besides, Christ in dying 'surely hath borne our griefs and carried our sorrows', and removed 'the curse of the law, being made a curse for us'. His mission was to introduce mercy, not sacrifice. Go up and refute Him if I don't come.[13]

At the meeting Parke read his paper to an audience of only 25 colleagues. The minute book made no reference at all to any religious element in his argument,[14] and only in some additional comments included in his pamphlet (published a year later) did Parke develop his religious views—which did not include the 'curse' argument.[15] By this time Simpson had already published his *Answer to the religious objections advanced against the employment of anaesthetic agents in midwifery and surgery*.[16] Thus Parke's religious arguments, at least in public form, appeared as a consequence of Simpson's 'Answer' rather than as its cause.

That Parke's religious philosophy included the concept of pain as not merely ordained by God, but actually constituting one of His blessings, is made clear by a statement towards the end of his pamphlet. 'You do not *really* bless a woman by removing the pains of labour—her *true* blessing flows from lifting up her heart to God, and asking for humility and strength to bear them. Over and over again, have I seen such faith rewarded, with far more comfort than chloroform could give'.[17]

Only one other 'religious' pamphlet on the subject was published at this time, Dr Protheroe Smith's *Scriptural Authority for Mitigation of the Pains of Labour*[18] (see Section 3.3 below). Of these three works, Simpson's has been the source of almost all subsequent accounts and comments.

2. Religious opposition to anaesthesia

It has been widely held by modern commentators that the greatest opposition to obstetric anaesthesia was that from religious sources. Subsequent to Simpson's death, reference to these 'religious objections' was first made in print in 1873 by Duns in his biography of Simpson,[19] although he failed to quote any specific evidence other than Simpson's own pamphlet. Indeed, when citing 'communications from patients', at least one of the ladies quoted by Duns averred that prior to reading Simpson's pamphlet she would not have had such objections herself in any case.[20]

---

[13] J. Y. Simpson, Postscript to letter to Mr Waldie of Liverpool dated 14 November 1847. In *Memoir of Sir J. Y. Simpson*, J. Duns (Edinburgh, 1873), 215–6. The reference to Isaiah is clearly incorrect. Possibly it was intended to refer to Isaiah 55. 13.

[14] Liverpool Medical Institution, *Minutes of Ordinary Meetings*, 9th Session (1847-8). Thursday, 25 November 1847.

[15] Parke (footnote 10).

[16] J. Y. Simpson, *Answer to the Religious Objections Advanced Against the Employment of Anaesthetic Agents in Midwifery and Surgery* (Edinburgh, 1847).

[17] Parke, footnote 10. Parke also included on the cover of his pamphlet the text 'Despise not the chastening of the Lord—Heb. xii, 5'.

[18] P. Smith, *Scriptural Authority for the Mitigation of the Pains of Labour by Chloroform and other anaesthetic Agents* (London, 1848).

[19] J. Duns, *Memoir of Sir James Y. Simpson* (Edinburgh, 1873). This is both a helpful and a potentially misleading work. Duns was an old friend of Simpson's and also particularly interested in recording 'Sir Jame's religious history'. He was learned both in science and religion and sought to reconcile these two areas of study.

[20] Ibid., 261.

Twenty-three years later Simpson's daughter Eve repeated the story, again without any precise reference other than to her father's pamphlet.[21] Eve Blantyre Simpson was born in 1856, eight years after the religious 'debate', and she was aged only 14 when her father died, so that she could have had no more than indirect knowledge of the affair.

Also writing in 1896, A. D. White, in his *History of the Warfare of Science with Theology and Christendom*, claimed that 'From pulpit after pulpit Simpson's use of chloroform was denounced as impious and contrary to Holy Writ; texts were cited abundantly, the ordinary declaration being that to use chloroform was "to avoid one part of the primeval curse on woman"'.[22] However, White's only cited source was Duns's biography; surprisingly, he did not even mention Simpson's own pamphlet on the subject.[23]

Whatever the origin of the allegation that religious objections to obstetric anaesthesia existed at the time of its introduction, it has been repeated many times by modern commentators. Although not all of these need be taken seriously, there remain sufficient references by authoritative authors for the allegation to have achieved historical credence.[24]

2.1. *References in periodical literature*

In an attempt to find direct evidence of 'religious' objections, a detailed study has been made of eighty-four contemporary newspapers and periodicals of British and North American origin as well as the *Acts of the General Assembly of the Church of Scotland* (including abridgements of the Proceedings) and the *Acts and Proceedings of the General Assembly of the Free Church of Scotland*.

The periodical material studied included thirty-five items of primarily religious or theological nature and forty-nine general magazines and reviews, and extended from the date of the first recorded use of anaesthesia in surgery (October 1846) to December 1849, eighteen months after Simpson claimed that religious opposition had 'ceased among us'.[25] As a result of this search, which extended to every issue of each of the eighty-four items for the period given, only seven references to religion in connection with anaesthesia were found, all of which were reviews (four of them specifically concerned with Simpson's pamphlet): none was critical of the procedure and five of them (including the only two found in theological periodicals) supported the use of obstetric anaesthesia and Simpson's stand on this.[26]

---

[21] E. B. Simpson, *Sir James Y. Simpson* (Edinburgh, 1896), pp. 63–4.

[22] A. D. White, *A History of the Warfare of Science with Theology in Christendom* (London, 1896). Reprinted New York: Dover Books, 1960, II, 63.

[23] White referred to an 'ancient and time-honoured belief in Scotland' opposing the concept of obstetric anaesthesia, and supported this by a distorted report of a 300-year-old case of alleged witchcraft which was entirely irrelevant. Subsequently, a number of twentieth-century commentators have resurrected this case uncritically and used it as 'evidence for the existence of mid-nineteenth-century prejudice against the practice. See, for example: R. F. Miller, *Triumph Over Pain* (New York, 1938). Translated by B. Paul and C. Paul, p. 334. V. Robinson, *Victory Over Pain* (New York, 1946), p. 201. F. Prescott, *The Control of Pain* (London, 1964), p. 31.

[24] For example, A. R. Simpson, 'The Jubilee of Anaesthetic Midwifery', *Transactions of the Glasgow Obstetrical and Gynaecological Society*, (1898), 1, 1–26, p. 17.

[25] J. Y. Simpson, letter to Protheroe Smith dated 8 July 1848. Published as an appendix to P. Smith, see Smith (footnote 18), 44.

[26] *Edinburgh Evening Courand*, 30 January 1847; *Edinburgh Weekly Journal*, 22 December 1847; *MacPhail's Edinburgh Ecclesiastical Journal*, 4 (1848), 417–26; *The Witness*, 29 December 1847; *Athenaeum*, 19 February 1848, no. 1060, p. 189; *North American Review*, 68 (1849), p. 311; *North British Review*, 7 (1847), 169–206.

The Scottish newspapers studied contained *inter alia* very detailed reports of meetings of both the established and free church synods and assemblies. It would thus seem reasonably certain that, at least until a year after Simpson wrote his reply to the religious objections to anaesthesia, no such objections had in fact been made publicly at any church gathering of importance in Scotland, in any of a wide range of theological publications of various denominational sympathies, nor in any of a large number of British or North American reviews and other periodicals.

2.2. *Objections made privately*

Simpson was in the habit of retaining not only most of the correspondence received by him, but also copies of many of the letters which he wrote himself. A few of Simpson's papers are held by the National Library of Scotland, but the majority are in the library of the Royal College of Surgeons of Edinburgh where, until recently, they have lain unsorted.[27] Examination of both these collections has revealed only two references to religious objections to obstetric anaesthesia which have not appeared amongst Simpson's published papers; these, and the published comments, are quoted below. Of Simpson's published comments only two are apposite:

(i) In his *Answer to the Religious Objections* ...—published eleven months after the first use of ether in obstetrics—Simpson referred to having heard patients and others strongly object to the superinduction of anaesthesia in labour, by the inhalation of Ether or Chloroform, on the assumed ground, that an immunity from pain during parturition was contrary to religion and the express commands of Scripture. Not a few medical men have, I know, joined in this same objection, and have refused to relieve their patients from the agonies of childbirth, on the allegation that they believed that their employment of suitable anaesthetic means for such a purpose would be unscriptural and irreligious.[28]

(ii) In a letter to Protheroe Smith (published by the latter as an appendix to his pamphlet) Simpson said only seven months later:

Here, in Edinburgh, I never now meet with any objections on this point, for the religious, like the other forms of opposition to chloroform, have ceased among us. But in Edinburgh matters were very different at first; I found many patients with strong religious scruples on the propriety of the practice. Some consulted their clergymen. One day, on meeting the Rev. Dr H—, he stopped me to say that he was just returning from absolving a patient's conscience on the subject, for she had taken chloroform during labour, and so avoided suffering, but she had felt unhappy ever since, under the idea that she had done something very wrong and sinful. A few among the clergy themselves, for a time, joined in the cry against the new practice. I have just looked up a letter which a clergyman wrote to a medical friend, in which he declares that chloroform is (I quote his own words) 'a decoy of Satan, apparently offering itself to bless woman: but, in the end', he continues 'it will harden society, and rob God of the deep earnest cries which arise in time of trouble for help'.[29]

---

[27] The work of cataloguing this huge and important collection has recently been completed by the College Librarian, Dr I. Simpson Hall, to whom I am indebted for access to some of the correspondence, and for permission to reproduce some of this which has not appeared in print elsewhere.

[28] Simpson (footnote 16), 3.

[29] Simpson (footnote 25), 43.

On this evidence the whole religious argument appears to have occupied less than eighteen months. It will be noted further that Simpson's comments both in 1847 and 1848 referred primarily to objections raised by some patients themselves and by their medical attendants. Only 'a few among the clergy themselves' were said to have had doubts.

This latter point is strengthened by an aside in Simpson's pamphlet in which he referred to an exchange between his friend Professor Miller (Professor of Surgery in the University of Edinburgh) and the Reverend Dr Chalmers (Moderator of the Free Church of Scotland and a former Moderator of the establish Kirk). Simpson said,

> my friend Professor Miller informs me, that when reluctantly consenting to write the elaborate article on Etherization, which he afterwards penned for the North British Review (No. for May 1847),[30] he stated to the late Dr Chalmers, who solicited him to undertake the task, that if he 'wrote the medical Dr Chalmers should himself write the theological part'. Dr Chalmers at once professed that he did not see any theological part pertaining to it. Mr Miller then explained to him, that some had been urging objections against the use of ether in midwifery on the ground of its so far improperly enabling women to avoid one part of the primeval curse. At last when Mr Miller was enabled to convince him that he was in earnest in saying that such ground *had* been taken, Dr Chalmers thought quietly for a minute or two, and then added, that if some 'small theologians' really took such an improper view of the subject, he would certainly advise Mr Miller not to 'heed them' in his article. Dr Chalmers' mind was not one that could take up or harbour the extraordinary idea, that, under the Christian dispensation, the God of Mercy should wish for, and delight in, the sacrifice of women's screams and sufferings in childbirth.

That such an eminent divine as Chalmers [31] regarded this issue as one for 'small theologians' makes it clear that support for anti-anaesthetic views cannot have had much currency amongst ministers of the church, whatever the outlook of some laymen.

That some lay persons should have questioned the propriety of the new procedure is not surprising, but it is clear that at least some ministers—including the very learned—were prepared to defend anaesthesia as not being contrary to Christian teaching. The allegation by one clergyman that chloroform was a 'decoy of Satan' which would 'rob God of the deep earnest cries which arise in time of trouble for help' would seem to be exceptional, for apart from a subsequent remark by Parke,[32] no other such comment has come to light.

---

[30] The article referred to was a review article published anonymously, and based upon three sources: J. Robinson (footnote 2); J. Y. Simpson. (footnote 4); and the medical periodicals *passim*. It appeared as article VII in *The North British Review*, 7 (1847), 169–206, and contained no reference to 'any possibility of religious objections to anaesthesia, in midwifery or elsewhere.

[31] Thomas Chalmers was one of the most notable figures in nineteenth-century Scottish church life. Born in 1780 and brought up as a strict Calvinist, Chalmers was licensed as a preacher at the age of 19, and became Professor of Moral Philosophy at St Andrews University in 1823 and of Divinity at Edinburgh University in 1828; he became Moderator of the General Assembly of the Free Church of Scotland, which position he held, together with the Chair of Divinity at New College, Edinburgh, until his death in 1847. Chalmers was the author of one of the eight Bridgewater Treatises and a recent assessment of him has averred that 'his theology was Calvinistic, with the stress rather on the needs of man than on the election of God' (*Oxford Dictionary of the Christian Church*, London, 1958, p. 261). If true, this may have affected his attitude to the propriety of anaesthesia.

[32] Parke (footnote 10). 12.

A more typical response appears to have been that of the Reverend Thomas Boodle of Virginia Water in Surrey. Writing to Simpson after reading his pamphlet, Boodle said that 'it has so far relieved my mind from the serious objections I had entertained that I am very anxious for further information and particulars in respect to the safety and expediency of its adoption in midwifery as a means of mitigating the pangs of labour'.[33] Here was a mind readily set at rest upon the religious issue and worried only about medical implications.

Simpson later wrote that following publication of his own pamphlet he had 'received a variety of written and verbal communications from some of the best theologians and most esteemed clergymen here and elsewhere, and all churches, Presbyterian, Independent, Episcopalian, etc.—approving of the views which I had taken'.[34] Perhaps he was more aware of the real reason for some individual doubts than he was prepared to admit publicly, for in the original draft of his letter to Protheroe Smith,[35] Simpson had written that 'all religious opposition to chloroform has entirely ceased among us, if we except an occasional remark on the point from some caustic old maid whose prospects of using chloroform are for ever passed, or a sneer from some antiquated lady who grieves and grudges that her daughters should not suffer as their mother was obliged to suffer before them'.[36] This passage was omitted from the final letter and one can well see why a successful obstetrician, moving in high social circles, might feel that discretion was likely to be preferable upon such a point. However, the fact that Simpson wrote such a comment at all shows that he was aware of other reasons for some private objections to anaesthesia.

Whether 'all religious opposition' had, in fact, ceased, as Simpson claimed in July 1848, is not entirely clear. A number of modern commentators have suggested that it only ceased with the use of chloroform by Queen Victoria at the birth of Prince Leopold on 7 April 1853.[37] Evidence for religious opposition after 1848 is almost entirely limited to such secondary sources, but there is no doubt that the Queen did receive chloroform in 1853—and approved of its use.[38]

For the decade following 1848, only two references to the religious aspect have been discovered. The first is in a letter written on 15 June 1852 by the Reverend Charles Kingsley to Lord —. Kingsley said:

> Let me thank you most cordially for your hint about chloroform. As for 'forbidden ground', can there be forbidden ground between husband and husband; or between two human beings who wish to diminish by one atom the

[33] T. Boodle, letter to J. Y. Simpson, dated 14 January 1848. MS in collection of Royal College of Surgeons, Edinburgh. Hitherto unpublished. Quoted by permission of the Librarian.

[34] Simpson (footnote 25), 44.

[35] J. Y. Simpson, draft of letter to Dr Protheroe Smith. Undated, but known to be early 1848. MS in collection of Royal College of Surgeons, Edinburgh. Hitherto unpublished. Quoted by permission of the Librarian.

[36] A similar view was expressed in an undated letter to Simpson from a Dr R. Malcolm of Edinburgh, who said: 'I have repeatedly found the mothers of my patients object to anaesthesia—as if they grudged that their daughters should not experience the same sufferings as themselves—but I have uniformly found them afterwards as grateful as their daughters for the relief administered'. (Hitherto unpublished letter in an uncatalogued recent acquisition of Simpson correspondence in the National Library of Scotland, Accession No. 5683.)

[37] See, for example, V. S. Thatcher, History of Anaesthesia (Philadelphia, 1953), p. 16; R. Calder, The Life Savers (London, 1961), p. 142; F. Prescott, The Control of Pain (London, 1964), p. 33; R. S. Atkinson, James Simpson and Chloroform (London, 1973), p. 76.

[38] Queen Victoria's Diary. Entry for 22 April 1853. This passage is quoted by K. B. Thomas in The Development of Anaesthetic Apparatus (London, 1975), p. 233.

amount of human suffering? . . . It is a real delight to my faith, as well as to my pity, to know that the suffering of childbirth can be avoided. . . . The popular superstition that it is the consequence of the fall I cannot but smile at—seeing it is contradicted by the plain words of the text which is quoted to prove it—'I will greatly *multiply* thy sorrow and thy conception', ... It being yet a puzzle to me, as a Cambridge man, how the multiplication of 0 can produce a number. $0 \times A$ used to $= 0$, did it not?[39]

This letter is difficult, for the text is incomplete and unclear and the letter to which it is a reply is missing. It is possible to interpret Kingsley as thanking his correspondent for factual information about anaesthesia while gently ridiculing the 'popular superstition' that labour pains were 'a consequence of the fall', no direct comment being made on the propriety or otherwise of their alleviation. Equally one may interpret him as indicating the existence of a 'popular superstition' which rejected chloroform as a means of diminishing 'that suffering of childbirth' to which he referred. If this was the case the question then arises, what did Kingsley mean by 'popular'? Certainly the evidence referred to above indicates that anti-anaesthetic views on religious grounds had never been commonly referred to publicly. It is not clear, therefore, whether Kingsley was or was not hinting that 'popular superstition' was opposed to the alleviation of suffering in parturition at this time.

The second reference occurred in a book published as late as 1855. In his *Chloroform; its properties and safety in childbirth*, Dr E. W. Murphy, after commenting upon Simpson's arguments, went on to say that 'even at the present moment, there are pious persons whose judgement is shaken by this interpretation of Scripture, who look upon Aetherisation as sinful'.[40] The implication was that no more than a very few individuals held such opinions and certainly, following Queen Victoria's example two years previously, there was no evidence of any popular feeling upon this point. Indeed, Murphy later merely commented that 'anaesthesia is now generally used in midwifery as well as in surgery and the only controversy that remains for discussion is whether chloroform or sulphuric aether is best for the purpose'.[41]

2.3. *Religious opposition secondary to medical objections*
Although religious objections to obstetric anaesthesia arose in medical writings on the subject, there are very few examples of this. Apart from Parke,[42] only three medical authors appear to have become involved in religious arguments.

(i) *G. T. Gream*, in his pamphlet on *The Misapplication of Anaesthesia in Childbirth*, referred briefly to some religious objections, saying of Simpson's pamphlet that he was 'of opinion it does not contain one single argument to prove that there is authority for allaying the pains of labour'.[43] He then proceeded to make a case that anaesthesia and intoxication were synonymous and 'justly esteemed a crime by the laws of God and Man'.

[39] C. Kingsley, *Charles Kingsley: His Letters and Memories of His Life*, edited by 'his wife', 4th edn (London, 1877), I, 326.
[40] E. W. MURPHY, *Chloroform: its Properties and Safety in Childbirth* (London, 1855), pp. 3–4.
[41] E. W. Murphy, *Lectures on the Principles and Practice of Midwifery*, 2nd edn (London, 1862), p. 562.
[42] Parke (footnote 10).
[43] G. T. Gream, *The Misapplication of Anaesthesia in Childbirth* (London, 1849), p. 7.

However, Gream had missed Simpson's point, for the latter had not sought to prove that Scripture positively authorized the relief of suffering in labour (the reality of which suffering Gream tacitly conceded), but that nowhere did Scripture forbid it.

(ii) *Charles Meigs*, Simpson's greatest opponent on the medical aspects of obstetric anaesthesia, was reticent upon the religious arguments, merely doubting 'any process, that the physician sets up, to contravene the operation of those natural and physiological forces that the Divinity has ordained us to enjoy or suffer'.[44]

(iii) *W. P. Montgomery* of Dublin was, perhaps, the medical opponent whom Simpson believed to be most strongly opposed to him on the religious issue—yet Montgomery vehemently denied this and opposed Simpson only upon what he called the 'indiscriminate' use of anaesthetics during labour.

In his pamphlet Simpson had said that he had been informed that 'in another medical school, my conduct in introducing and advocating the super-induction of anaesthesia in labour has been publicly denounced *ex cathedra* as an attempt to contravene the arrangements and decrees of Providence, hence reprehensible and heretical in its character, and anxiously to be avoided and eschewed by all properly principled students and practioners'.[45] This apparently referred to Professor Montgomery, who took grave exception. In a hitherto unpublished letter to Simpson, dated 27 December 1848, Montgomery fully refuted the allegation, and this is worth quoting *in extenso*.

Referring to two letters which Simpson had apparently received and sent to Montgomery for comment, the latter referred to a

> '*Dublin man*' who reported my opinion on the 'religious objections'—on which subject you say you were induced to write your 'Answer' by being informed that I was publicly advocating these so called 'Religious objections' and that I had denounced you ex cathedra as acting in an unchristian way in advocating the abrogation of pain in labour by anaesthesia—and that the only ground you had for thinking that I did so was hearing it 'very casually from a Dublin Man' I really feel astonished that *you*, who must know as well as any one, how constantly what a lecturer says is misunderstood or misrepresented, could thus admit on mere hearsay evidence a position to which you attached sufficient importance to induce you to take the trouble of writing a formal reply to arguments which never were made use of by me—I never advocated or countenanced either *in public* or *in private* the so called '*Religious objections*' to anaesthesia in labour, but invariably rejected that objection and many and many a time have had the trouble of shewing patients the utter untenableness of such an objection—as is perfectly well known to every one here.[46]

That Montgomery took such trouble to dissociate himself from 'religious' objections, while maintaining certain medical objections to obstetric anaesthesia, suggests that he was probably speaking the truth. Indeed, in a later paper he said explicitly: 'I attach no value to what are called the "religious objections" to the use of this remedy'.[47]

[44] Meigs (footnote 3), 353.
[45] Simpson (footnote 16), 3.
[46] W. F. Montgomery, letter to J. Y. Simpson, dated 27 December 1848, unpublished. MS in collection of the Royal College of Surgeons, Edinburgh. Quoted by permission of the Librarian. The punctuation of Montgomery's letter has been left unaltered.
[47] Dublin Quarterly Journal of Medical Science, 7 (1949), p. 335.

Montgomery did criticize Simpson, however, for the use of the two texts on the title page of his pamphlet (see Section 3.2 below) which were said to be (respectively) taken out of context and a *non sequitur*: he also said of Simpson's suggestion that the removal of Adam's rib was the first surgical operation with anaesthesia: 'A cause which requires such assistance as this, one would suppose, must be in great need of support'. Montgomery's position was that, while not himself holding religious objections to obstetric anaesthesia, he defended the right of others to hold them.

It might be concluded that, although religious objections were referred to by medical opponents of anaesthesia, this was infrequent. It may be more significant to note the readiness with which Simpsson assumed such behaviour on the part of colleagues apparently innocent of the charge.

3. The defence against religious objections

3.1. *James Young Simpson*

It has generally been held that Simpson was a deeply religious man. While this is a true generalization it is less often appreciated that Simpson's 'conversion' to active Christianity was a phenomenon of his later life, and that until 1861–62 his Christian virtues were probably no greater than those of many of his colleagues.[48]

Writing of the period following Simpson's acquisition of the Edinburgh Chair of Midwifery in 1839, Duns commented that 'up to this period, there is scarcely a trace among Dr Simpson's papers and correspondence of the least interest in religious matters....In a word, there was that baptized heathenism which often becomes the broken reed on which noble and richly-endowed minds are content to lean.[49] After his marriage (also in 1839) Simpson attended St Stephen's Church in Edinburgh where he fell under the evangelical influence of the minister, Dr William Muir, and 'began to think about religion, but without any efforts to become religious'.[50] When the disruption of the Church of Scotland occurred in May 1843, and 474 ministers and many laymen seceded to form a Free Church of Scotland, Simpson joined with them.

Simpson's eldest child died in 1844 aged 4 and another daughter died in infancy in 1847, events which certainly caused him to think more closely of the Almightly. Also the illness and death from cancer in 1848 of his childhood friend John Reid moved him deeply, and Duns dated Simpson's own growing interest in religion from this latter event and time.

Simpson's first recorded comments on theology were his concern about Parke's views[51] and the subsequent publication of his pamphlet *Answer to the Religious Objections*...in 1847.[52] This latter document—an impressive piece of Biblical exegesis—was prepared by a man who had no theological background or training, and one is bound to wonder whether Simpson consulted any theologians over its

---

[48] See Duns (footnote 19).
[49] Ibid., 125–6.
[50] Ibid., 127.
[51] Simpson (footnote 13).
[52] Simpson (footnote 16).

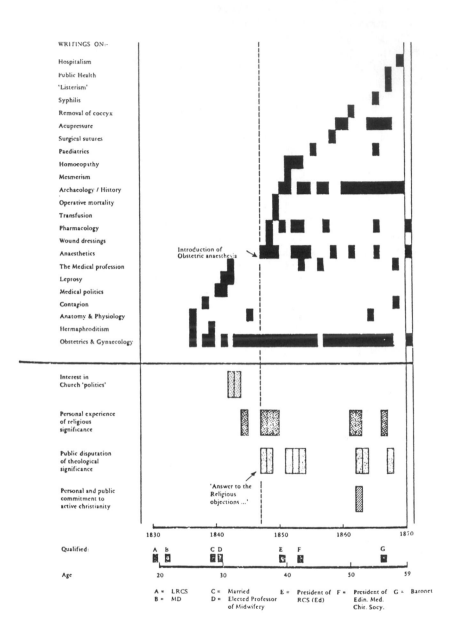

WRITINGS ON:-

Hospitalism
Public Health
'Listerism'
Syphilis
Removal of coccyx
Acupressure
Surgical sutures
Paediatrics
Homoeopathy
Mesmerism
Archaeology / History
Operative mortality
Transfusion
Pharmacology
Wound dressings
Anaesthetics
The Medical profession
Leprosy
Medical politics
Contagion
Anatomy & Physiology
Hermaphroditism
Obstetrics & Gynaecology

Introduction of
Obstetric anaesthesia

Interest in
Church 'politics'

Personal experience
of religious
significance

Public disputation
of theological
significance

Personal and public
commitment to
active christianity

'Answer to the
Religious
objections ...'

1830   1840   1850   1860   1870

Qualified:
A   B   C D   E   F   G

Age
20   30   40   50   59

A = LRCS   C = Married   E = President of   F = President of   G = Baronet
B = MD   D = Elected Professor   RCS (Ed)   Edin. Med.
                    of Midwifery   Chir. Socy.

72

preparation.[53] Although avowedly written 'during a day's confinement to my room—when convalescing from the prevailing influenza',[54] the pamphlet bears all the marks of considerable forethought and preparation.

The progress of Simpson's religious interests in this period are placed in the context of his professional life in Figure 1.[55] It will be noted that Simpson's *Answer to the Religious Objections* ...(and the subsequent development of his arguments in a letter to Protheroe Smith)[56] came at a time when he was starting to develop interests in many other subjects now that his professional future was secure. The year 1847 marked a watershed in Simpson's career: outside his own professional concern with obstetrics, anaesthesia was only one of his many interests, but it happened to coincide that year with the growth of his attention to religion. What would be more natural than the juxtaposition of the two subjects in Simpson's mind, resulting in a study of their supposed inter-relationship?

3.2. *Simpson's defence*

Simpson's pamphlet *Answer to the Religious Objections advanced against the employment of Anaesthetic Agents in Midwifery and Surgery* was published in December 1847 in Edinburgh, and a second edition of 1,000 copies was printed in 1848. The pamphlet bore on its cover two texts from the New Testament—'For every creature of God is good, and nothing to be refused, if it be received with thanksgiving' (I Timothy 4. 4) and, 'Therefore to him that knoweth to do good and doeth it not, to him it is Sin' (James 4. 17)—and these texts seem to have summed up Simpson's philosophy.

A further element entered into Simpson's argument, however, and formed a major part of his thesis: the accuracy (or inaccuracy) of translation of the scripture which pronounced the primeval curse which he believed lay at the core of the problem. He also refuted the view that medical men were 'not entitled to put the activity and consciousness of the mind of any patient in abeyance, for the mere purpose of saving that patient from any bodily pain or agony' by noting that the use of opium and other narcotics to render patients unconscious was long-established medical practice, and even quoted Genesis 2. 21 as precedent for the use of anaesthesia in surgery by God Himself: 'And the Lord God caused a deep sleep to fall upon Adam; and he slept; and he took one of his ribs, and closed up the flesh instead thereof'.

Simpson's arguments reveal a peculiar mixture of erudite philosophy and simple, homespun Christian faith. Whereas his case for more accurate translation of the Hebrew text was convincing, the likening of the making of a woman from Adam's rib to a surgical operation with anaesthesia drew upon Simpson a certain amount of ridicule.

---

[53] It has not been possible to trace any relevant correspondence between Simpson and his friend, the Rev. Dr Thomas Chalmers, Moderator of the General Assembly of the Free Church of Scotland, or any other minister. Sources searched include T. Chalmers, *Selection from the Correspondence of Thomas Chalmers,* edited by N. Hanna (Edinburgh, 1853); the catalogue of manuscripts in the library of the Royal College of Physicians, Edinburgh; the collection of Simpson correspondence in the Royal College of Surgeons. Edinburgh; the manuscript collection of the National Library of Scotland (including a recent acquisition of uncatalogued correspondence of J. Y. Simpson—Accession No. 5683); and the catalogue of manuscripts in the library of New College, Edinburgh (of which Chalmers was Principal and Professor of Divinity from 1843 until his death in 1847).

[54] Simpson (footnote 25).

[55] Figure 1 was compiled from information given in Duns's biography (footnote 19) and K. F. Russell and F. M. C. Forster's *A List of the Works of Sir James Young Simpson, 1811–1870* (Melbourne, 1971), which is the most complete bibliography of Simpson yet to appear.

[56] Simpson (footnote 25).

It is interesting to conjecture where Simpson obtained his theological ideas and the knowledge of Hebrew which was implied in his comments on Biblical translation. Concerning the theology it seems reasonable to suppose that Simpson at least referred to one or more Bible commentaries,[57] of which at that time there were certainly eight reasonably accessible. Of these, five made no comment on the implications of Genesis 3. 16, other than to note briefly the fact that the 'sorrow' of pregnancy was punishment for the sin of Eve,[58] while two others (those of Scott[59] and Henry[60]) may be held to support a tenuous case for religious objections to obstetric anaesthesia, and which Simpson might have used as a guide to points requiring answers.

Only Candlish might have given Simpson grounds for refuting the necessity of pain in parturition when he wrote of the consequences of the fall that 'provision is made for their alleviation in the meantime, and their entire removal at last'.[61] Candlish was minister of St George's Church in Edinburgh and his commentary on Genesis was published in 1843; it is most probable that Simpson was aware of it and was encouraged by it in viewing the 'curse' as neither permanent nor irremovable. There is no record of any correspondence between Simpson and Candlish, however.

Concerning Simpson's views on the Hebrew of the Old Testament, it is possible to reconstruct his sources with some certainty. He obviously used a Hebrew Old Testament—although which particular edition is not known—but he also made passing reference to two other books, Tregelles's translation of Gesenius's *Hebrew and Chaldee Lexicon to the Old Testament Scriptures*,[62] and Wigram's *The Englishman's Hebrew and Chaldee Concordance of the Old Testament*,[63] published in 1846 and 1843 respectively. It was clearly from these two works that Simpson abstracted the philological information used in the third and fourth sections of his pamphlet. Simpson's comment in his pamphlet that 'In the Old Testament, above twenty different terms or nouns in the original Hebrew text are translated by the single term or noun "sorrow" in the English text'[64] is an observation which can be made directly from Wigram's concordance,[65] and his examples are exactly those of Wigram. Similarly Simpson's definitions of certain words are direct quotations from Gesenius's lexicon.

Simpson had a good command of Latin and had studied Greek,[66] but there is no record of his every having studied Hebrew. The exposition in his pamphlet, when

---

[57] The manuscript catalogue of books in J. Y. Simpson's personal library (in the possession of the Royal College of Physicians, Edinburgh) contains no entry for any Bibles, Commentaries, or other theological works (apart from Row's *History of the Kirks of Scotland*). The 2200 entries are nearly all of medical works published up to 1853, and probably are not inclusive of all of Simpson's books. I am indebted to the Librarian of the Royal College for allowing me to study this catalogue.

[58] J. Hewlett, *Commentaries and Annotations on the Holy Scriptures* (London, 1816); F. Close, *The Book of Genesis Considered and Illustrated* (London, 1826); J. Brown, *The Self-Interpreting Bible* (Glasgow, 1839); S. Patrick, *A Commentary on the Historical Books of the Old Testament* (London, 1842); J. Calvin, *Commentaries on the First Book of Moses called Genesis*, translated by J. King, I (Edinburgh, 1847).

[59] T. Scott, *The Holy Bible ... with Explanatory Notes* (London, 1788).

[60] M. Henry, *An Exposition of all the Books of the Old and New Testaments* (Edinburgh, 1810).

[61] R. S. Candlish, *Contributions towards the Exposition of the Book of Genesis* (Edinburgh, 1843), p. 99.

[62] W. Gesenius, *Hebrew and Chaldee Lexicon to the Old Testament Scriptures*, translated by S. P. Tregelles (London, 1846), p. 646 b (2).

[63] *The Englishman's Hebrew and Chaldee Concordance of the Old Testament*, edited by G. V. Wigram (London, 1843).

[64] Simpson (footnote 16), 11.

[65] Wigram, footnote 63, 1639. There are actually 27 such terms.

[66] He was one of the last candidates for the Edinburgh M.D. to be examined in Latin; for his Greek, see Duns (footnote 19), 22–3.

compared with Gesenius and Wigram, bears all the hallmarks of an intelligent layman's utilization of reference books in a subject with which he was not familiar, and Simpson's philogy was indeed criticised by a very distinguished Hebrew scholar as being imperfect.[67]

Early in 1848 Simpson was approached by Dr Protheroe Smith of London for advice on the subject of religious objections to obstetric anaesthesia. He wrote a lengthy letter to Smith, who published it as an appendix to the pamphlet which he himself was writing on the subject. Simpson's letter elaborated 'some points on which, if I had had time, I would perhaps have more insisted on'.[68] An unpublished draft for this letter indicates that, despite the writer's reference to it as a 'few hurried notes', the letter was carefully written, several times revised and polished, and the subject of very deliberate and considered thought.[69] The final letter was dated 8 July 1848 and was primarily concerned with emphasizing the arguments from philology in Simpson's original pamphlet, with an additional appeal to physiology.

Criticism was also made of practitioners who, in seeking to take the 'curse' in Genesis 3.16 literally, were acting illogically in attempting to practise medicine in general, and midwifery in particular, and thus breaching the curse in its other aspects.

3.3. *Protheroe Smith and his defence*
Dr Protheroe Smith published his pamphlet *Scriptural Authority for the Mitigation of the Pains of Labour, by Chloroform, and other anaesthetic agents* in the second half of 1848. Smith said little that was new. He repeated arguments which Simpson had already used but he wrote with a different object. Simpson's pamphlet had sought to show that there was no scriptural reason against obstetric anaesthesia, whereas Smith sought to produce positive Biblical authority for the procedure.

Protheroe Smith had trained at St Bartholomew's Hospital in London and first qualified in 1833. He graduated MD at Aberdeen in 1844, but although he travelled to Aberdeen to be examined,[70] there is no indication whether at that (or any other) time he ever met Simpson. In 1842 Smith founded the first hospital for women in Britain and about 1847–8 became a lecturer in Midwifery and Diseases of Women at St Bartholomew's Hospital.

Protheroe Smith was a staunch Evangelical Christian and almost certainly a member of the Church of England.[71] His theology was inclined to the dispensationalism which was then beginning to be taught and his arguments in favour of obstetric anaesthesia included this aspect of Christian belief.[72]

Smith's approach to the anaesthesia debate was to query 'what is truth', answering with a quotation from the gospels—'Thy word is truth' (John 17. 17). Upon this assumption he decided to 'submit the question at issue to the test of Holy writ, and the

---

[67] G. R. Noyes, Letters to Professor W. Channing, dated 3 February and 22 Feburary 1848. In W. Channing, *A Treatise on Etherization in Childbirth* (Boston, 1848), pp. 144–5, 146–8.
[68] Simpson (footnote 25).
[69] Simpson (footnote 35).
[70] Aberdeen University (King's College). Minutes of Court, 11 and 31 July 1844.
[71] In 1848, J. Y. Simpson, in his letter to Smith, referred to some letters he had received from 'one of your most exalted and most esteemed episcopal dignitaries' (Smith, footnote 18, 44).
[72] Smith (footnote 18), 18: 'Believing, then, that a knowledge of the *dispensational* character of God's dealing with man is essential to the clear perception of my argument, I shall venture here to enlarge a little on this subject . . .'

41-page pamphlet contained over 190 biblical references—not all of which are strictly apposite.

Having repeated most of Simpson's arguments, Smith stated that the Old Testament law was replaced by Christ who, by His death, redeemed all mankind and (quoting the Church of England Communion Service) 'by His one oblation of himself once offered He made a full, perfect, and sufficient sacrifice, oblation, and satisfaction for the sins of the whole world'. From this, Smith argued, it followed that as sin was the ground upon which the primeval curse had existed, in Christ's expiation of the sins of mankind 'Even the primal curse has been in a measure, deprived of its terrors by that "one Sacrifice for sins for ever"'.

Whether Smith had any effect in allaying qualms over the implications of obstetric anaesthesia cannot be known. By the time that he wrote, the conflict appeared to be virtually over and his pamphlet was not subsequently mentioned in the literature. However, it was the only original work on this subject ever to be published in England.

3.4. Miscellaneous writings

A few other medical writers referred briefly to this subject. Dr J. T. Conquest, a noted London obstetrician, included a section on 'the use of chloroform' in his *Letters to a Mother*, first published in 1848, giving strong support to its use in obstetrics and quoting substantially from Simpson's pamphlet.[73] Conquest was a religiously-minded man (he was responsible for an edition of *The Bible with 20,000 Emendations*) and a firm admirer of Simpson.[74]

Of possibly greater signficance was a section in an American textbook published in 1848 at about the same time as Protheroe Smith's pamphlet. Channing's *A Treatise on Etherization in Childbirth* reviewed the whole subject of obstetric anaesthesia, and ten pages were devoted to 'The Religious Objection to Etherization'.[75] As with Conquest's book this work contained little new, but this was the only American text in which religious objections to anaesthesia were studied by an obstetrician.[76] Channing cited Simpson's arguments, and had also sought the views of a theologian on the subject. Professor G. R. Noyes,[77] whom Channing consulted twice, believed that in reading Genesis 3. 16, 'the common mode of understanding the verse must be retained'.

Noyes disagreed with Simpson's exercises in philology (his own translation of Genesis 3. 16 would read: 'I will greatly increase the painfulness of thy conception. In pain shalt thou bring forth children'), but commented that:

> No one will pretend, that there is anything preceptive in Genesis 3. 16. It is of the nature of prediction. But the duty of relieving distress is the express dictate of nature and revelation. It would seem, therefore, to be wisdom to follow the

[73] J. T. Conquest, *Letters to a Mother on the Management of Herself and Her Children* (London, 1848), 4th edn (1852), pp. 42–54.
[74] Ibid., Dedication, p.v.
[75] Footnote 67.
[76] Channing was Professor of Midwifery and Medical Jurisprudence in the University at Cambridge, Massachusetts.
[77] George Rapall Noyes (1798–1868) was a Unitarian clergyman, who held the dual post of Professor of Hebrew and Oriental Languages and Lecturer on Biblical Literature and Theology, at the Harvard Divinity School. He was described in the *Dictionary of American Biography* (London, 1934), xiii, 587–8, as 'one of the ablest Biblical scholars of his day'.

dictates of nature and revelation, and leave predictions and threatenings to be fulfilled by Him who made them.[78]

This suggestion that 'No one will pretend, that there is any thing *preceptive* in Genesis 3. 16' is interesting in the light of the suggestion (made *infra*) that religious objections to anaesthesia were more imagined than real. It is possible that not many people did make this 'pretence', but it was the possibility that they may which underlay the whole debate.

A particularly interesting contribution to the debate, which has apparently been lost sight of/for the whole of this century, was an unpublished thesis by one of Simpson's own students, Francis John de Quincey,[79] which contained some comments by his father, Thomas de Quincey.[80]

Written in March 1849 (i.e. some fifteen months after Simpson's pamphlet) the thesis—predictably—largely followed Simpson's own arguments, although one or two additional points were well made. In particular de Quincey noted that, followed to its logical conclusion, a literal interpretation of the primeval curse would imply forbidding embryotomy and the caesarian operation, so that a woman with a contracted pelvis must be allowed to die undelivered because she is guilty of the sin of having a contracted pelvis; a sin which is certainly not under her control; and the punishing of which would seem to war with the attributes of infinite wisdom, justice and love, which we regard as the brightest characteristics of the deity.[81]

Both the de Quinceys were clear as to the real reason for apparent religious objections. The son referred to 'a large class of mankind, who considering the words *old* and *good* as synonymous, can admire nothing that has not upon it the dust of forty generations; and to whom novelty is a mere rock of offence'. His father was more blunt. He asked 'is there any real religious scruple at the bottom of these objections? Is it not a jealousy of Professor Simpson's great discovery that *really* speaks through this jesuitical masquerade of conscientious scruples?'

4. The anaesthesia 'conflict'

Simpson's attitude to anaesthesia—especially in obstetrics—was one of keen enthusiasm and he was deeply involved in its defence against all the medical and other objections which were voiced. Protheroe Smith, who was the first to use anaesthetics in midwifery in England, was 'a man of marked religious views, of the Evangelical school' who 'made those views prominent in every relationship of his life'.[82]

It may be questioned to what extent the attention given to religious objections arose from a mis-judgement of the situation in the minds of Simpson and Smith. With this

---

[78] Footnote 67, p. 148.
[79] F. J. de Quincey, *On the Religious Objections to the use of Chloroform in Obstetric Medicine*, M.D. Graduation thesis, University of Edinburgh (1849). MS in Edinburgh University Library, 85 pp. 4to., p. 47. This thesis was cited by A. R. Simpson in 'The Jubilee of Anaesthetic Midwifery', *Transactions of the Glasgow Obstetrical and Gynaecological Society*, 1 (1898), Papers 17–81. It has not been referred to since and, on recent enquiry, Edinburgh University Library claimed to have no knowledge of it. A search instigated in 1975 at the request of the present author uncovered the thesis, which was uncatalogued. A further copy was at one time in the library of J. Y. Simpson, but it cannot be found in the collection of his books which is now in the possession of the Royal College of Physicians, Edinburgh.
[80] This was Thomas de Quincey (1785–1859), the famous prose writer and 'opium-eater', who lived in Edinburgh from 1828 until his death. See *Dictionary of National Biography*.
[81] Footnote 79, p. 27. Nevertheless, this attitude was sometimes adopted. See T. Radford, 'Cases of Laceration of the Uterus, with Remarks', *Transactions of the Obstetrical Society of London*, 8 (1867), pp. 150–213; Case 4, pp. 158–60.
[82] Anon. Obituary notice, *The Lancet*, 1889, i, 770, and *British Medical Journal*, 1 (1889), 849.

possibility in mind it is suggested that the apparent 'religious conflict' arose through an order of events approximately as follows.

Smith may have had doubts voiced to him concerning the religious propriety of annulling labour pains and, in the course of reporting his first cases early in 1847[83] he briefly expanded upon this point, perhaps because of his 'marked religious views'. Simpson, also a man with a growing interest in religion, was disturbed by his conversations with Parke in October 1847.[84] Following upon this came Smith's comments and perhaps similar queries made privately in his own practice. Being both a prolific author and a keen defender of anaesthesia, Simpson produced a pamphlet defending obstetric anaesthesia from attacks on religious grounds. This was written partly for general defensive purposes and partly to clear Simpson's own mind on the theology of the practice, as this was currently his other main interest. So little was the actual religious opposition, however, that six months later Simpson could report his belief that 'any objections on this point ... have ceased among us'.

Smith was, perhaps, so impressed by Simpson's pamphlet defending the procedure that, moved by his own religious views, he went a stage further and wrote a pamphlet claiming positive 'Scriptural Authority for' the practice. Smith asked Simpson for advice and, although the latter regarded the problem as no longer a live issue, he wrote a reply which expanded his original views slightly. It is clear that, by this time, Simpson believed that the comments of at least some of his patients sprang more from envy and frustration than from genuine religious doubts.[85] Following Smith's 1848 pamphlet the 'debate' was not aired again publicly, although a few private doubts may have lingered.[86]

This explanation also fits the evidence when one looks beyond Britain. With only one exception, no reference at all has been found to the existence of any religious objections to anaesthesia either in Europe or America. The exception (Channing's *Treatise on Etherization in Childbirth*)[87] was clearly stimulated by Simpson's pamphlet—which Channing quoted extensively—and the implication in Channing's writing was that it was that pamphlet which had planted the idea in America.

Both America and Britain shared an extensive period of evangelical revival during the nineteenth century. The fact that the social climate of neither country gave rise to religious objections to anaesthesia, other than by a very few individuals, suggests that such views were not widespread. In short, despite a spirited battle between the protagonists and opponents of anaesthesia upon medical, physiological, and even moral grounds,[88] the religious issue was never a real factor in this particular medical development; nor was the anaesthesia question a factor in the mainstream of nineteenth century religious belief.

Virtually every contemporary writer who referred to religious views upon anaesthesia did so (i) following the publication of Simpson's pamphlet on the subject and (ii) based his comments almost entirely upon it. It is possible that many historians reading Simpson's pamphlet and Duns's biography (for long the standard source for information on Simpson) which referred uncritically to it, have approached the subject

[83] P. Smith, 'On the Employment of Ether by Inhalation in Obstetric Practice', *The Lancet*, 1847, i, 452–57.

[84] Parke (footnote 10).

[85] Simpson (footnote 35).

[86] See Kingsley (footnote 39), and Murphy (footnote 40).

[87] Footnote 67.

[88] A. D. Farr, 'Early Opposition to Obstetric Anaesthesia', *Anaesthesia*, 35 (1980), 896–907.

with a preconceived expectation of conflict and have written accordingly, without sufficient critical assessment of the actual extent of religious opposition. Some few objections were certainly raised privately but it is Simpson's defence—rather than any actual objection—which has been noticed by almost every commentator since.

The two men who did consider the relief of pain and religious belief to be connected—Simpson and Smith—were from what might be termed 'the left wing' of the Christian church: a Calvinist and an Evangelical Anglican. While this might have predisposed their minds to consideration of any subject in terms of scriptural authority it did not similarly move any of the countless other medical practitioners brought up within these (and similar) denominational beliefs to action upon this one point. One is bound to see religious beliefs on the propriety of anaesthesia as essentially personal, therefore, and it is indeed probable that, had Simpson not been the prominent and charismatic figure that he was, the whole controversy would have passed with little notice and this particular area of (apparent) conflict long since forgotten.

That anaesthesia received only a cautious welcome from the medical profession (on other grounds) and that a few medical practitioners introduced a religious (or more often, a moral) element into their arguments, may well have reinforced the impression of a regular dispute upon religious grounds. Constant repetition of this theme over the last hundred years has so impressed the public with the reality of a 'religious conflict' over anaesthesia that it is probable that what is, in fact, no more than an artifact of historiography has become sanctified as a historical 'fact'—a 'conflict' which actually never existed.

Acknowledgments

I am grateful to the Royal College of Surgeons of Edinburgh, and in particular to the College Librarian Dr I. Simpson Hall, for access to some of the hitherto unpublished correspondence of Sir James Young Simpson, and for permission to reproduce certain items of this for the first time.

REVISIONS/REPORTS

Birthing and Anesthesia: The Debate over Twilight Sleep

Judith Walzer Leavitt

"At midnight I was awakened by a very sharp pain," wrote Mrs. Cecil Stewart, describing the birth of her child in 1914. "The head nurse . . . gave me an injection of scopolamin-morphin. . . . I woke up the next morning about half-past seven . . . the door opened, and the head nurse brought in my baby. . . . I was so happy."[1] Mrs. Stewart had delivered her baby under the influence of scopolamine, a narcotic and amnesiac that, together with morphine, produced a state popularly known as "twilight sleep." She did not remember anything of the experience when she woke up after giving birth. This 1914 ideal contrasts with today's feminist stress on being awake, aware, and in control during the birthing experience. In 1914 and 1915, thousands of American women testified to the marvels of having babies without the trauma of childbirth. As one of them gratefully put it, "The night of my confinement will always be a night dropped out of my life."[2]

I am grateful to William J. Orr, Jr., and Susan Duke for their assistance in the preparation of this study. I would also like to thank Mari Jo Buhle, Norman Fost, Susan Friedman, Lewis Leavitt, Elaine Marks, Regina Morantz, and Ronald Numbers for their comments on earlier drafts of this paper.

1. Testimony quoted in Marguerite Tracy and Mary Boyd, *Painless Childbirth* (New York: Frederick A. Stokes Co., 1915), pp. 188–89. For a thorough account of the twilight sleep controversy in America, see Lawrence G. Miller, "Pain, Parturition, and the Profession: The Twilight Sleep in America," in *Health Care in America: Essays in Social History*, ed. Susan Reverby and David Rosner (Philadelphia: Temple University Press, 1979), pp. 19–44.

2. Tracy and Boyd, p. 198.

[*Signs: Journal of Women in Culture and Society* 1980, vol. 6, no. 1]
© 1980 by The University of Chicago. 0097-9740/81/0601-0012$01.00

From the perspective of today's ideology of woman-controlled births, it may appear that women who want anesthesia sought to cede control of their births to their doctors. I will argue however, that the twilight sleep movement led by women in 1914 and 1915 was not a relinquishing of control. Rather, it was an attempt to gain control over the birthing process. Feminist women wanted the parturient, not the doctor or attendant, to choose the kind of delivery she would have. This essay examines the apparent contradiction in the women's demand to control their births by going to sleep.

The Process

The attendants, location, and drugs or instruments used in American women's birthing experiences varied in the early decades of the twentieth century. America's poorer and immigrant women delivered their babies predominantly at home, attended by midwives who seldom administered drugs and who called physicians only in difficult cases. A small number of poor women gave birth in charity or public hospitals where physicians attended them. Most upper- and middle-class women, who had more choice, elected to be attended by a physician, usually a general practitioner but increasingly a specially trained obstetrician, rather than a midwife. At the turn of the twentieth century, these births, too, typically took place in the woman's home; however, by the second decade of the century, specialists, aided partly by the twilight sleep movement, were moving childbirth from the home to the hospital.[3]

Physicians used drugs and techniques of physical intervention in many cases, although the extent cannot be quantified accurately. In addition to forceps, physicians relied on opium, chloroform, chloral, cocaine, quinine, nitrous oxide, ergot, and ether to relieve pain, expedite labor, prevent injury in precipitous labors, control hemorrhage, and prevent sepsis.[4] In one study of 972 consecutive births in Wisconsin, physicians used chloroform during the second stage of labor in half of their cases and forceps in 12 percent.[5] The reports indicate that drugs and instruments may have made labors shorter but not necessarily more enjoyable. Because most drugs could not be used safely throughout the labor and delivery, either because they affected muscle function or because they were dangerous for the baby, women still experienced pain. The use of forceps frequently added to discomfort and caused perineal tears, complicating postdelivery recovery. Maternal mortality remained

3. For more information on childbirth practices in this period, see Judy Barrett Litoff, *American Midwives: 1860 to the Present* (Westport, Conn.: Greenwood Press, 1978).

4. J. F. Ford, "Use of Drugs in Labor," *Wisconsin Medical Journal* 3 (1904–5): 257–65.

5. Ibid.

high in the early decades of the twentieth century, and childbirth, whether attended by physicians or midwives, continued to be risky.[6]

Most women described their physician-attended childbirths as unpleasant at best. Observers of the declining birthrates among America's "better" classes worried that the "fear of childbirth has poisoned the happiness of many women"[7] and caused them to want fewer children. One woman told her doctor that her childbirth had been "hell. . . . It bursts your brain, and tears out your heart, and crashes your nerves to bits. It's just like hell, and I won't stand it again. Never."[8] In scopolamine deliveries, the women went to sleep, delivered their babies, and woke up feeling vigorous. The drug altered their consciousness so that they did not remember painful labors, and their bodies did not feel exhausted by their efforts.[9] Both the women who demanded scopolamine and the doctors who agreed to use it perceived it as far superior to other anesthesia because it did not inhibit muscle function and could be administered throughout the birthing process. It was the newest and finest technique available—"the greatest boon the Twentieth Century could give to women," in the words of Dr. Bertha Van Hoosen, one of its foremost medical advocates.[10]

However, women's bodies experienced their labors, even if their minds did not remember them. Thus observers witnessed women screaming in pain during contractions, thrashing about, and giving all the outward signs of "acute suffering." Residents of Riverside Drive in New York City testified that women in Dr. William H. W. Knipe's twilight sleep hospital sent forth "objectionable" noises in the middle of the night.[11]

A successful twilight sleep delivery, as practiced by Dr. Van Hoosen at the Mary Thompson Hospital in Chicago, required elaborate facilities and careful supervision. Attending physicians and nurses gave the first

6. See, e.g., Dorothy Reed Mendenhall ("Prenatal and Natal Conditions in Wisconsin," *Wisconsin Medical Journal* 15 [1917]: 353–69), who reported, "The death rate from maternity is gradually increasing in Wisconsin, as it is throughout the United States" (p. 364). Dr. Mendenhall also noted that death rates for physician-attended births were higher than for midwife-attended births in Wisconsin (p. 353). I would like to thank Dale Treleven for calling this article to my attention.

7. Mary Boyd, "The Story of Dammerschlaf: An American Woman's Personal Experience and Study at Freiburg," *Survey* 33 (1915): 129.

8. Quoted in Russell Kelso Carter, *The Sleeping Car "Twilight," or Motherhood without Pain* (Boston: Chapple Publishing Co., 1915), pp. 10–11.

9. Scopolamine is an alkaloid found in the leaves and seeds of solanaceous plants. It is a sedative and a mild analgesic as well as an amnesiac, causing forgetfulness of pain rather than blocking the pain sensation. For obstetrical twilight sleep, scopolamine was administered with morphine—the most active alkaloid of opium—in the first dose and alone for subsequent doses.

10. Bertha Van Hoosen, *Scopolamine-Morphine Anaesthesia* (Chicago: House of Manz, 1915), p. 101.

11. *New York Times* (June 9, 1917), p. 13.

injection of scopolamine as soon as a woman appeared to be in active labor and continued the injections at carefully determined intervals throughout her labor and delivery. They periodically administered two tests to determine the effectiveness of the anesthesia: the "calling test," which the parturient passed if the doctor could not arouse her even by addressing her in a loud voice, and the "incoordination test," which she passed if her movements were uncoordinated. Once the laboring woman was under the effects of scopolamine, the doctors put her into a specially designed crib-bed to contain her sometimes violent movements (see fig. 1). Van Hoosen described the need for the bed screens: "As the pains increase in frequency and strength, the patient tosses or throws herself about, but without injury to herself, and may be left without fear that she will roll onto the floor or be found wandering aimlessly in the corridors. In rare cases, where the patient is very excitable and insists on getting out of bed. . . . I prefer to fasten a canvas cover over the tops of the screens, thereby shutting out light, noise and possibility of leaving the bed.[12] When delivery began, attendants took down the canvas crib and positioned the patient in stirrups, familiar in modern obstetrical services. Van Hoosen advised the use of a continuous sleeve to ensure that patients did not interfere with the sterile field (see fig. 2). The canvas crib and the continuous sleeve were Van Hoosen's response to a common need in twilight sleep deliveries: a secure, darkened, quiet, contained environment.

The Events

Twilight sleep became a controversial issue in American obstetrics in June 1914, when *McClure's Magazine* published an article by two laywomen describing this newly popular German method of painless childbirth.[13] In the article, Marguerite Tracy and Constance Leupp, both visitors at the Freiburg women's clinic, criticized high-forceps deliveries (which they called the common American technique) as dangerous and conducive to infection. They contrasted these imperfect births to the safety and comfort of twilight sleep. The new method was so wonderful that women, having once experienced it, would "walk all the way [to Germany] from California" to have their subsequent births under twilight sleep. The physicians at the Freiburg clinic thought the method was best suited for the upper-class "modern woman . . . [who] responds to the stimulus of severe pain . . . with nervous exhaustion and paralysis of the will to carry labor to conclusion." They were less certain

12. Van Hoosen, p. 42.
13. Marguerite Tracy and Constance Leupp, "Painless Childbirth," *McClure's Magazine* 43 (1914): 37–51.

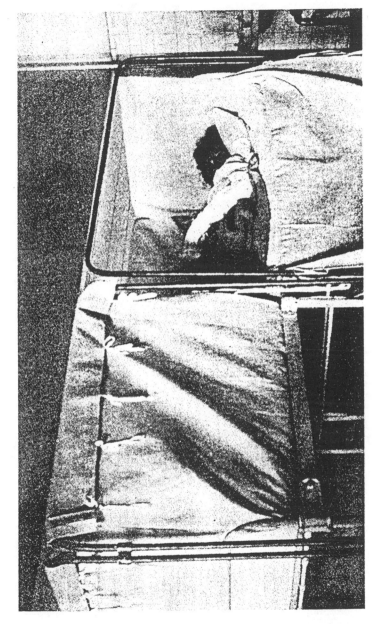

Fig. 1.—Patient in crib-bed waiting for examination. (Source: Bertha Van Hoosen. *Scopolamine-Morphine Anaesthesia* [Chicago: House of Manz, 1915], p. 48.)

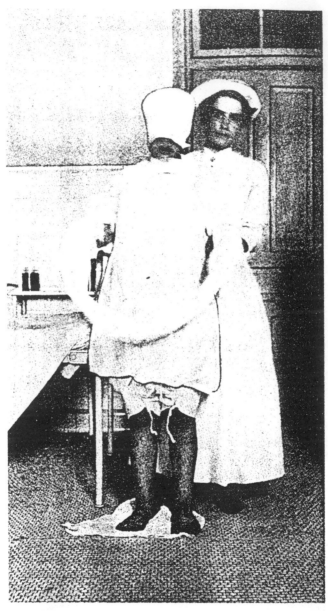

FIG. 2.—Gown with continuous sleeve. (Source: Bertha Van Hoosen, *Scopolamine-Morphine Anaesthesia* [Chicago: House of Manz, 1915], p. 88.)

about its usefulness for women who "earn their living by manual labor" and could tolerate more pain.[14]

The women who took up the cause of twilight sleep concluded that it was not in general use in this country because doctors were consciously withholding this panacea. Physicians have "held back" on developing painless childbirth, accused Mary Boyd and Marguerite Tracy, two of the most active proponents, because it "takes too much time." "Women alone," they asserted, "can bring Freiburg methods into American obstetrical practice."[15] Others echoed the call to arms: journalist Hanna Rion urged her readers to "take up the battle for painless childbirth. . . . Fight not only for yourselves, but fight for your . . . sex."[16] Newspapers and popular magazines joined the chorus, advocating a widespread use of scopolamine in childbirth.[17]

The lay public's anger at the medical profession's apparent refusal to adopt a technique beneficial to women erupted into a national movement. The National Twilight Sleep Association, formed by upper-middle-class clubwomen,[18] was best epitomized by its leaders. They included women such as Mrs. Jesse F. Attwater, editor of *Femina* in Boston; Dr. Eliza Taylor Ransom, active women's rights advocate and physician in Boston; Mrs. Julian Heath of the National Housewife's League; author Rheta Childe Dorr of the Committee on the Industrial Conditions of Women and Children; Mary Ware Dennett of the National Suffrage Association (and later the National Birth Control League); and Dr. Bertha Van Hoosen, outspoken women's leader in medical circles in Chicago.[19] Many of these leaders saw the horrors of childbirth as an

---

14. Ibid., p. 43. For the same sentiment among American physicians, see, e.g., John O. Polak, "A Study of Scopolamin and Morphine Amnesia as Employed at Long Island College Hospital," *American Journal of Obstetrics* 71 (1915): 722; and Henry Smith Williams, *Painless Childbirth* (New York: Goodhue Co., 1914), pp. 90–91. The classic descriptions of the ideal scopolamine delivery are Bernhard Kronig, "Painless Delivery in Dammerschlaf " (1908); and Carl J. Gauss, "Births in Artificial Dammerschlaf" (1906) and "Further Experiments in Dammerschlaf" (1911), all translated and reprinted in Tracy and Boyd (n. 1 above), pp. 205–308.

15. Mary Boyd and Marguerite Tracy, "More about Painless Childbirth," *McClure's Magazine* 43 (1914): 57–58.

16. Hanna Rion, *Painless Childbirth in Twilight Sleep* (London: T. Werner Laurie Ltd., 1915), p. 239; see also her "The Painless Childbirth," *Ladies Home Journal* 31 (1914): 9–10.

17. See, e.g., "Is the Twilight Sleep Safe—for Me?" *Woman's Home Companion* 42 (1915): 10, 43; William Armstrong, "The 'Twilight Sleep' of Freiburg: A Visit to the Much Talked of Women's Clinic," *Woman's Home Companion* 41 (1914): 4, 69; *New York Times* (September 17, 1914), p. 8; (November 28, 1914), p. 2.

18. On women's clubs and clubwomen, see Mary P. Ryan, *Womanhood in America: From Colonial Times to the Present* (New York: New Viewpoints, 1975), pp. 227–32; Edith Hoshino Altbach, *Women in America* (Lexington, Mass.: D.C. Heath & Co., 1914), pp. 114–21; William L. O'Neill, *Everyone Was Brave: A History of Feminism in America* (Chicago: Quadrangle Books, 1969), pp. 107–68; Sheila M. Rothman, *Woman's Proper Place: A History of Changing Ideals and Practices, 1870 to the Present* (New York: Basic Books, 1978), pp. 63–93.

19. Carter, pp. 174–75.

experience that united all women: "Childbirth has for every woman through all time been potentially great emergency."[20] Dr. Ransom thought that the use of twilight sleep would "create a more perfect motherhood" and urged others to work "for the betterment of womenkind."[21] Because they saw it as an issue for their sex, not just their class, and because many of the twilight sleep leaders were active feminists, they spoke in the idiom of the woman movement.[22]

The association sponsored rallies in major cities to acquaint women with the issue of painless childbirth and to pressure the medical profession into adopting the new method. In order to broaden their appeal, the association staged meetings "between the marked-down suits and the table linen" of department stores where "the ordinary woman" as well as the activist clubwoman could be found.[23] At these rallies, women who had traveled to Freiburg testified to the wonders of twilight sleep (see fig. 3). "I experienced absolutely no pain," claimed Mrs. Francis X. Carmody of Brooklyn, displaying her healthy baby at Gimbels. "An hour after my child was born I ate a hearty breakfast. . . . The third day I went for an automobile ride. . . . The Twilight Sleep is wonderful." Mrs. Carmody ended with the familiar rallying cry: "If you women want it you will have to fight for it, for the mass of doctors are opposed to it."[24]

Department-store rallies and extensive press coverage brought the movement to the attention of a broad segment of American women. Movement leaders rejoiced over episodes such as the one in which a "tenement house mother . . . collected a crowd" on a street corner where she joyfully told of her twilight sleep experience.[25] Many working-class women were attracted to twilight sleep not only because it made childbirth "pleasanter" but because they saw its use as "an important cause of decreased mortality and increased health and vitality among the mothers of children."[26] Some feared, however, that twilight sleep would remain a "superadded luxury of the wealthy mother" because it involved so much physician time and hospital expense.[27] Although different motivations propelled the physician-advocates who believed twilight sleep was safe, middle- and upper-class women who wanted the newest

20. Tracy and Boyd, p. 145.
21. Eliza Taylor Ransom, "Twilight Sleep," *Massachusetts Club Women* 1 (1917): 5. I am grateful to Regina Markell Morantz for this reference.
22. The connections between clubwomen and suffrage or other women's issues are explored in Altbach, pp. 114–15; O'Neill, pp. 49–76, 146–68; Ryan, pp. 230–49; and Eleanor Flexner, *Century of Struggle: The Woman's Rights Movement in the United States* (New York: Atheneum Publishers, 1970), pp. 172–92. The term "woman movement," in the nineteenth and early twentieth centuries, described the movement to better women's condition, including, but not limited to, the drive for suffrage.
23. Tracy and Boyd, p. 145.
24. Quoted in *New York Times* (November 18, 1914), p. 18.
25. Tracy and Boyd, p. 145.
26. Clara G. Stillman, "Painless Childbirth," *New York Call* (July 12, 1914), p. 15.
27. Sam Schmalhauser, "The Twilight Sleep for Women," *International Socialist Review* 15 (1914): 234–35. I am grateful to Mari Jo Buhle for this and the previous reference.

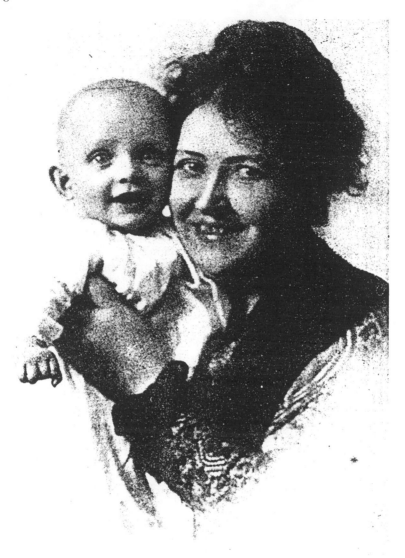

Fig. 3.—Mrs. Francis Xavier Carmody and "Charlemagne," born in Freiburg. (Source: Marguerite Tracy and Mary Boyd, *Painless Childbirth* [New York: Frederick A. Stokes Co., 1915], p. 143.)

thing medicine had to offer, and working-class women who wanted simple relief from childbed suffering, they were all united by their common desire to make childbirth safer and easier for women.

Van Hoosen emerged as the most avid advocate of twilight sleep in the Midwest. She received her M.D. from the University of Michigan

Medical School and worked at the New England Hospital for Women and Children in Boston before setting up practice in Chicago in 1892. Her enthusiasm for the method came from two sources: her strong commitment to the best in obstetrical care and her equally strong commitment to women's rights. Through her use of scopolamine in surgery and obstetrics, she became convinced that twilight sleep offered women a "return of more physiological births" at the same time that it increased the efficiency of physicians, giving them "complete control of everything."[28] She guided many other physicians to the twilight sleep method.[29] In terms of safety and comfort, she could not imagine a better method of birthing.

Increasingly, doctors began to deliver twilight sleep babies. Some traveled to Germany to learn the Freiburg technique and subsequently offered it to both private and charity patients.[30] A few physicians even became enthusiastic about the possibilities of twilight sleep. "If the male had to endure this suffering," said Dr. James Harrar of New York, "I think he would resort very precipitously to something that might relieve the . . . pain."[31] Dr. W. Francis B. Wakefield of California went even further, declaring "I would just as soon consider performing a surgical operation without an anesthetic as conducting a labor without scopolamin amnesia. Skillfully administered the best interest of both the mother and the child are advanced by its use."[32] Another physician listed its advantages: painless labor, reduction of subsequent "nerve exhaustion that comes after a prolonged hard labor," better milk secretion, fewer cervical and perineal lacerations, fewer forcep deliveries, less strain on the heart, and a "better race for future generations" since upper-class women would be more likely to have babies if they could have them painlessly.[33] There was also, it was claimed, an "advantage to

28. Bertha Van Hoosen, *Petticoat Surgeon* (Chicago: Pellegrini & Cudahy, 1947), pp. 282–82.

29. See, e.g., Bertha Van Hoosen, "A Fixed Dosage in Scopalamine-Morphine Anaesthesia," *Woman's Medical Journal* 26 (1916): 57–58; and "Twilight Sleep in the Home," ibid., p. 132.

30. For early American trials, see William H. Wellington Knipe, " 'Twilight Sleep' from the Hospital Viewpoint," *Modern Hospital* 2 (1914): 250–51; A. M. Hilkowich, "Further Observations on Scopalamine-Narcophin Anesthesia during Labor with Report of Two Hundred (200) Cases," *American Medicine* 20 (1914): 786–94; William H. Wellington Knipe, "The Freiburg Method of Dammerschlaf or Twilight Sleep," *American Journal of Obstetrics* 70 (1914): 364–71; and James A. Harrar and Ross McPherson, "Scopolamine-Narcophin Seminarcosis in Labor," *Transactions of the American Association of Obstetricians and Gynecologists* 27 (1914): 372–89.

31. Quoted during discussion of Rongy, Harrar, and McPherson papers, *Transactions of the American Association of Obstetricians and Gynecologists* 27 (1914): 389.

32. W. Francis B. Wakefield, "Scopolamine Amnesia in Labor," *American Journal of Obstetrics* 71 (1915): 428. For more of this kind of enthusiasm, see also Elizabeth R. Miner, "Letter and Report of Nineteen Cases in Which 'Twilight' Was Used," *Woman's Medical Journal* 26 (1916): 131.

33. Ralph M. Beach, "Twilight Sleep," *American Medicine* 21 (1915): 40–41.

the child: To give it a better chance for life at the time of delivery; a better chance to have breast-feeding; a better chance to have a strong, normal mother."[34]

Despite the energy and enthusiasm of the twilight sleep advocates, many American doctors resisted the technique. They lashed out against the "pseudo-scientific rubbish" and the "quackish hocus-pocus" published in *McClure's*[35] and simply refused to be "stampeded by these misguided ladies."[36] These physicians did not believe that nonmedical people should determine therapeutic methods; it was a "question of medical ethics."[37] Other physicians refused to use scopolamine because they feared its dangers either to the mother or the child. The *Journal of the American Medical Association* concluded that "this method has been thoroughly investigated, tried, and found wanting, because of the danger connected with it."[38]

Because the evidence about safety was mixed, many doctors were frustrated in their attempts to find out whether scopolamine was harmful or safe for use in obstetrics. Earlier experience with the unstable form of the drug led some to refuse to try scopolamine again, although at least one pharmaceutical company had solved the problem of drug stability by 1914. "The bad and indifferent results which were at first obtained by the use of these drugs we now know to have been due entirely to overdosage and the use of impure and unstable preparations," concluded one physician in a report on his successful results with 1,000 twilight sleep mothers in 1915.[39] Dr. Van Hoosen had successfully performed surgery on 2,000 patients with the help of scopolamine by 1908[40] and began using the drug routinely in deliveries in 1914. She concluded after 100 consecutive cases that scopolamine, properly administered, "solves the problems of child-bearing" and is safe for mother and child.[41] But the medical literature continued to express concern

34. Bertha Van Hoosen, *Scopolamine-Morphine Anaesthesia*, p. 101. Some physicians reported success using twilight sleep at home, but most thought the method best suited to hospital deliveries.

35. Quoted from the *Journal of the American Medical Association* in "Another 'Twilight Sleep,'" *Literary Digest* 50 (1915): 187; W. Gillespie, "Analgesics and Anesthetics in Labor, Their Indication and Contra-Indications," *Ohio Medical Journal* 11 (1915): 611.

36. "Twilight Sleep Again," *American Medicine* 21 (1915): 149.

37. "'Twilight Sleep' in the Light of Day," *Scientific American* 79, suppl. 2041 (1915): 112. See also the *New York Times* (October 20, 1914), p. 12; (November 28, 1914), p. 12; (February 5, 1915), p. 10; (February 11, 1915), p. 8.

38. *Journal of the American Medical Association* (June 6, 1914), quoted in "'Twilight Sleeps' and Medical Publicity," *Literary Digest* 49 (1914): 60.

39. Ralph M. Beach, "Twilight Sleep: Report of One Thousand Cases," *American Journal of Obstetrics* 71 (1915): 728.

40. Frederick A. Stratton, "Scopolamine Anesthesia," *Wisconsin Medical Journal* 8 (1908–9): 27.

41. Van Hoosen, *Scopolamine-Morphine Anaesthesia*, p. 101.

about the possible ill effects of a breathing irregularity in babies whose mothers had been given scopolamine and morphine late in labor.[42] Doctors trying to understand the evaluation of twilight sleep must have been confused. In one journal, they read that the procedure was "too dangerous to be pursued," while another journal assured them that scopolamine, when properly used during labor, "has no danger for either mother or child."[43] Increasingly, by 1915, medical journals published studies that at least cautiously favored twilight sleep (the January 1915 issue of *American Medicine* published nine such articles),[44] although they frequently ran editorials warning of the drug's potential dangers and stressing the need for caution. Practicing physicians faced a dilemma when pregnant women demanded painless childbirth with scopolamine.[45]

While physicians debated the desirability of using scopolamine in 1914 and 1915, the public, surer of its position, demanded that twilight sleep be routinely available to women who wanted it. Hospitals in the major cities responded to these demands and to physicians' growing interest in the method by allowing deliveries of babies the Freiburg way.[46] In order to gain additional clinical experience, and possibly in response to some women's requests, some doctors used twilight sleep in hospital charity wards. But the technique was most successful in the specialty wards there upper- and middle-class patients increasingly gave birth and hospital attendants and facilities were available. By May 1915, *McClure's Magazine*'s national survey reported that the use of twilight

42. This condition, called "oligopnea," usually resolved after a few hours, but it was frightening to observe, especially for attendants who had no experience with it (Gauss, "Further Experiments in Dammerschlaf," p. 302).

43. See discussion of the Polak paper (n. 14 above) in *American Journal of Obstetrics* 7 (1915): 798; and Hilkowich, p. 793.

44. *American Medicine* 21 (1915): 24–70.

45. See, e.g., the discussion following Knipe's paper (n. 30 above) in the *American Journal of Obstetrics* 70 (1914): 1025. For articles with positive conclusions, see John Osborn Polock, "A Study of Twilight Sleep," *New York Medical Journal* 101 (1915): 293; Robert T. Gillmore, "Scopolamine and Morphine in Obstetrics and Surgery," *New York Medical Journal* 102 (1915): 298; William H. Wellington Knipe, " 'Twilight Sleep' from the Hospital Viewpoint," p. 250; W. Francis B. Wakefield, "Scopolamin-Amnesia in Labor," *American Journal of Obstetrics* 71 (1915): 428; Samuel J. Druskin and Nathan Ratnoff, "Twilight Sleep in Obstetrics—with a Report of 200 Cases," *New York State Journal of Medicine* 15 (1915): 152; Charles B. Reed, "A Contribution to the Study of 'Twilight Sleep,' " *Surgery, Gynecology and Obstetrics* 22 (1916): 656. For a negative conclusion, see Joseph Louis Baer, "Scopolamin-Morphin Treatment in Labor," *Journal of the American Medical Association* 64 (1915): 1723–28. The actual dangers of the drug varied according to dosage and timing, and it is impossible for the historian to assess the events accurately without individual case records. Any drug can be dangerous if misused, and the variability in advance about scopolamine suggests that some disasters occurred with it.

46. E.g., see *New York Times* (August 22, 1914), p. 9; and (September 10, 1914); and the American hospitals mentioned in Tracy and Boyd.

sleep, although still battling for acceptance, "gains steadily" around the country.[47]

Because of the need for expertise and extra care in administration of scopolamine, the twilight sleep movement easily fed into widespread efforts in the second decade of the twentieth century to upgrade obstetrical practice and eliminate midwives.[48] Both the women who demanded the technique and the doctors who adopted it applauded the new specialty of obstetrics. Mary Boyd desired to put an end to home deliveries when she advocated twilight sleep for charity patients: "Just as the village barber no longer performs operations, the untrained midwife of the neighborhood will pass out of existence under the effective competition of free painless wards."[49] Not only did scopolamine advocates try to displace midwives, but they also regarded general practitioners as unqualified to deliver twilight sleep babies. "The twentieth century woman will no more think of having an ordinary practitioner attend her in childbed at her own home," said two supporters, "she will go to a [twilight sleep] hospital as a matter of course."[50] Specialists agreed that "the method is not adapted for the general practitioner, but should be practiced only by those who devote themselves to obstetrics."[51] Eliza Taylor Ransom went so far as to recommend the passage of a federal law forbidding "anyone administering scopolamine without a course of instruction and a special license."[52]

Some obstetricians used this issue to discredit their general practitioner colleagues and the midwives who still delivered large numbers of America's babies. Another factor that might have pushed obstetricians to support twilight sleep was that births under scopolamine could be managed more completely by the physician. As one succinctly put it, anesthesia gave "absolute control over your patient at all stages of the game. . . . You are 'boss.' "[53] Physicians' time at the bedside could even be used for other pursuits. "I catch up on my reading and writing," testified one practitioner, "I am never harassed by relatives who want me to tell them things."[54]

47. Anna Steele Richardson's survey was reported in the *New York Times* (May 10, 1915), p. 24.

48. Litoff (n. 3 above), pp. 69–70.

49. Mary Boyd, "The Story of Dammerschlaf," *Survey* 33 (1914): 129. See the same statement in Boyd and Tracy, p. 69.

50. Constance Leupp and Burton J. Hendrick, "Twilight Sleep in America," *McClure's Magazine* 44 (1915): 172–73. The argument about expertise appeared repeatedly (see, e.g., William H. W. Knipe, "The Truth about Twilight Sleep," *Delineator* 85 [1914]: 4). Twilight sleep women were aware that theirs was an expensive demand. They expected the cost of physician-attended childbirth to jump from twenty-five to eighty-five dollars (Tracy and Boyd, p. 180).

51. Druskin and Ratnoff, p. 1520.

52. *New York Times* (April 30, 1915). p. 8.

53. Quoted from the *New Orleans Medical and Surgical Journal* in Miller (n. 1 above), p. 24.

54. Van Hoosen, *Petticoat Surgeon*, p. 282.

93

The Issue of Control

How do we explain the seeming contradictions in this episode in medical history? Why did women demand to undergo a process which many physicians deemed risky and in which parturients lost self-control? Why did some physicians resist a process that would have given women an easier birthing experience and would have reinforced physicians' control over childbirth in a hospital environment?

Several factors contributed to the open tensions about the use of twilight sleep. One was safety. Many physicians rejected scopolamine because they did not have access to facilities like those at the Mary Thompson Hospital or because they believed the drug too risky under any circumstances. Because of the variability among physicians' use of scopolamine and the contradictory evidence in the professional journals, we know that safety was a guiding motivation of many physicians. However, this is not enough to explain physician reluctance since so many doctors administered other drugs during labor despite questionable safety reports.[55] Differing perceptions about pain during childbirth also contributed to the intensity of feeling about twilight sleep in 1914 and 1915. Although many physicians believed that women's "extremely delicate nervous sensibilities" needed relief, others were reluctant to interfere with the natural process of childbirth. One anti–twilight sleep physician argued, "when we reflect that we are dealing with a perfectly healthy individual, and an organ engaged in a purely physiological function . . . I fail to see the necessity of instituting such a measure in a normal labor and attempt[ing] to bridge the parturient woman over this physiological process in a semi-conscious condition."[56] Women perceived, too, that some physicians used anesthesia only for "suffering when it becomes a serious impediment to the birth process."[57] However, women who had suffered greatly, or whose friends had suffered greatly, actively sought relief from their "physiological" births: They thought pain in itself a hindrance to a successful childbirth experience and "demanded" that their physicians provide them with more positive, less painful, experiences in the future.[58]

Both sides in the twilight sleep debate grappled with a third important question: whether the women or the attendants should determine

55. Fifty percent of 100 general practitioners surveyed in rural districts and small towns in Wisconsin indicated that they used ergot during labor, although its use was blamed for "a very large per cent of necessary operations for repair of injuries to the floor and pelvic organs of the female patient" (Ford [n. 4 above], p. 257).

56. Dr. Francis Reder, during a discussion of Rongy, Harrar, and MacPherson papers, *Transactions of the American Association of Obstetricians and Gynecologists* 27 (1914): 386.

57. Tracy and Boyd, p. 149.

58. For physicians' perceptions of "demanding" women, see, e.g., the discussion following the Rongy and Harrar papers, *Transactions of the American Association of Obstetricians and Gynecologists* 27 (1914): 382–83.

and control the birthing process.[59] The women who demanded that doctors put them to sleep were partially blind to the safety issue because the issue of control (over pain, bodily function, decision making) was so important to them. Control became important when doctors refused to allow women "to receive the same benefits from this great discovery that their sisters abroad are getting."[60] Twilight sleep advocates demanded their right to decide how they would have their children. Tracy and Boyd articulated this issue: "Women took their doctor's word before. They are now beginning to believe . . . that the use of painlessness should be at *their* discretion."[61] Although women were out of control during twilight sleep births—unconscious and needing crib-beds or constant attention to restrain their wild movements—this loss of control was less important to them than their determination to control the decision about what kind of labor and delivery they would have. Hanna Rion, whose influential book and articles had garnered support for the method, wrote:

> In the old-fashioned days when women were merely the blindfolded guardians of the power of child-bearing, they had no choice but to trust themselves without question in the hands of the all-wise physician, but that day is past and will return no more. Women have torn away the bandages of false modesty; they are no longer ashamed of their bodies; they want to know all the wondrous workings of nature, and they demand that they be taught how best to safeguard themselves as wives and mothers. When it comes to the supreme function of childbearing every woman should certainly have the choice of saying *how* she will have her child.[62]

Twilight sleep women wanted to control their own births by choosing to go to sleep. They were not succumbing to physicians or technology but were, they thought, demanding the right to control their own birthing experiences.

This feminist emphasis on control over decision making appears in the writings and lectures of the twilight sleep movement; its followers sought simple relief from pain.[63] Many leaders were active suffragists

---

59. Other contributing factors cannot be developed here. Growing professionalization and specialization with medicine produced tensions among groups of doctors that surfaced during this debate. The method's German "origins" invalidated it with many Americans during the war years. My emphasis here on the issue of control is not meant to minimize these and other factors. However, because others, especially Lawrence Miller (n. 1 above) have explored the general outlines, I have focused on the previously unanalyzed question of decision-making power. Its importance, I think, is indicated by the intensity in the women's arguments on this issue.

60. Letter from "Ex-Medicus" in *New York Times* (November 28, 1914), p. 12.

61. Tracy and Boyd, p. 147 (emphasis in original).

62. Rion (n. 16 above), p. 47.

63. Tracy and Boyd claimed "four to five million" twilight sleep followers, obviously an exaggeration (p. 144).

whose commitment to twilight sleep was rooted in their belief in women's rights.[64] Although these activists agreed with most physicians that birth should increasingly be the domain of the obstetricians and that women should not suffer unnecessarily, they disagreed vehemently about who should decide what the birthing woman's experience would be. They clearly and adamantly wanted women to have the right to decide their own method of birthing.[65]

In the face of advancing obstetrical technology, many physicians wanted to retain their traditional professional right and duty to decide therapy on the basis of their judgment about the medical indications. They refused to be "dragooned" into "indiscriminate adoption" of a procedure that they themselves did not choose.[66] Even the doctors who supported twilight sleep believed that in the final analysis, the method of childbirth was "a question for the attending man and not the patient to decide."[67] It was principally this question of power over decision making that separated the movement's proponents from its opponents.

The Decline

In the very successes of the twilight sleep movement lay the seeds for its demise. Pressured by the clubwomen's associations and their own pregnant patients, doctors who had not been trained in the Freiburg method delivered babies with scopolamine. There was an enormous variation in the use of the drug, its timing through labor, the conditions in which the woman labored, and the watchfulness of attendants. As its advocates had feared, problems emerged when scopolamine was not properly monitored in a hospital setting. Following reports of adverse effects on the newborn, the drug fell into ill repute, and some hospitals that had been among the first to use it stopped administering it routinely.[68]

Those physicians who continued to advocate twilight sleep believed that accidents were due to misuse of the Freiburg method and not to the drug itself. Commenting on its discontinuation at Michael Reese Hospital in Chicago, Dr. Bertha Van Hoosen noted that "it is . . . probable that this adverse report demonstrates nothing more than the inexperience of the people using this anesthetic."[69] Dr. Ralph Beach agreed that "there is no doubt that all of the bad results which have been reported due to this

64. See, e.g., *New York Times* (November 28, 1914), p. 12.

65. See esp. Tracy and Boyd, Rion, Ransom (n. 21 above), and Van Hoosen (n. 10 above).

66. *New York Times* (September 26, 1914), p. 10.

67. Dr. Arthur J. Booker in his remarks defending Van Hoosen's use of scopolamine, quoted in Van Hoosen, *Scopolamine-Morphine Anaesthesia*, p. 12.

68. *New York Times* (April 24, 1915), p. 10; (April 30, 1915), p. 8; (May 29, 1915), p. 20; (August 25, 1915), p. 10; (August 16, 1916), p. 7.

69. Van Hoosen, "A Fixed Dosage" (n. 29 above), p. 57.

method, are due to an improper technic, or the administration of unstable preparations."[70] Simultaneously, in 1915, some hospitals expanded their obstetric services to offer twilight sleep, and others began cutting back its use. Either because they judged the drug dangerous or because they did not use it correctly, some hospitals found the method too troublesome to administer on a routine basis to all patients. Most reached a compromise and continued to use scopolamine during labor's first stage (when it was deemed safe), thus preempting their patients' protests without compromising their medical beliefs. A second inhibitory factor appeared in August 1915 when Mrs. Francis X. Carmody, one of the country's leading exponents of twilight sleep, died during childbirth at Long Island College Hospital in New York. Although doctors and her husband insisted that her death was unrelated to scopolamine, it nonetheless harmed the movement.[71] Mrs. Carmody's neighbor started a new movement to oppose twilight sleep, and women became more alert to the question of safety than they had been.[72] Doctors and some former twilight sleep advocates, emphasizing the issues of safety and difficulty of administration, began exploring other methods of achieving painless childbirth.[73]

The obstetric literature after 1915 indicates that twilight sleep did not die in that year. The women's movement may have failed to make scopalamine routinely available to all laboring women, but it succeeded in making the concept of painless childbirth more acceptable and in adding scopolamine to the obstetric pharmacopoeia. In fact, obstetricians continued to use scopolamine into the 1960s during the first stage of hospital births.[74] The use of anesthesia (including scopolamine) in childbirth grew in the years after 1915, since women, aware of the possibility of painlessness, continued to want "shorter and less painful parturition" and since physicians felt they could disregard these desires "only at great risk to [their] own practice."[75]

The attempt by a group of women, including some feminists, to control their birthing experiences backfired. The medical profession retained the choice of birth procedures and perhaps gained additional

70. Beach (n. 33 above), p. 43.
71. *New York Times* (August 24, 1915), p. 7.
72. Ibid. (August 31, 1915), p. 5.
73. See, e.g., Frank W. Lynch, "Nitrous Oxide Gas Analgesia in Obstetrics," *Journal of the American Medical Association* 64 (1915): 813.
74. See, e.g., Henry Schwarz, "Painless Childbirth and the Safe Conduct of Labor," *American Journal of Obstetrics and Diseases of Women and Children* 79 (1919): 46–63; and W. C. Danforth and C. Henry Davis, "Obstetric Analgesia and Anesthesia," *Journal of the American Medical Association* 81 (1923): 1090–96.
75. See the assessment of anesthesia used in childbirth in New York Academy of Medicine Committee on Public Health Relations, *Maternal Mortality in New York City: A Study of all Puerperal Deaths 1930–1932* (New York: Commonwealth Fund, 1933), p. 113; see also Joyce Antler and Daniel M. Fox, "Movement toward a Safe Maternity: Physician Accountability in New York City, 1915–1940," *Bulletin of the History of Medicine* 50 (1976): 569–95.

control as a result of this episode. Partial acceptance by the profession quieted the lay revolt, and women lost the power they had sought. Ironically, by encouraging women to go to sleep during their deliveries, the twilight sleep movement helped to distance women from their bodies. Put to sleep with a variety of drugs, most parturient women from the 1920s to the 1960s did not experience one of their bodies' most powerful actions and thus lost touch with their own physical potential.[76] The twilight sleep movement helped change the definition of birthing from a natural home event, as it was in the nineteenth century, to an illness requiring hospitalization and physician attendance. Parturient feminists today, seeking fully to experience childbirth, paradoxically must fight a tradition of drugged, hospital-controlled births, itself the partial result of a struggle to increase women's control over their bodies.

History of Medicine Department and *Women's Studies Program*
University of Wisconsin—Madison

76. The legacy for the parent-infant bond and for subsequent child development is explored in M. H. Klaus and J. H. Kennell, *Maternal Infant Bonding: The Impact of Early Separation or Loss on Family Development* (St. Louis: C. V. Mosby Co., 1976). For a feminist perspective on women's missing their deliveries, see Adrienne Rich, *Of Woman Born: Motherhood as Experience and Institution* (New York: W. W. Norton & Co., 1976).

Pain, 19 (1984) 321–337
Elsevier

PAI 00676

Review Article

The Myth of Painless Childbirth
(The John J. Bonica Lecture)

Ronald Melzack

Department of Psychology, McGill University, Montreal, Que. (Canada)

(Received 29 March 1984, accepted 30 March 1984)

We are all familiar with John Bonica's magnificent contributions to the management and understanding of acute and chronic pain. But some people are not aware
that John is also a world authority on obstetrical anesthesia. He developed a special
interest in obstetrical problems early in his career, after his wife Emma had a
near-disastrous experience with improperly administered ether anesthesia during the
birth of their first child. He worked hard at acquiring skill and expertise in
administering epidural analgesia, and subsequently organized the first 24-h medical
anesthesia service for obstetrics in the United States. After two decades of experience, he wrote the 2-vol set *Principles and Practice of Obstetric Analgesia and
Anesthesia* [4] which is an acknowledged modern medical classic. Every aspect of
childbirth is addressed with the same thoughtfulness, insight and meticulous detail
that are characteristic of John's books and papers on chronic pain. John has
repeatedly argued [5,6] that labor is often extremely painful and that severe,
prolonged pain can be dangerous to women with cardiovascular problems and to the
fetus whose oxygen supply may be at risk during protracted, complicated deliveries.
My recent work supports John's contention that most women suffer severe pain
during labor.

The promise of painless childbirth

Fernand Lamaze's popular book, *Painless Childbirth: Psychoprophylactic Method*
[15], contained the explicit promise that prepared childbirth training would abolish
labor pain. My research [20,21], however, shows that the promise is not fulfilled:
pain is diminished but remains severe. Nevertheless, the prepared childbirth movement, despite its unwarranted emphasis on the self-control of pain, makes a valid
point: childbirth is often treated by obstetricians and anesthetists as just another
medical problem, 'an appropriate occasion for maximum surgical and chemical

0304-3959/84/$03.00 © 1984 Elsevier Science Publishers B.V.

intervention' [16, p.2]. As a result, prospective mothers and fathers may lose all say in a situation that should be emotionally fulfilling and a happy, memorable event. The problem, as Judith Lumley and Jill Astbury [16] point out in their excellent book *Birth Rites, Birth Rights*, is that the emphasis on pain in the prepared childbirth movement has obscured recognition of the psychological individuality of each mother and her unique anxieties, expectations, problems and needs. The time has come to put the field in perspective so that obstetricians, anesthesiologists and prepared childbirth trainers can work together toward the common goal of achieving physical safety *and* psychological fulfillment.

A brief history

Labor has been portrayed as a fearsome, painful, life-threatening event since the earliest recorded history and has held that status until this century [4]. When the anesthetic effects of ether and chloroform were discovered in the mid-1800's, many members of the British clergy argued strenuously that this human intervention in the miracle of birth was a sin against the will of God. If He had wished labor to be painless, He would have created it so. Queen Victoria, undaunted by the clergy, chose one day to use an anesthetic during labor and the clergy's position crumbled. Anesthetics were subsequently used increasingly for labor pain, and the concurrent drop in mortality and morbidity in both mother and infant were attributed, in part at least, to the absence of pain which permitted the midwife or obstetrician to work unhindered in difficult labors.

All this changed in the mid-1900's. Dick-Read's book, *Childbirth Without Fear* [9], and Lamaze's book, *Painless Childbirth: Psychoprophylactic Method* [15], rapidly led to the belief that labor is not inherently painful. Basically, these writers believe that fears about birth are learned and are a by-product of civilization. These fears, they propose, lead during labor to muscle tension which is the cause of pain during uterine contractions. The pain enhances the fears, which in turn increase the tension, and thus a vicious circle is set up. Clearly, the only way to break the circle is by proper training, and the Lamaze prescription of breathing exercises, relaxation, distraction of attention and loving care by spouse and trainer is supposed to produce the desired result of 'painless childbirth.' Implicit in all of this is the assumption that if labor *does* become painful, it is the fault of the mother for not having learned the training regimen properly. Not only does the prospective mother face pain, then, but the pain itself becomes a token of failure. The mother is now burdened with a sense of guilt for having betrayed her own expectations as well as those of her husband and her trainer [16].

Prepared childbirth training: some assumptions

Explicit in 'prepared childbirth training' are a number of simple assumptions: first, animals show no evidence of pain during labor so that pain in women must therefore be learned through fear and tension; second, natural physiological processes (such as breathing or urination) are painless and, since childbirth is a natural process, it must also be painless; third, women in primitive cultures (who have presumably not been taught to be afraid of childbirth) have painless births.

All 3 assumptions are wrong. First, the pelvis of the upright human female is so much more complex, anatomically, than that of lower 4-legged animals that the entire birth process itself has increased greatly in complexity. The pelvis of a female sheep, for example, is large and relatively simple while the pelvis of the female human is broad and curved forward, with large weight-bearing muscles and ligaments that may impede the expulsion of the fetus [3] (Fig. 1). Second, during labor, intense contractions of smooth muscle and stretched or torn tissues of sensitive, richly innervated organs in the pelvic floor and perineum [4,13] would be expected to produce pain. Third, serious studies of primitive cultures show, without the shadow of a doubt, that labor pain is felt by women in all cultures. If inadequate observations and preconceived notions are set aside [26], it is abundantly clear that labor pain is felt universally and is often extremely severe. Every culture has invented chants, incantations. rituals and pseudomedical practices in the attempt to counteract labor pain. The image of the primitive woman having her baby painlessly is pure myth [4,10,26,29].

One assumption that is clearly correct, however, is that women in labor are subject to intense fears and anxieties related to their ability to bear the pain, the possibility of medical complications, and the baby's health [5,16]. Methods such as prepared childbirth training (PCT), which are designed to reduce fear, anxiety and tension, should, theoretically, also decrease pain. Yet the effects of PCT are still controversial. While several studies [25,31,33] have shown that relaxation, distraction and other components of PCT diminish pain, other studies [8,12,24] report that PCT has no demonstrable effects on pain itself but simply decreases the emotional reactions to pain.

A major cause of this controversy has been the lack of adequate methods to measure pain. Recently, however, the McGill Pain Questionnaire has provided a new approach to the measurement of the intensity and qualities of pain [18,19].

Relative intensity of labor pain

In the first study my colleagues and I carried out [21], we were astonished by the high intensity of pain suffered by most women in labor. Fig. 2 shows the mean pain scores for trained and untrained primiparas and multiparas. It is evident that the average scores for labor pain are exceeded only by those for causalgia in chronic-pain patients and amputation of a digit in acute-pain patients. It is higher than average pain scores reported by patients with chronic low-back pain, pain in non-terminal cancer patiens, arthritic pain and other forms of chronic and acute pain that are universally acknowledged to be severe. Although there are obvious limitations to comparing pains of such widely different origins and implications for the future life of the patients, it is nevertheless clear that, at the very least, labor pain ranks among

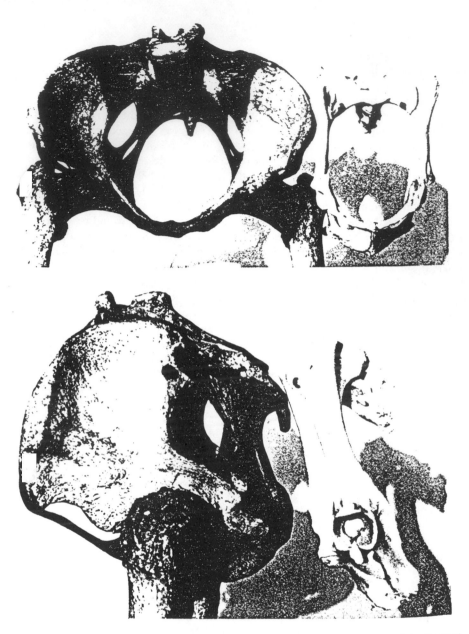

Fig. 1. Comparison of the pelvic structure of the human female and the ewe, whose infants have the same average birth weight as human infants. Beischer and Mackay [3, p. 22] note that 'The human pelvis is a bony basin not a mere bony ring as in the ewe. In animals the sacrum is not directly opposite the pubic symphysis and during birth the fetus does not have to pass both bones simultaneously. The effect of the erect posture is to push the pubes upwards (via the femoral heads) and the sacrum downwards (effect of the weight of the trunk) — hence the mechanical difficulties of human parturition.' The pelvic brim of the human is 11 cm × 13 cm and of the sheep is 12 cm × 9 cm. Frontal (top) and lateral (bottom) views are shown. (Reprinted by kind permission of Dr. N.A. Beischer and Dr. E.V. Mackay [3]. Copright Holt-Saunders Pty. Ltd.)

the most intense pains recorded with the McGill Pain Questionnaire.

While the average intensity of labor pain is extremely high, there is a wide range in pain scores (Fig. 3). Among primiparas, 9.2% had scores in the lower third of the range: 2–11 (very mild pain); 12–21 (mild pain). In the middle third, 29.5% had scores of 22–31 (moderate pain) and 37.9% had scores of 32–41 (severe pain). The remaining 23.4% had scores in the top third (42–62) of the range. Pain scores as high as these are usually described as unbearable, intolerable or extremely severe and, indeed, 25% of primiparas labeled their pain as 'horrible' or 'excruciating' on a brief intensity scale of the MPQ. This distribution is in excellent agreement with the pain scores described by Nettelbladt et al. [24] for a group of 78 primiparas: 28% reported moderate pain, 37% had severe pain and 35% had intolerable pain.

Multiparas have lower pain scores (Fig. 3): 24.1% had scores in the lower third of the range, while 29.6% had moderate pain, 35.2% had severe pain, and only 11.1% had scores in the top third of the range. Still, 46.3% of multiparas — a sizeable number — had scores rated as severe or extremely severe.

The intensity is also reflected in the large number of words chosen by the women to describe their pain [21]. The following *sensory* words were chosen by 33% or more of the combined sample of primiparas and multiparas: sharp, cramping, aching, throbbing, stabbing, hot, shooting, heavy. Among *affective* descriptors, the word tiring was chosen by 49% of women and exhausting by 36%. The *evaluative* word intense was chosen by 52%, and the *miscellaneous* word tight by 44%.

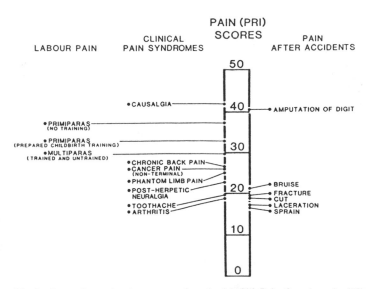

Fig. 2. Comparison of pain scores, using the McGill Pain Questionnaire [18], obtained from women during labor [21] and from patients in a general hospital pain clinic [18] and an emergency department [22]. The pain score for causalgic pain is reported by Tahmoush [34]. The Pain Rating Index (PRI) represents the sum of the rank values of all the words chosen from 20 sets of pain descriptors [18].

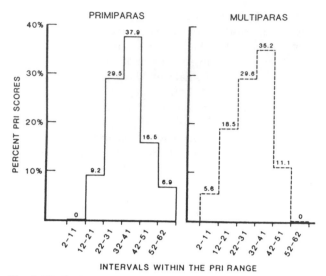

INTERVALS WITHIN THE PRI RANGE

Fig. 3. Distribution of Pain Rating Index (PRI) scores for primiparas and multiparas in 6 intervals of the total PRI range recorded by Melzack et al. [21].

TABLE I

CORRELATES OF LABOR PAIN

Significant correlations between personal variables and scores in the Pain Rating Index (PRI) subclasses of the McGill Pain Questionnaire. Based on data from 87 primiparas and 54 multiparas [21].

	Pearson correlation coefficient	P value (2-tailed)
PRI — sensory		
Socioeconomic status	−0.29	0.02
PRI — affective		
Previous delivery	−0.22	0.01
Husband in room	+0.30	0.04
Menstrual difficulties	+0.25	0.01
PRI — evaluative		
Previous delivery	−0.20	0.02
PRI — miscellaneous		
Socioeconomic status	−0.40	0.002
Age	−0.24	0.006
Previous delivery	−0.21	0.02
Menstrual difficulties	+0.22	0.02
PRI — total		
Socioeconomic status	−0.34	0.006
Previous delivery	−0.24	0.005
Menstrual difficulties	+0.21	0.04

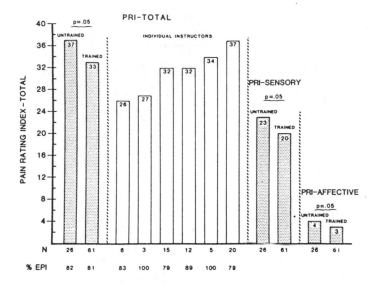

Fig. 4. Left: mean PRI scores obtained by untrained and trained primiparas [21]. Center: the average PRI scores of trained women categorized by individual prepared-training instructors. Right: mean PRI scores for the sensory and affective descriptor sets of the MPQ. The percentages of women who received an epidural block are indicated at the bottom.

Some correlates of labor pain

Several important variables — some expected, some not — were found to correlate with labor pain [21]. Table I shows that socioenconomic status and age are negatively correlated with pain, confirming earlier reports [8,14,24]. This is not a surprise since women of higher socioeconomic status tend to have children when they are older [14], and are more likely to attend prepared childbirth training classes which, as we shall soon see, tend to diminish pain intensity.

The positive correlations (in Table I) between several measures of labor pain and menstrual difficulties are particularly interesting. There is strong evidence that women who have dysmenorrhea produce excessive amounts of prostaglandins, which trigger uterine contractions [17]. Drugs that inhibit prostaglandin synthesis also diminish menstrual pain. Because of the positive correlation between menstrual and labor pain, it is conceivable that women who suffer severe labor pain may also produce excessive prostaglandins during labor.

Another correlation in Table I is surprising and interesting — the affective descriptor category shows that pain scores were higher when the husband was in the case-room than when he was absent. This may reflect genuinely higher affective pain scores or may be due to a deliberate choice of descriptors in the attempt to impress the husband or express anger at him. Whatever the reason, the finding seems not to be spurious. Wallach [36] found a similar effect in an independent study.

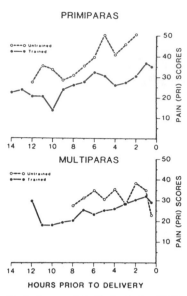

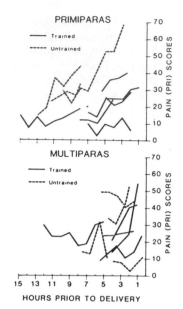

HOURS PRIOR TO DELIVERY

HOURS PRIOR TO DELIVERY

Fig. 5. Average Pain Rating Index (PRI) scores reported by primiparas and multiparas at successive hours prior to delivery [20]. Pain scores, shown separately for trained and untrained women, were assigned to the nearest hour for purposes of calculation.

Fig. 6. Individual Pain Rating Index (PRI) scores reported by primiparas and multiparas at successive hours prior to delivery [20]. Pain scores, shown separately for trained and untrained women, were assigned to the nearest hour for purposes of calculation.

Effects of prepared childbirth training

Fig. 4 shows the mean pain scores of primiparas who received prepared childbirth training and those who did not. The results of training by individual instructors are also shown. In all cases the training consisted of a series of classes that included instruction in obstetric physiology, breathing exercises and relaxation techniques. Clearly there was considerable variability in the scores obtained during labor among different instructors' groups.

Primiparas who elected to have prepared childbirth training had significantly lower pain scores than those who received no training (Fig. 4). Not only the total mean pain score but also the sensory and affective scores were significantly lower. However, the average scores of the women who received training were still very high. For example, the training by instructor 1 was clearly the most effective, yet the mean total pain score for the 6 patients in her group was about the same as those for outpatients with chronic back pain and cancer (Fig. 2). Most important is the fact that although instructor 1 strongly encouraged her patients to forego an epidural block, 5 of the 6 women specifically requested one late in labor. Interestingly, the percentages of women who had epidural blocks (shown at the bottom of Fig. 4) are remarkably uniform across all the groups.

Variability of labor pain

Perhaps the most striking feature of the data presented so far is the astonishing individual variability of the pain. This is even clearer in a second study [20] in which 79 women (42 primiparas; 37 multiparas) received several successive questionnaires at hourly intervals until they entered the delivery room, or had an epidural block, or asked the experimenter to stop. Fig. 5 shows the averaged pain curves for trained and untrained women. Although these curves indicate a gradually rising pain intensity, graphs of pain scores obtained from individual women reveal a high level of variability as labor progresses (Fig. 6). Instead of the idealized rising curve usually seen in obstetrical texts [11], which reflects the group scores shown in Fig. 5, there is a remarkable variety of patterns. Some women show the expected rising curve. Others show rises and falls in pain level. Some women have extremely high levels of pain early in labor, while others, up to the time of delivery, show fairly low, constant pain scores. Incomplete curves in Fig. 4 are due to refusal by the women to continue because they were exhausted or they wanted an epidural block.

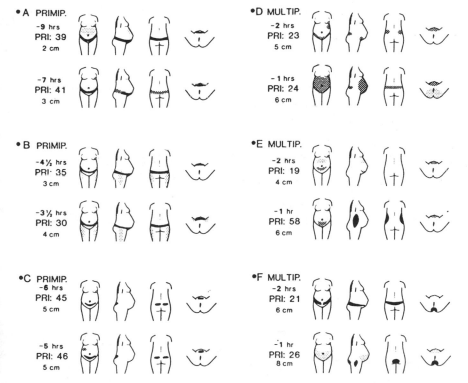

Fig. 7. Spatial distribution of pain in 6 women at various time-points before delivery [20]. The PRI scores and extent of cervical dilation are indicated. Pain intensity is indicated by: stipple — mild; cross-hatch — moderate; black — severe.

The high level of individual variability is also reflected in the spatial distribution of pain (Fig. 7). The typical, idealized distributions depicted by Bonica [6] may reflect average events in a large population but hide the considerable variability among individual women shown in Fig. 7. Some women have widespread pain over a large part of the abdomen, back and perineum, while others have discrete painful areas.

Weight, height and other physical variables

The emphasis on psychological factors in recent years has led to the neglect of physical variables. It is evident in Table II that the normal-weight/height ratio contributes significantly to the pain scores of primiparas. That is, the heavier the mother per unit of height, the higher the pain scores. The same variable contributed to the pain scores of multiparas but, in addition, heavier mothers and mothers with heavier babies also had higher pain scores. However, the relatively low correlation coefficients, though statistically significant, reflect the high degree of variability of all measures related to labor.

TABLE II

SIGNIFICANT CORRELATIONS BETWEEN PHYSICAL VARIABLES AND PAIN INDICES

All correlations shown are significant at $P < 0.05$. NS = not significant; PRI = Pain Rating Index; S = sensory; A = affective; E = evaluative; M = miscellaneous; T = total. The pain indices are derived from the McGill Pain Questionnaire.

	Primiparas		Multiparas	
	N		N	
Mother				
Height	57	NS	41	NS
Normal weight	72	NS	43	PRI(E): $r = 0.30$
				PRI(M): $r = 0.43$
				PRI(T): $r = 0.30$
Normal weight/height	57	PRI(S): $r = 0.23$	40	PRI(E): $r = 0.27$
		PRI(A): $r = 0.23$		PRI(M): $r = 0.36$
		PRI(T): $r = 0.27$		
Weight gain	60	NS	35	NS
Weight gain				
Height	47	NS	35	NS
Baby				
Weight	82	NS	51	PRI(S): $r = 0.27$
				PRI(M): $r = 0.24$
				PRI(T): $r = 0.29$
Gestational age	74	NS	44	NS

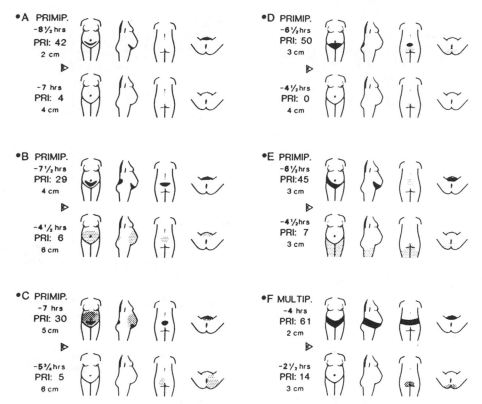

Fig. 8. Changes in spatial distribution of pain in 6 women before and after a successful epidural block [20]. The number of hours before delivery, the PRI and the extent of cervical dilation are indicated. Pain intensity is indicated as in Fig. 7.

Epidural blocks

We examined the effectiveness of epidural blocks in two studies [20,21]. In the first, 31 women completed the McGill Pain Questionnaire before and after administration of the anesthetic. The block was judged to be ineffective by three (10%) of the patients. In those in whom the block was effective (eliminating the sharp, shooting qualities of the pain) the mean total pain score was 27.9 before the block and 8.0 and 7.6 respectively 30 and 60 min after administration of the anesthetic. In the women in whom the block was ineffective the mean score before administration of the anesthetic was 32.6; the score dropped to 12 after 30 min but then rose to 35 0.5 h later despite continued administration of the agent.

In the second study [20], the effects of epidural blocks were studied in 12 women. The blocks were ineffective in 4 (33%). Pain scores decreased by an average of 89% in the women with an effective epidural, but increased by an average of 9% after an ineffective block. There was no clear-cut relationship between pain intensity and

332

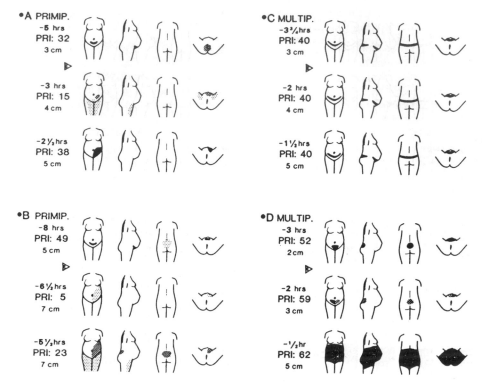

Fig. 9. Changes in spatial distribution of pain in 4 women before and after an unsuccessful epidural block [20]. The number of hours before delivery, the PRI and the extent of cervical dilation are indicated. Pain intensity is indicated as in Fig. 7.

spatial distribution of pain after an effective epidural block (Fig. 8). Fig. 9 reveals the unpredictable changes in pain distribution produced by an ineffective block (probably because the catheter or the patient was positioned incorrectly). The failure rate of 33% in epidural blocks is unusually high. Previous studies [4,21,28] have found a failure rate of about 10%. The high percentage is likely due to the inexperience of the anesthetists involved at the time, several of whom were just beginning their residency in anesthesiology. This variability of the effectiveness of anesthesiologists is not to be dismissed more lightly than the variability of effectiveness of prepared childbirth trainers.

The need for a balanced approach

The most striking feature of these data is that, on the average, labor pain ranks among the severest forms of pain recorded with the McGill Pain Questionnaire. Prepared childbirth training was consistently associated with lower levels of pain.

However, the training did not produce dramatic reductions in pain, even though the women elected to have the training and therefore represented a self-selected sample with positive attitudes. The most effective training in our study – by an instructor who uses the orthodox Lamaze technique – was associated with an average pain reduction of about 30%, but most of the patients in her group still found the pain so intense that they requested an epidural block despite the instructor's bias against it. These results show that the title of Lamaze's book, *Painless Childbirth* [15], is misleading. Although the pain is diminished, the reduction is not nearly as large as the title suggests.

These observations should be interpreted in a positive sense, however. The fact that the current training procedures have statistically significant effects on pain is encouraging and indicates that psychological preparation is valuable. That the pain reduction is relatively small indicates a need for further development of these obviously useful procedures.

The results emphasize the need for a balanced view of the roles of prepared childbirth training and epidural block in labor. While many proponents of natural childbirth believe it is highly desirable to have delivery without epidural block or other forms of anesthesia, cerain facts must be kept in mind. Many women have intense pain, which is invariably associated with reflex increases in blood pressure, oxygen consumption, and the liberation of catacholamines — all of which may adversely affect uterine blood flow. Bonica [5,6] cites recent evidence which suggests that epidural analgesia diminishes these reflex effects. Indeed, epidural anesthesia increases uterine blood flow, especially in patients with pregnancy-induced hypertension, toxemia and other disorders that decrease placental function [5,6]. On the other hand, since epidural analgesia eliminates the reflex urge to bear down, it is associated with a higher rate of forceps deliveries [4,15]. Moreover, unless the administrator is extremely careful, accidental puncture of the dura may occur with consequent post-puncture headache [4]. Furthermore, if the epidural block is ineffective, the woman is generally disappointed, angry and fearful.

These pros and cons must be considered without losing sight of the fact that many women have such severe pain that they request an epidural block even when the training instructor has advised against it. When this happens the woman may feel that she has failed herself, her husband and her instructor. Furthermore, if the woman is not psychologically prepared for the possibility of needing an epidural block she may be emotionally disturbed by the sudden prospect of this procedure. Obviously anesthetics may not be necessary for women who have low levels of pain (9% of the primiparas and 24% of the multiparas in this study), but most have high levels. There are many causes of pain during childbirth, such as intense muscle contraction and stretching or tearing of cervical, vaginal and other tissues [4]. Astbury [1] recently reported a major reason why women should be prepared for the possibility of intense pain during childbirth: those whose expectations of labor are violated by the actual labor experience report more severe pain.

The intensity of the feelings of guilt, anger and failure in some women when they anticipate a 'natural, painless birth' and are then confronted with such severe pain or complications that they require an epidural or a cesarian section has recently been documented. Dr. Donna Stewart [32] reports that some women become miserable, depressed, even suicidal, may lose interest in sex and in their marriage, and may require psychotherapy. In some cases [32], the husbands of women who anticipated 'natural' births required psychotherapy after intense feelings of nausea at the sight of blood or seeing their wives in such terrible pain. They experienced a profound sense of guilt and helplessness, and needed therapy for impotence, phobias and depression.

Toward a new approach

The decision to administer and receive an epidural block must be based on full awareness of many considerations. Because so many women have severe pain and request an epidural block it seems reasonable that information on anesthetic procedures should be included in prepared childbirth training. Fortunately the training philosophy does not preclude epidural or pudendal blocks [4] and therefore could be used to prepare the mother for anesthetic procedures, which are often a source of fear and anxiety (as are many medical procedures). The purpose of the dialogue between mother, instructor and physician is to provide the most comfortable and safest labor for both mother and infant. Prepared childbirth training and obstetric anesthesia are compatible, complementary procedures aimed at assisting women in childbirth to suffer less fear, anxiety and pain.

It is now amply clear that there are no panaceas to abolish labor pain. The Dick-Read [9] and Lamaze [15] procedures have limited effectiveness. The Leboyer method to prevent a 'violent birth' has no demonstrable effects [23], and the concept of 'early bonding' has fallen by the wayside [7]. The recent enthusiasm for birthing chairs has also begun to wane in light of convincing evidence that women in the later stages of labor actually prefer to lie down rather than sit because it is more confortable [27]. Even epidural blocks may fail, forcing women to cope with deep disappointment in addition to pain.

Where does this leave us? The evidence, taken together, indicates the necessity for an honest presentation of information. Lumley and Astbury [16] make a powerful case for the need to present a prospective mother with information that will match with what actually happens during labor. They found that, compared to an untrained group of women, women who attended prepared childbirth classes actually acquired unrealistic expectations regarding pain and, as a consequence, developed negative attitudes toward themselves, toward childbirth, as well as toward doctors and nurses. These women perceived their pain in a context that made them judge themselves as failures. Lumley and Astbury [16, p. 52] conclude that 'it seems psychologically dangerous to provide women with a model of childbirth which avoids all mention of pain and, furthermore, sees pain as a form of psychological failure.'

The enormous individual differences in every parameter described above lead to the same conclusion reached by Lumley and Astbury: it is absurd to treat all women and all labors in the same way. Women should be informed that the 'average' labor is a statistical concept and many women will have patterns of pain that deviate from this concept. In short, any prepared childbirth training course should spend considerable time preparing the prospective mother for possible deviations from the 'average,' preparing her for the possibility that she may (or may not) need an epidural block, a forceps delivery, a cesarian section. To do otherwise may lead to psychological trauma of sufficient seriousness to require psychotherapy [32].

The studies described here underscore individual differences — extraordinary variability in every aspect of pain — and these differences should be the basis of an honest relationship between a prospective mother and her medical and paramedical helpers. By allowing women to understand why certain procedures are taken and by presenting them with realistic expectations, the possibility of disappointment, guilt and a sense of failure are diminished. Prepared childbirth instructors are in a position to present this information to prospective mothers and by replacing dogma by facts they increase the chances that the mother will feel that unique kind of psychological fulfillment and joy that should attend the miracle of birth.

The major aim of the prepared childbirth movement should be to do just what the name of the movement implies: to *prepare* the mother-to-be to cope with the possibilities that may confront her at the time of birth. She should know not only the typical or 'average' event but many of the variations as well so that she is not caught off guard should the unexpected occur. The movement's emphasis on pain — perhaps the least tractable aspect of labor — has been misleading and unfortunate. The future of the movement lies in the striking advances in psychology, particularly in the field of individual differences — in responses to anxiety and stress, in the development and use of coping strategies, in the tendency to attribute control over events to one's self or to others [2,30,35]. The prepared childbirth movement needs to recognize the importance of the uniqueness of each individual and to tailor training programs to suit the needs of each woman. This, it seems to me, is the surest way to a birth with the kind of dignity and rich, personal fulfillment that should accompany such a miraculous event.

In conclusion, decades of reasearch on labor pain by many investigators lead inevitably to the thesis that lies at the heart of this lecture: prepared childbirth training and skillfully administered epidural analgesia are compatible, complementary procedures that allow recognition of the individuality of each woman. In this perspective, a woman in labor stops being a 'statistic' and becomes a unique person who can be prepared to cope with an event which is often extremely painful and, at the same time, one of the most fulfilling peak experiences in her life.

Acknowledgements

Invited address delivered on Award of the Fourth John J. Bonica Lecturership sponsored by the Eastern Pain Association, Inc., with a grant from Bristol Laboratories.

It is a pleasure to thank my colleagues and assistants who worked with me in carrying out the studies that are described in this lecture: Dr. Robert A. Kinch, Dr.

Perle Feldman and Dr. Paul Taenzer, as well as Lucy Melzack, Patricia Dobkin and Mary Lebrun.

The research was supported by Grant A7891 from the Natural Sciences and Engineering Research Council of Canada.

References

1 Astbury, J., Labour pain: the role of childbirth education, information and expectation. In: C. Peck and M. Wallace (Eds.), Problems in Pain, Pergamon, London, 1980, pp. 245–252.
2 Barber, J. and Adrian, C., Psychological Approaches to the Management of Pain, Brunner/Mazel, New York, 1982.
3 Beischer, N.A. and Mackay, E.V., Obstetrics and the Newborn, Saunders, Philadelphia, PA, 1976.
4 Bonica, J.J., Principles and Practice of Obstetric Analgesia and Anesthesia, Davis, Philadelphia, PA, Vol. 1, 1967, Vol. 2, 1969.
5 Bonica, J.J., Obstetric Analgesia and Anesthesia, World Federation of Societies of Anesthesiologists, Amsterdam, 1980.
6 Bonica, J.J., Labour pain. In: P.D. Wall and R. Melzack (Eds.), Textbook of Pain, Churchill-Livingstone, Edinburgh, 1984.
7 Brody, J.E., Influential theory of birth 'bonding' losing supporters, New York Times, reprinted in The Gazette, Montreal, April 2 (1983) 1-5.
8 Davensport-Slack, B. and Boylan, C.H., Psychological correlates of childbirth pain, Psychosom. Med., 36 (1974) 215–223.
9 Dick-Read, G., Childbirth Without Fear, Harper, New York, 1944.
10 Freedman, L.Z. and Ferguson, V.M., The question of 'painless childbirth' in primitive cultures, Amer. J. Orthopsychiat., 20 (1950) 363–379.
11 Friedman, E.A., Labor: Clinical Evaluation and Management, Appleton-Century-Crofts, New York, 1978.
12 Javert, C.T. and Hardy, J.D., Measurement of pain intensity in labor and its physiologic, neurologic and pharmacologic implications, Amer. J. Obstet. Gynec., 60 (1950) 552–563.
13 Krantz, K.E., Innervation of the human uterus, Ann. N.Y. Acad. Sci., 75 (1959) 770–785.
14 Kubista, E., Kucera, H., Salzer, H. und Reinhold, E., Einfluss des Sozialstatus auf Schwangerschaft, Geburt und Wochenbett, Wien. med. Wschr., 127 (1977) 341–346.
15 Lamaze, F., Painless Childbirth: Psychoprophylactic Method, Regnery, Chicago, IL, 1970.
16 Lumley, J. and Astbury J., Birth Rites, Birth Rights, Sphere Books, Melbourne, 1980.
17 Marx, J.L., Dysmenorrhea: basic research leads to a rational theory, Science, 205 (1979) 175–176.
18 Melzack, R., The McGill Pain Questionnaire: major properties and scoring methods, Pain, 1 (1975) 277–299.
19 Melzack, R. (Ed.), Pain Measurement and Assessment, Raven Press, New York, 1983.
20 Melzack, R., Kinch, R.A., Dobkin, P., Lebrun, M. and Taenzer, P., Severity of labour pain: influenced of physical as well as psychological variables, Canad. med. Ass. J., 130 (1984) 579–584.
21 Melzack, R., Taenzer, P., Feldman, P. and Kinch, R.A., Labour is still painful after prepared childbirth training, Canad. med. Ass. J., 125 (1981) 357–363.
22 Melzack, R., Wall, P.D. and Ty, T.C., Acute pain in an emergency clinic: latency of onset and descriptor patterns related to different injuries, Pain, 14 (1982) 33–43.
23 Nelson, N.M., Enkin, M.W., Saigal, S., Bennett, K.J., Milner, R. and Sackett, D.L., A randomized clinical trial of the Leboyer approach to childbirth, New Engl. J. Med., 302 (1980) 655–660.
24 Nettelbladt, P., Fagerstrom, C.-F. and Uddenberg, N., The significance of reported childbirth pain, J. psychosom. Res., 20 (1976) 215–221.
25 Norr, K.L., Block, C.R., Charles, A., Meyering, S. and Meyers, E., Explaining pain and enjoyment in childbirth, J. Hlth Soc. Behav., 18 (1977) 260–275.
26 Reid, D.E. and Cohen, M.E., Evaluation of present day trends in obstetrics, J. Amer. med. Ass., 142 (1950) 615–622.

27 Roberts, J., Melasanos, L. and Mendez-Bauer, C., Maternal positions in labor: analysis in relation to comfort and efficiency, Birth Defects (Orig. Art. Ser.), 17 (1981) 97–128.

28 Shnider, S.M. and Levinson, G., Anesthesia for Obstetrics, Williams and Wilkins, Baltimore, MD, 1979.

29 Stanton, M.E., The myth of 'natural' childbirth, J. Nurs. Midwif., 24 (1979) 25–29.

30 Sternbach, R.A. (Ed.), The Psychology of Pain, Raven Press, New York, 1978.

31 Stevens, R.J. and Heide, F., Analgesic characteristics of prepared childbirth techniques: attention focussing and systematic relaxation, J. psychosom. Res., 21 (1977) 429–438.

32 Stewart, D.E., Psychiatric symptoms following attempted natural childbirth, Canad. med. Ass. J., 127 (1982) 713–716.

33 Stone, C.I., Demchik-Stone, D.A. and Horan, J.J., Coping with pain: a component analysis of Lamaze and cognitive-behavioral procedures, J. psychosom. Res., 21 (1977) 451–456.

34 Tahmoush, A.J., Causalgia: redefinition as a clinical pain syndrome, Pain, 10 (1981) 187–197.

35 Turk, D.C., Meichenbaum, D. and Genest, M., Pain and Behavioral Medicine: a Cognitive Behavioral Perspective, Guilford Press, New York, 1983.

36 Wallach, H., Psychological and Physiological Childbirth-Related Variables Affecting Pain of Labour, Unpublished Master's Thesis, Lakehead University, 1982.

115

Cesarean Sections

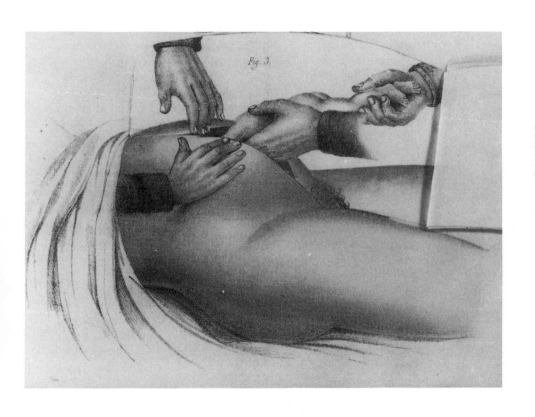

Fig. 3.

XXXVIII. *The* Cæsarean Operation *done with Success by a Midwife*; *by Mr.* DUNCAN STEWART, *Surgeon in* Dungannon *in the County of* Tyrone, Ireland.

THE Histories of the *Cæsarean Operation* being so few, I send you the following.

Alice O Neal, aged about 33 Years, Wife to a poor Farmer near *Charlemont*, and Mother of several Children, in *January* 1738-9 took
her

her Labour-pains; but could not be delivered of her Child by feveral Women who attempted it. She remained in this Condition twelve Days; the Child was judged to be dead after the third Day. *Mary Donally,* an illiterate Woman, but eminent among the common People for extracting dead Births, being then called, tried alfo to deliver her in the common Way: And her Attempts not fucceeding, performed the *Cæfarean Operation,* by cutting with a Razor firft the containing Parts of the *Abdomen,* and then the *Uterus* ; at the Aperture of which fhe took out the Child and *Secundines.* The upper Part of the Incifion was an Inch higher, and to a Side of the Navel, and was continued about fix Inches downwards in the Middle betwixt the right *Os Ilium* and the *Linea alba.* She held the Lips of the Wound together with her Hand, till one went a Mile and returned with Silk and the common Needles which Taylors ufe: With thefe fhe joined the Lips in the Manner of the Stitch employed ordinarily for the *Hare-lip,* and dreffed the Wound with Whites of Eggs, as fhe told me fome Days after, when led by Curiofity I vifited the poor Woman who had undergone the Operation. The Cure was completed with Salves of the Midwife's own compounding.

In about twenty feven Days, the Patient was able to walk a Mile on Foot, and came to me in a Farmer's Houfe, where fhe fhewed me the Wound covered with a Cicatrice ; but fhe complained of her Belly hanging outwards on the Right-fide, where I obferved a Tumor as large

VOL. V. H h as

as a Child's Head ; and she was distressed with the *Fluor albus*, for which I gave her some Medicines, and advised her to drink the Decoctions of the vulnerary Plants, and to support the Side of her Belly with a Bandage. The Patient has enjoyed very good Health ever since, manages her Family-affairs, and has frequently walked to Market in this Town, which is six Miles Distance from her own House.

Art. II.—*History of a successful case of Cæsarean Operation.*—
By John L. Richmond, M. D. of Newton, Ohio.

On the 22d of April 1827, I was called to visit a Miss E.
C. in labour; on my arrival at the house, I found she had been
in labour about 30 hours. Two midwives had been called,
but neither of them could give any account of the case, except that "she had fits and the pains did no good."

On examination, I found that the os externum, had suffered
no dilatation, and there was no fœtal tumour in the pelvis,
except when the pain was on, when there was a kind of
pressing down of the uterus and the contents of the pelvis.
The uterus presented a smooth tumour towards the superior
extremity of the vagina, which seemed only to be felt through
the anterior part of the vagina, and the anterior part appeared to form an acute angle with the posterior, immediately
in the hollow of the sacrum, and a little posterior to the tumour.

She lay, by spells, comparatively easy; when her pains
came on, they continued for a short space of time, nearly
regular or natural, but in twenty or thirty seconds were
transfered to the stomach, and immediately terminated in
general convulsions, which continued from three to five minutes, and were succeeded by alarming faintings, which lasted
from ten to twenty minutes. The system was much exhausted, the pulse depressed, and not the least advantage had
yet resulted from all she had suffered.

My first object was, to prevent the convulsions and to recruit the system; for which purpose I gave laudanum and
sulphuric ether, and applied flannel wet with hot spirits to
the feet. These measures produced considerable mitigation
of the convulsions, but the fainting increased. I had no recourse to cordials, for these could not be obtained. I was
seven miles from home, and had but few medicines with me.
I spent four hours in fruitless attempts, either to recruit my
patient or to ascertain the exact condition of the mother, or
the presentation of the child. The vagina seemed a kind of

123

sack, the extremity of which could easily be reached with the finger, but nothing like a uterus, could be felt, except a tumour above, which was felt through the vagina; under these circumstances, finding my patient fast sinking, I requested advice, which, however, could not be obtained, on account of high water in the Little Miami and the darkness of the night.

I informed the patient and her friends, of the only means by which I could conceive of relief; this was at once consented to as affording some hopes of life.

After doing all in my power for her preservation, and feeling myself entirely in the dark as to her situation, and finding that whatever was done, must be done soon, and feeling a deep and solemn sense of my responsibility, with only a case of common pocket instruments, about one o'clock at night, I commenced the CAESAREAN SECTION. Here I must take the liberty to digress from my subject, and relate the condition of the house, which was made of logs that were green, and put together not more than a week before. The crevices were not chinked, there was no chimney, nor chamber floor. The night was stormy and windy, insomuch, that the assitants had to hold blankets to keep the candles from being blown out. Under these circumstances it is hard to conceive of the state of my feelings, when I was convinced that the patient must die, or the operation be performed.

I commenced the operation, by making an incision through the integuments, down to the *linea alba* from the umbilicus, to within an inch and a half of the pubis. I then made a short incision through the tendon, about one third of the way from the lower extremity of the other, and introducing my finger, I found that the omentum was much in the way, as she was very fat. I introduced the blade of a crooked pair of scissors, and crowding the omentum up with my finger, cut first up and then down. During this part of the operation, the hæmorrhage was very trifling. I presume not exceeding four or five ounces.

As soon as the tension of the abdominal muscles was taken off, the convulsions subsided, and the patient became composed and tranquil. The uterus then presenting, I proceeded to divide it in the same manner as I had done the *linea alba.* I made the incision from as low down as I could, to near the fundus uteri; the incision passed immediately over the placenta. This incision produced considerable hæmorrhage, which however, soon partially subsided and I, then, divided the placenta, by making a small incision in it, and then lacerating it, which I thought would occasion less hemorrhage than to cut the whole of it. I then suffered all the blood to escape that I could, while the whole cavity of the abdomen was filled; and wiped away all I could, before trying to remove the child.

The child lay with the back presenting to the incision, the head resting on the superior strait of the pelvis; the uterus and placenta being thus divided, the contraction of the former were rapid, and the latter soon became entirely detached. As soon as the gush of blood partially subsided, I commenced my efforts to remove the child; but as it was uncommonly large, and the mother very fat, and having no assistance, I found this part of my operation more difficult than I had anticipated. My first endeavor was to raise the child sufficiently towards the stomach, to bring the head from under the pubis; but this I was unable to do, by any force which appeared to me safe to exert. I then made several vain attempts to raise the breech. After which I endeavored to pass my hand around the child, and get hold of the feet, but this the patient could not endure; and thinking the danger of the mother very great; and believing or supposing, that the child was dead from the detachment of the placenta; and considering, at all events, that a childless mother, was better than a motherless child, I determined to do all I could for the preservation of the mother. Accordingly I made a transverse incision across the back of the foetus, near the upper lumbar vertebræ, and the muscles of the back being divided, it formed an angle instead of a curve, by which means I was enabled, easily to extract it. The placenta, being entirely detached from the uterus, was at once removed, and the blood carefully wiped out of the uterus and all the surrounding parts properly cleansed.

I now determined to make, if possible, some discovery in relation to the *orificium uteri*. I accordingly passed my hand into the uterus; and, by examining carefully, I found an apperture which, to the touch, from within, did not seem to bear any resemblance to a natural orifice. I introduced the finger of the other hand, into the vagina and could not bring them into contact with each other—there seemed to be a kind of tube, leading from the uterus, to within about three fourths of an inch of the *meatus urinarius* into which I could not pass my finger at the upper extremity, to any distance, and not at all below. I then dressed the wound in the common manner, with sutures and adhesive straps, leaving about two inches of the lower extremity open.

She now lay perfectly easy and went to sleep. I kept her in one position for four days, keeping the bowels open with saline purges and injections. The lochial discharge commenced in about eight hours, and continued for five days: some discharge also occured from the open part of the incision. That part of the wound which was closed, adhered by the first intention. I suffered her to take no nourishment but weak gruel. On the seventh day, I closed the lower part of the wound; but finding, on the twelfth, that an accumulation had taken place in the cavity of the abdomen, I opened a small orifice from which a large quantity of black very offensive blood and water, was discharged. I then introduced a female catheter, and with a pint syringe, threw in three pints of warm water with a small quantity of soap in it, and drew it back with the syringe, after the manner of a stomach pump; this I repeated six successive days, when the water which was injected ceased to be coloured and the orifice was suffered to close. The patient never complained of pain during the whole course of the cure. She commenced work in twenty-four days from the operation, and in the fifth week walked a mile and back the same day.

One circumstance I cannot forbear relating. As I was syringing out the abdomen, as above mentioned, a neighboring woman, standing by my side, said to her what makes you laugh? to which she replied, because it feels so queer. I looked to her face and she was laughing.

I have made a recent examination of this patient, *per-vaginam*, and the condition of the vagina remains as above described, only it is now more shallow than it was when the uterus was raised into the abdomen; the whole depth of the vagina is now only two thirds of a fingers length, the orifice, or abnomral *os tincæ*, would not be discovered by the most minute examiner, who was not apprised of its situation. The anterior coat of the vagina now feels like a kind of septum, passing obliquely upward from before backward, leaving, I think, about one and a half inches between it and the forchet. I should think, if it were possible, that it is an unnaturally situated hymen. Here is as much room for others to theorize on the physiology of conception as for me. She has been married since and lived two years with a husband, during which time she tells me that she suffered great inconvenience on account of the shallowness of the vagina, but no conception has taken place. She suffers no inconvenience from the abdominal cicatrix, it being perfectly firm.

Newton, Hamilton county, Ohio, Feb. 1830.

———

Special Article

THE RÔLE OF FRONTIER AMERICA IN THE DEVELOPMENT OF CESAREAN SECTION

NICHOLSON J. EASTMAN, M.D., BALTIMORE, MD.

(From the Department of Obstetrics, the Johns Hopkins University and Hospital)

WITH the present year the so-called modern era of cesarean section concludes its first half-century; and were one asked in what respect obstetrics has advanced most conspicuously during these five decades, one might fittingly point to the revolutionary changes which have occurred in the indications, the technic, and the prognosis of the cesarean operation. Throughout the greater part of the nineteenth century, cesarean section was the most fatal of surgical procedures. In Great Britain and Ireland, the maternal mortality from the operation had mounted in 1865 to the appalling figure of 85 per cent. In Paris, during the ninety years ending in 1876, not a single successful cesarean section had been performed. The results in Germany, Austria, and Italy were so poor that the newly introduced operation of Porro, which included hysterectomy as well as removal of the child, was superceding the old and almost universally fatal cesarean section; the Porro procedure, it was claimed, saved more than half of the women subjected to it. As late as 1887, Harris noted that cesarean section was actually more successful when performed by the patient herself, or when the abdomen was ripped open by the horn of an infuriated bull. He collected nine such cases from the literature with five recoveries, and contrasted these with twelve cesarean sections performed in New York City during the same period, with only one recovery. In the face of such results, it is not surprising that many obstetricians of the nineteenth century doubted the wisdom of ever resorting to cesarean section, and predicted that the operation would shortly lapse into desuetude.

The turning point in the evolution of cesarean section was clear-cut and decisive. It was the appearance in 1882 of a monograph by Max Sänger, then a twenty-eight-year-old assistant of Credé in the University Clinic at Leipzig. The title of the work, ''Der Kaiserschnitt bei Uterusfibromen nebst vergleichender Methodik der Sectio Caesarea und der Porro-Operation,'' scarcely suggested its real purpose, which was to recommend in cesarean section the routine employment of carefully placed uterine sutures. ''The salient consideration in the proposed improvement of the classical cesarean section,'' he urges, ''is without doubt the treatment of the uterine wound''; and through two hundred pages he evolves, amplifies and substantiates this same theme. The history of the uterine suture, the advantage of the buried uterine suture, the best material for sutures—these were a few of the many aspects of the subject which received detailed attention. In particular, Sänger deprecated the growing tendency to abandon the old classical cesarean section in favor of the new Porro procedure, since he believed that careful coaptation of the uterine wound with sutures would obviate all difficulties and permanently establish the superiority of the older operation. Such views were new, for neither in Europe nor in England had uterine sutures been considered necessary. His opinions were at variance, moreover, with the dictates of the most experienced operators of the time—and, let us remind ourselves, Sänger's experience had been limited to but one successful case. His contentions, however, were supported by such carefully documented evidence, and his facts marshalled in such a logical and convincing manner, that the justice of his claims was apparent. Confirmation of his convictions followed quickly. Within a few years uterine suture was generally recognized as an indispensable part of cesarean section and forthwith the modern operation came into being.

The long neglect of so simple an expedient as uterine suture in cesarean section was not the result of oversight but was due to a deep-rooted belief that sutures in the uterus were superfluous as well as harmful. In 1770, Andre Levret, the foremost obstetrician of eighteenth century Paris, had taught that uterine sutures in cesarean section ''were not only prejudicial but were absolutely useless because of the prodigious contractions which the uterine muscle undergoes following delivery.'' This view that sutures would cut through the uterine muscle and thus defeat their

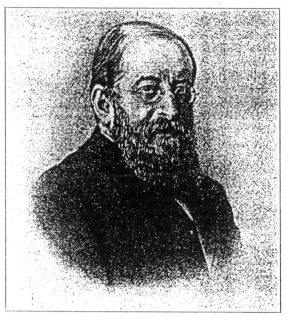

MAX SÄNGER
1853-1903

own end became widespread and was reflected a hundred years later in the unique work of the Italian surgeon, Silvestri, who sought to obviate this untoward result by employing elastic suture material. In 1874 he and his assistant, Veyer, reported two cases of cesarean section in which rubber bands were used for suturing the uterus. Another compelling argument against the use of uterine sutures was the copious suppuration which followed the suturing of abdominal wounds, a fact which naturally deterred surgeons from hazarding similar procedures in the uterus. In the main textbooks of the period, uterine suture was rarely mentioned, and, if so, but incidentally. Thus, Blundell, in his ''Principles and Practice of Obstetric Medicine,'' published in 1840, dismissed the subject with the remark that ''sutures to the uterus have not hitherto been in general employ.'' Similarly, Caseau, in his ''Traité théorique et practique de l'art des accouchements,'' which was enjoying wide popularity even as late as Sänger's time, commented briefly that ''the uterine wound needs no treatment other than to keep it clean.''

In other words, throughout the greater part of the nineteenth century, the uterine suture in cesarean section had been in general disrepute. It is true that, in a few isolated cases, it had been used both in Europe and in England, but these instances were not at all illustrative of Sänger's conception, for in them sutures had been employed usually to stop bleeding rather than to unite the wound; as Sänger points out, they were really ligatures. Thus, in the earliest recorded case of cesarean section in which uterine sutures were used, that of Lebas of Mouilleron, reported in 1769, three sutures were inserted, but avowedly for the sole purpose of controlling dangerous hemorrhage. Even this use of uterine suture, however, was so rare that Hasse, in 1856, could find in the literature only six cases in which uterine suture had been employed; and in general it seems clear that at the time Sänger's monograph appeared, neither Europe nor England had had any appreciable experience with this procedure. If, now, in conjunction with this fact, it is also recalled that Sänger's own experience with the uterine suture in cesarean section had been limited to one case, the question arises: whence came Sänger's idea? What were the sources of that carefully documented evidence in favor of the uterine suture? Who were his forerunners? The answer to this question Sänger, himself, states frankly and without reserve. As we have seen, his predecessors were certainly not his colleagues in the sophisticated medical centers of Europe, but were—oddly enough—certain pioneer surgeons working in the outposts of the American frontier. And, without wishing to detract in the slightest from the greater credit due to Sänger, it is the purpose of this article to recall the almost forgotten contributions of these Americans to cesarean section.

The rôle of nineteenth century America in the development of cesarean section was two-fold. It comprised, in the first place, the introduction and the perfection of the silver wire uterine suture, which, as Sänger later pointed out, constituted a turning point in the evolution of the operation; it consisted, secondly, in demonstrating the importance of that axiom of modern obstetrics, namely, cesarean section to be safe, must be done early in labor.

The conception and development of the silver wire suture in cesarean section was wholly an American achievement. In December, 1852, Frank E. Polin, a well known surgeon of Springfield, Kentucky, was consulted in the case of a certain Mary Brown, who had become exhausted from forty hours of labor, the dystocia being due apparently to a hydrocephalic child. Polin performed a cesarean section and closed the uterine incision with silver wire sutures; the patient survived, later bore two infants spontaneously, and was still in good health thirty years later. The details of the operation are scantily reported, and just what prompted Polin to employ sutures in the uterus, and particularly silver wire sutures, is not clear. It is significant, however, that in the January preceding Polin's operation, there appeared the celebrated paper of J. Marion Sims on the use of silver wire sutures in vesicovaginal fistula, and, although Sims did not mention the use of silver wire in cesarean section, it appears that his general idea bore fruit at the hands of the Kentucky surgeon. Polin did not record his case in the literature so that during the ensuing decade and a half, his experience was apparently forgotten. Between the years 1867 and 1880, however, uterine sutures were employed in sixteen cesarean operations in the United States, and in nine instances, at least, the material used was silver wire.

These early American surgeons were correct in believing that the silver wire suture offered them certain peculiar advantages in cesarean section. In the first place it did not require removal. As Sims himself had demonstrated in various abdominal operations, silver wire could be left in the tissues indefinitely as an innocuous buried suture with ''no inflammation, no suppuration, no cutting out of sutures, no gaping or retraction of flaps, and therefore no necessity for disturbing

TABLE I. TABLE SHOWING THE EARLY AMERICAN CASES OF CESAREAN SECTION IN WHICH UTERINE SUTURES WERE EMPLOYED
(Translated from Sänger)

CASE NO.	DATE	OPERATOR	AGE AND RACE	INDICATION FOR OPERATION	LENGTH OF LABOR, CONDITION OF PATIENT	KIND AND NUMBER OF SUTURES	OUTCOME MOTHER	CHILD
1	1852	Frank E. Polin	36 White	Hydrocephalus	40 hours. Exhausted	Silver wire sutures	Lived	Lived
2	1867	T. Beers-Townsend	16 Black	Contracted Pelvis	62 hours	3 Hemp sutures. Also 5 ligatures	Lived	Lived
3	1867	D'Aquin and Brickell	23 Creole	Stricture of Cervix and Vagina	10 days. Restless. Pulse 144	6 silver wire sutures	Lived	Died
4	1869	Sager	35 White	Contracted Pelvis (Dwarf)	9 hours. Sick. Has always used crutches	4 silver wire sutures	Died	Lived
5	1870	Pahul de Marmon & Rodenstein	40 White	Contracted Pelvis	44 hours. Exhausted	1 uterine suture	Died	Lived
6	1870	T. A. Foster	40 White	Eclampsia	2 weeks (?). Having convulsions	10 silk sutures	Died	Lived
7	1871	J. U. L. Quackenbush	30 White	Contracted Pelvis (Dwarf)	3 days. Exhausted	2 silver wire sutures	Died	Died
8	1872	E. C. Griffin	37 White	Fibromyomata	No definite pains but exhausted	1 silk suture	Died	Died
9	1874	T. Gaillard Thomas	30 White	Fibromyomata uteri	Few hours in labor. Attempts at version and craniotomy	Silver sutures	Died	Died
10	1875	Jones & Kline	35 White	Sacral exostosis (Dwarf)	38 hours. Exhausted	1 silk suture	Lived	Lived
11	1875	S. S. Lungren	29 White	Contracted Pelvis (Dwarf)	Few hours. Membranes intact	5 silver wire sutures	Lived	Lived
12	1876	O. B. Barber	17 White	Contracted Pelvis (Dwarf)	Early operation	3 silver wire sutures	Died	Lived
13	1877	E. W. Jenks	24 White	Contracted Pelvis Shoulder presentation	7 days. Exhausted	4 silver wire sutures	Lived	Died
14	1877	G. E. Walton	19 White	Contracted Pelvis	Long labor. Already sick; abscess in flank; cough; diarrhea. Attempt at forceps	1 silver wire suture	Died	Lived
15	1878	R. G. Curtin	20 Black	Contracted pelvis (Dwarf)	24 hours. Membranes intact	7 carbolized catgut sutures	Died	Lived
16	1880	S. S. Lungren	34 White	Patient same as in Case No. 11	Contracted pelvis. Previous cesarean section	3 silver wire sutures 9 horse-hair sutures	Lived	Lived
17	1880	M. Baker	34 White	Fibromyomata uteri	60 hours	4 silk sutures	Lived	Lived

the dressing till all is firmly united and permanently well.'' This Utopian picture of wound healing was in welcome contrast to the prolonged ordeal of suppuration and sloughing which in those days followed the use of silk, linen and hemp. Particularly in cesarean section, in those few early cases in which uterine sutures had been employed, the irritation and suppuration caused by nonmetallic sutures were so intense that the early removal of the stitches was thought imperative. To this end various expedients had to be devised. Sometimes the ends of the sutures were left long and were allowed to extrude from one end of the abdominal wound; more frequently the lower angle of the abdominal incision was intentionally left open so that the uterine sutures might later be inspected and fished out by sight; some authors even advised that the ends of the sutures be brought out through the vagina and subsequently withdrawn through that outlet. This difficulty in regaining the uterine sutures was, indeed, one of the chief obstacles to their general use. Furthermore, the prevalent practice of removing the uterine sutures on the third or fourth day postpartum prevented their serving any real purpose in effecting permanent coaptation of the uterine edges, and it is not surprising that subsequent autopsy studies on such cases revealed conditions identical with those in which no sutures at all had been employed. In patients who died before removal of the silk or linen sutures, it was commonly observed either that the stitches had cut through the tissues or that the knots had slipped, and in either event the sutures were found dangling loose in the suppurating wound. But all these difficulties, which had seemed so inseparably associated with the insertion of nonmetallic material into the uterus, promised to vanish with the advent of silver wire.

The pertinent facts concerning the seventeen American operations in which uterine sutures were used, are listed in the accompanying table. As is noted in the legend, the table is a translation of one occurring in Sänger's monograph. That Sänger saw fit to collect and tabulate these cases in such detail and that he gave them such prominence in his study, is clear enough evidence of the important rôle they played in the evolution of his hypothesis. It may also be noted that no more convincing proof of Sänger's wholehearted fairness and generosity could be desired than this enthusiastic tribute to his American predecessors. The maternal mortality among the sixteen cases in which the suture material was specified, was 50 per cent, a figure decidedly better than that reported in England for cesarean section and slightly lower than that recorded by the most experienced surgeons on the Continent. Most of these patients had been in labor for days; all of them had been subjected to repeated and lengthy vaginal examinations and in many instances, vain attempts had been made to deliver the women by forceps or craniotomy before the cesarean operation was undertaken. In view of the desperate condition of the patients, indeed, it seems doubtful whether classical cesarean section today would offer such a group a much better outlook. Sänger, however, was interested not so much in studying the gross mortality rate as in the correlation between the maternal outcome and the number and kind of uterine sutures which had been employed; and on the basis of the American statistics he was able to show that the prognosis in cesarean section improved in proportion to the number of uterine sutures used, particularly in those cases treated with silver wire.

It is true that in some of the earlier cases in the group, uterine sutures were employed primarily for hemostasis, but even in these cases, it soon became evident to the operators that the sutures also fostered better wound healing, prevented the escape of lochial fluids into the peritoneal cavity and decreased the likelihood of puerperal peritonitis. Thus, in the earliest of the American cases to be recorded, that reported by Brickell in 1869, the several advantages of the uterine suture are clearly set forth:

"A most important observation was that of the failure of the uterus to contract fully on its own cavity after the ovum was removed. Indeed, the organ had to be freely manipulated to make it contract even moderately. Not only did the blood continue to flow freely from the large wound inflicted, but one side of the flaccid organ absolutely fell in, and had to be lifted up to pass the sutures. . . . .

"The remedy for this hemorrhagic condition is, so far as I am aware, novel. With the exigency before us, there could not be a doubt in my mind as to the remedy, and it is seen that not only was the hemorrhage promptly arrested by close adaptation of the cut surfaces of the uterus but the collapsion of the organ was in this way relieved, and the wires have up to this moment proved wholly innocuous. I find in this part of the operation the most interesting point of all. I have long been of the opinion that in all probability the majority of deaths from cesarean section were the result of bleeding from the uterine walls into the cavity of the abdomen—the bleeding itself depressing the woman, and the effused blood lighting up peritonitis. Moreover, I have thought that concomitant with this bleeding was the gaping condition of the wound, the consequent absence of healing by first intention, and the strong invitation to metritis and septicemia. I have often resolved in my own mind to sew up the uterus in case I should be called on to operate, no matter how well it might contract at the time of operation; and on the ground that even the most vigorous uterus, after a normal delivery, is liable to expand and bleed, and in case of the section being made and our sewing up the abdomen over a womb we see to be well contracted, we cannot say that such secondary expansion will not occur; indeed, I contend that we have the right to expect the shock of operation to produce such expansion, and if the organ be not secured by sutures the result must ever be disastrous. I am satisfied that it may be theoretically and practically asserted true surgery to apply the metallic suture to the uterus in all such cases. The innocuous nature of the metallic suture is every day proved in surgery, and there can be no reason for apprehending the danger from its application in every case of cesarean section.''

To other American surgeons, the study of the uterine wound, when examined possibly years later at autopsy or at a subsequent operation, afforded further evidence of the value of the uterine suture. Thus, in 1880, S. S. Lungren, a Toledo surgeon, had occasion to perform a cesarean section on a patient who had undergone the same operation five years before. In commenting on the condition of the uterine scar, Lungren observed that ''contrary to expectations, no adhesions were found between the uterine and abdominal walls. The uterus was freely movable. . . . . The silver sutures were seen under the peritoneum as bright as when placed there five years previously.'' The theoretical advantages of the uterine suture were likewise clear to Lungren, as the following passage shows:

"′. . . . the sutures being introduced partly through the uterus, the peritoneal surfaces are retained in contact until union takes place, and all danger of escape of (lochial) fluids averted. This method of introducing the sutures is the more necessary, for as soon as the incision is made and the contents of the womb extracted, eversion of the lips of the wound takes place to a great degree, the external edges being bevelled off; and as soon as absorption commences below in the interior, the slit would be enlarged, affording ready exit to the fluids. To obviate such results was the aim in the introduction of sutures.''

Another zealous advocate of the uterine suture in cesarean section was Charles F. Rodenstein of Westchester, New York, who as early as 1870 stated that ''the application of uterine sutures after every cesarean section will probably diminish the rate of mortality attending that operation.'' His view was founded on an examination of the records of four hundred cesarean operations performed since the beginning of the nineteenth century. In studying the postmortem findings, he was particularly struck with the frequency of such statements as these: ''the uterus was found open''; ''the edges of the wound gaped''; and ''the uterine incision did not close.'' He reached the inevitable conclusion that the majority of fatalities following cesarean section resulted from the escape of blood and lochia into the peritoneal cavity; but, he advised, ''by closing the wound with sutures, the danger of such unfortunate occurrences may be prevented.''

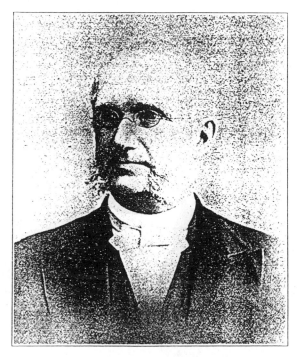

ROBERT P. HARRIS
1822-1899

The papers of Brickell, Rodenstein, Lungren and others, thus, leave little doubt as to the genuine enthusiasm with which many American surgeons pleaded for the use of the uterine suture in cesarean section. Some years before the appearance of Sänger's work, these men had appreciated the whole rationale of the uterine suture, had shown by their results its many practical advantages and had advocated its employment in every cesarean operation. Yet, it is questionable whether any of their individual reports, which were often brief and appeared for the most part in obscure medical journals, would ever have attracted European consideration if it had not been for the exhaustive studies of Robert P. Harris of Philadelphia, who must be regarded, at least so far as Europe was concerned, as the spokesman for the American surgeons. With unremitting energy he searched the whole country for every case of cesarean section which had been performed, tabulated the circumstances and details of each operation and between the years 1872 and 1881 published six lengthy statistical surveys covering the whole field of cesarean section in the United States. As Dr. Howard A. Kelly has noted, Harris was the most prominent obstetric statistician this country has ever known, his writings attracting attention both in Europe and in England. Indeed, one of his statistical studies on ectopic gestation involved him in an imbroglio with Lawson Tait, who called him a ''library surgeon.'' Other papers of Harris appeared in German and Italian medical periodicals. The influence which his writings on cesarean section exerted in European circles is amply attested by the fact that in Sänger's monograph his name appears more often than that of any other author, Zweifel, the leading German authority on cesarean section, not excepted. If it be granted then, that Sänger's acquaintance with cesarean section in the United States was derived from Harris' papers, what did the German author learn there concerning the American attitude toward the uterine suture? Did Harris recommend its routine employment? This question is important, since its answer explains Sänger's honest belief that he was the first to advise the routine use of this procedure. Harris did not advocate the insertion of uterine sutures in every cesarean section, but only in certain selected cases. In general, he was inclined to reserve his opinion, and as late as 1878 remarked that ''the experience of our country is as yet entirely too limited to determine whether the employment of the uterine suture is, or is not, an improvement in the method of operating. . . . . The fear has been that sutures in the uterus would greatly increase the danger of peritonitis; but the dangers to be encountered by using them are often not to be considered, in view of the greater risks in endeavoring to avoid their employment. In atony or hemorrhage at the time of the operation, there can be no question as to the better safety of the suture.'' It was thus, with faint praise, that the spokesman for the American surgeons reported his country's experience with the uterine suture in cesarean section.

But upon another important issue in cesarean section, Harris took a much firmer stand and was adamant in his insistence that cesarean section to be safe must be done early in labor. This one unifying theme runs throughout his writings; and whether he deals with ''cattle-horn cesarean section'' on the plains of the West or with the results of cesarean section in the hospitals of New York City, he invariably finds evidence in support of the ''timely operation.'' This teaching that cesarean section be performed early in labor has since proved to be the watchword to success in the operation, and as it was first announced clearly by American surgeons, it deserves recollection as one of the creditable contributions of this country to obstetrics.

It must be noted, however, that the advisability of early operation had already been suggested, at least, by Thomas Radford of Manchester, England. In 1865, this author analyzed all the recorded cases of cesarean section in Great Britain and Ireland and, after finding that the maternal mortality of the series was 85 per cent, advanced the opinion that better results might be obtained if the operation were performed earlier in labor as a procedure of choice rather than being delayed until it became one of necessity. He cites no figures to substantiate his opinion, however, and summarizes his views in the following two sentences: ''Notwithstanding all the preexisting dangers of cesarean cases, several recoveries have taken place. The favorable terminations ought to encourage us to hope, and indeed ought to inspire us with confidence, that if the operations were earlier performed, and on a different class of subjects, it would be attended with infinitely more success.'' Until the close of the nineteenth century in fact, it was still held that the most favorable time for performing cesarean section was at the end of the first stage of labor, an attitude prompted by the belief that the hemorrhage incident to incising the uterus would be minimized if the uterine muscle was in a very active state of contraction.

To perform cesarean section before the advent of labor was thought to be particularly dangerous and even after Bar of Paris, in 1888, had reported favorable results in cesarean operations done at this time, the practice was still regarded as hazardous. In view of this doctrine, the natural tendency to delay so dangerous an operation until it was clearly imperative met with general approval, and cesarean section remained an operation of last resort.

The first of Harris' papers attacking the evils of delay in cesarean section appeared in 1871, and from the beginning the author pleaded with compelling logic and vigor in behalf of the early operation. Some of the evidence upon which he based his contentions was unique. Thus, he called to mind, in the first place, that the first cesarean section to be performed upon a living woman was said to have been done in 1500 by a Swiss sow-gelder upon his wife, with happy results both for mother and child. The first authentic operation in the British Isles was one performed by a common midwife, Mary Dunally, upon a certain Alice O'Neal of Ireland, in 1739. The outcome was successful, although in the next thirty-seven cesarean sections performed by physicians in Great Britain between 1739 and 1845, only three women survived. The first recorded cesarean section in the United States was performed in 1822 by the patient herself, a fourteen-year-old quadroon servant, who made an ''L'' shaped incision through the abdominal wall and uterus while lying in a snow bank; she also recovered. Having noted these facts, Harris then extended his observations to more recent years and in studying the conditions in this country found that the mortality from the operation actually seemed to increase in direct proportion to the skill of the surgeon and the excellence of his equipment. For instance, the highest death rate was reported for New York City and State, where among twelve women subjected to cesarean section by surgeons and surgical accoucheurs of considerable eminence, but one mother survived. Some of the best results, on the other hand, came from the prairies of the West, where, as we have already noted, the outcome was often favorable even in cases in which the abdomen had been ripped open by the horn of a bull. Particularly gratifying were the figures reported from the plantations of Louisiana, where the mortality from the operation among the slave women was but twelve and one-half per cent, although in New Orleans three-quarters of the mothers subjected to cesarean section had died. Similarly, in the farm houses of Indiana, Ohio and Kentucky, the operation was frequently successful. From Mexico, Cuba, Jamaica, Martinique and Tortola, came reports of eight cases of cesarean section with seven maternal recoveries. Indeed, it seemed that the farther from civilization the operation was done, the greater the likelihood was of success. The truth of this paradox Harris emphasized even more strikingly by showing that in ''the open country'' of the United States, the maternal mortality from the operation was but 38 per cent, while in the towns and villages it was 65 per cent and rose still higher in the large cities. What could account for these inconsistencies? Were surgical skill and hospital care of no avail? Of course they were, answered Harris, but they could not offset the dangers caused by delaying the operation; and it was in the cities, Harris showed, that delay was most common, the delay which so often comes from multiplicity of counsel. In the open country, on the other hand, either by accident or by the boldness of ignorance, the operation was performed early in labor while the patients were still in good condition, and hence it was successful. Certainly, in the case of ''cattle-horn cesarean section,'' an accident that usually occurred before labor had even begun, such an interpretation was the only available one. Today, we might be inclined to supplement Harris' explanation with other factors, but in the main his tenets were sound; it was the countryside, the American frontier, which first demonstrated the safety of cesarean section.

Other types of cases were likewise grist for Harris' statistical mill and afforded additional evidence in favor of the "timely" operation. Thus, in cases of rupture of the uterus during labor, he found that abdominal delivery was a relatively safe procedure. One might think that this operation, performed after rupture of the uterus in order to remove the fetus and its secundines, would turn out to be a more severe and fatal operation than cesarean section, but such was not the case, and, as Harris pointed out, for two reasons. In the first place, where rupture of the uterus occurred, the necessity for a prompt operation was generally recognized both by the accoucheur and the surgeon; and secondly, the subjects of rupture were as a general rule in better condition than those who eventually subjected themselves to cesarean section. Still more convincing were the lessons which Harris drew from another class of patients; namely, those upon whom cesarean sections had been repeated. In such cases, the circumstances which had necessitated the previous operation usually made it clear that a natural labor would be impossible and accordingly cesarean section was decided upon at an early date and carried out either at the onset of labor or shortly after. Here, then, was a group of cases which exemplified *par excellence* the teachings which Harris had advanced, and, as he had predicted, the results were startling. Among nineteen operations performed on nine women, there were only three maternal deaths. By adding to these American statistics those of similar cases from other countries, it was shown by Lungren that a total of one hundred and nineteen operations had been done on forty-eight women with only eight maternal deaths, or in other words, with a maternal mortality of less than seven per cent, which in 1881 was an unheard of figure. So, by utilizing cases of various sorts from many sources, Harris, Lungren, and other American writers made it plain that cesarean section in this country was in general attended by a maternal mortality of about fifty per cent, but that when the operation was performed during the first twenty-four hours of labor, the mortality fell to twenty per cent, while in operations done at the onset of labor, as in repeated cesarean sections, it dropped to a level below ten per cent. It is not surprising, therefore, that Harris was such a fervent champion of the "timely" cesarean operation and that, somewhat before Sänger, he urged its superiority over the Porro procedure in the following words:

> "I do not feel that there is the same demand for a change in the United States, where the old operation has had so large a measure of success, especially when performed in a few hours after the commencement of labor. Let the cesarean operation be one of election and anticipation as the most successful Porro sections have been; let it be performed under carbolic spray; the abdominal cavity thoroughly cleansed from blood and amniotic fluid; the uterine wound, if need be, closed with silver wire; let a drainage tube be introduced, and the parts be dressed according to the methods of Keith and Lister; and we shall expect in this country to save more cases than has been done, in proportion, in any European hospital, under the Porro method."

However, in attempting to evaluate the accomplishments of these nineteenth century Americans, it is important not to lose historical perspective. After all, it was Sänger's study which dealt the final blow to the old cesarean methods. At a time when all of Europe was clamoring for the radical Porro procedure and England was turning to craniotomy, he proved to his colleagues on undeniable grounds the superiority of the conservative cesarean section; he not only advocated the routine use of aseptic uterine sutures, but showed in the minutest detail how to insert them; and by combining the scientific principles of wound coaptation with full Listerian technic, he created at one stroke the modern operation. But, to have furnished the supporting data for Sänger's hypothesis, to have devised and demonstrated the earliest successful type of uterine suture and to have shown for the first time the immeasurable value of the "timely" operation—these were certainly no mean achievements and may be recalled with pride as contributions of frontier America to cesarean section.

REFERENCES

Brickell: A Successful Case of Caesarean Section, New Orleans J. Med. **21:** 454-466, 1868. *Dibble:* A Successful Case of Caesarean Section, Med. Rec. **3:** 1-2, 1868. *Harris:* The Caesarean Operation in the United States, Am. Jour. Obst. **4:** 409-439, 622-663, 1872. *Harris:* The Operation of Gastro-Hysterotomy (True Caesarean Section), Viewed in the Light of American Experience and Success; With the History and Results of Sewing Up the Uterine Wound; and a Full Tabular Record of the Caesarean Operations Performed in the United States, Many of Them Not Hitherto Reported, Am. Jour. Med. Sc. **75:** 313-342, 1878. *Harris:* Lessons From a Study of the Caesarean Operation in the City and State of New York, and Their Bearing Upon the True Position of Gastroelytrotomy, Am. Jour. Obst. **12:** 82-91, 1879. *Harris:* Special Statistics of the Caesarean Operation in the United States, Showing the Successes and Failures in Each State, Am. Jour. Obst. **14:** 341-361, 1881. *Harris:* Does the Removal of a Foetus by Abdominal Section, After Rupture of the Uterus, Constitute a "Caesarean Section"? Am. Jour. Obst. **14:** 856-865, 1881. *Harris:* Cattle-Horn Lacerations of the Abdomen and Uterus in Pregnant Women, Am. Jour. Obst. **20:** 673-685, 1887. *Jenks:* Report of a Successful Case of Caesarean Section After Seven Days' Labor, With Some Comment Upon the Operation, Am. Jour. Obst. **10:** 606-612, 1877. *Kelly and Burrage:* American Medical Biographies, Baltimore, 1920. *Lungren:* A Case of Caesarean Section Twice Successfully Performed on the Same Patient, With Remarks on the Time, Indications, and Details of the Operation, Am. Jour. Obst. **14:** 78-94, 1881. *Radford:* Observations on the Caesarean Section and on Other Obstetric Operations, Manchester, 1865. *Rodenstein:* On the Introduction of Sutures Into the Uterus After Caesarean Section, Am. Jour. Obst. **3:** 577-582, 1871. *Sager:* Case of Delivery by Caesarean Section, Mich. Univ. Med. Jour. **2:** 385 393, 1871. *Sänger:* Der Kaiserschnitt bei Uterusfibromen nebst Vergleichender Methodik der Sectio Caesarea und der Porro-Operation, Leipzig, 1882. *Sims:* Silver Sutures in Surgery, New York, 1858. *Williams:* A Comparison Between the Caesarean Section and the High Forceps Operation, Am. Jour. Obst. **12:** 23-31, 1879. *Winckel:* Handbuch der Geburtshülfe, Munich, 1906, vol. 3, 669-810.

J. biosoc. Sci. (1980) 12, 353–362

BIRTHS BY CAESAREAN SECTION IN THE UNITED STATES OF AMERICA AND IN BRITAIN

COLIN FRANCOME* AND PETER J. HUNTINGFORD†

*Department of Social Science, Middlesex Polytechnic, The Burroughs, London
and † London Hospital Medical College, Turner Street, London

Summary. The rise in Caesarian section rates has been much greater in the United States than in Britain. This article analyses the reasons for these trends and finds they are not clearly related to good medical practice. It is concluded that it should be a cause for concern if rates rise above 6% of live births. In this case operations must be shown to be in the best interests of the mothers and their babies.

Introduction

The proportion of births by Caesarean section in the United States of America has almost tripled in 15 years. Data for New York State reflect the national situation. Whereas in 1963 only 4·3% of births were by Caesarean section (Burcmetta, 1974), the proportion had increased by 1972 to 6·9% and by 1977 to 14%. In 1978, 20 hospitals on Long Island, New York, on average carried out Caesarean section in 19·7% of the women delivered (Tarmey, 1979, personal communication). The use of Caesarean section has also increased in Britain, but in 1976 the rate was still only 6·5% (OPCS, 1979), which is less than half that for the United States. This article attempts to analyse the sociological and medical causes of this difference.

If the increase in Caesarean sections in the US is due to better medical practice, the result of more accurate diagnosis and better management of problems leading to healthier mothers and babies, then there would be a case for a comparable rise in the rate in Britain. However, if the US rise is due to other, non-medical, causes, a similar rise here would not necessarily be justified. It would not be the first time that operations have been carried out unnecessarily on a large scale and the error discovered only years later. One recalls the large increase in tonsillectomies which began in the late 1920s and persisted at a high rate for 30 years until an outbreak of poliomyelitis in the 1950s led to the postponement of many operations and eventually to the realization that, for the majority of children, the operation was not needed.

In this article it is argued that the increase in Caesarean section in the US and of obstetric intervention in general in Britain is due to non-medical factors, particularly the social structure of the medical profession and the nature of society

141

rather than to the medical needs of the individual woman, and that a serious attempt should be made to reduce the number of such interventions.

US experience

The overall increase in the Caesarean section rate in the US masks variations between hospitals and between different social groups. Table 1 shows that the Caesarean section rates of hospitals on Long Island in 1977 ranged from a low of 7·7% in Central Suffolk up to to 25·7% in Southampton. The rate has also increased: in 1971, in Nassau County Medical Center only 6·7% of births were by Caesarean section, but by 1977 the rate had increased two and a half times to 15·9%. The rate does not seem to be related to hospital size, so that there are small hospitals with both high and low rates. Neither does it seem to affect the perinatal and neonatal mortality rate. Nassau County Medical Center has the highest perinatal mortality rate but it also cares for a high proportion of socially deprived women. In the smallest hospitals there are few deaths in any one year and so the rate is likely to have a great annual fluctuation. The Syosset Hospital had only one death in 1977 to give the lowest neonatal mortality rate of 0·8 per 1000, whereas in 1976 there were ten neonatal deaths giving a rate of 7·6 per 1000. Larger hospitals with more births where the random fluctuations are likely to be smaller, still show differences in mortality that are not related to the rate of Caesarean section. The

Table 1. Caesarean section rates in hospitals on Long Island, New York, 1977

Hospital	% non-white women	No. of births	No. of Caesarean sections Primary*	Secondary†	No. of forceps deliveries	% by Caesarean section	Neonatal mortality/1000 live births
Central Suffolk	22·3	292	11	8	26	7·7	13·7
Glen Cove	6·8	673	120	48	175	24·9	1·5
Franklin General	4·2	784	50	39	365	11·4	8·9
Southampton	14·0	719	123	62	61	25·7	8·3
Brunswick General	26·1	827	91	38	219	15·6	9·7
Nassau County Medical Center	48·8	1417	153	72	337	15·9	32·5
Mid Island	1·1	1009	88	41	173	12·8	10·9
Syosset	6·8	1314	102	71	159	13·2	0·8
Smithtown General	6·0	1121	97	64	161	14·4	8·9
South Nassau	8·3	1442	91	62	508	10·6	11·8
Mercy	11·3	1589	152	103	542	16·0	7·6
Brookhaven Memorial	9·6	1672	104	93	166	11·8	8·4
St Johns Smithtown	1·4	1548	256	107	256	23·4	6·5
Nassau Mineola	10·7	1937	320	130	456	23·2	6·2
North Shore	8·1	3115	548	240	950	25·3	11·6
Southside	9·5	1904	197	119	561	16·6	7·4
Huntingdon	6·7	1909	205	144	211	18·3	4·7
St. Charles Good Samaritan	10·5	2344	217	117	402	14·2	5·5
St Charles	4·2	2237	243	150	306	17·6	7·2

* First Caesarean section.
† Repeat Caesarean section.

overall neonatal mortality rate for Long Island, 8·9 per 1000, was just 0·1 per 1000 lower than the average of New York State.

Underlying the wide variations in Caesarean section rates between hospitals are even greater differences between individual physicians. In Nassau Hospital, Mineola, one doctor had a personal Caesarean section rate of 9% for 1977, so others must have had rates greater than the average of 23% for the whole hospital.

In New York State the primary Caesarean section rate has been related to factors such as age, race, education and obstetric care (Zdeb, Therriault & Longrillo, in preparation). The Caesarean section rate for blacks and Puerto Ricans was 27% higher than it was for whites. There was little variation with age until 35 years, when it rose sharply, and in women over 40 years the Caesarean section rate was twice that for women aged 15–35 years. More educated women were likely to have a Caesarean section and this applied to both whites and non-whites. However, this effect seems to be age related. Highly educated women are more likely to postpone their childbearing, and when age is held constant the difference disappears.

Those women who had prenatal care from the first trimester were more likely to have a Caesarean section than those who started their prenatal care later or had none at all. Zdeb and his colleagues point out that this may be due to women at high risk seeking early treatment, but that this is unlikely to be the whole explanation. It is more probable that the hospitals encouraging early attendance have also adopted new techniques leading to a higher Caesarean section rate. Nulliparous women were three times as likely to have a primary Caesarean section as those who already had between one and three children. The rate rose again for the fifth child, although it remained well below the level for the nulliparous. In summary, this evidence shows that the woman on Long Island most likely to have a Caesarean section is highly educated and black having her first child after regular prenatal care from the beginning of pregnancy in Southampton Hospital.

British experience

In England and Wales (Table 2) there has been a steady decline in both maternal and perinatal mortality rates since 1963. Although there has been a rise overall in the amount of obstetric intervention from 1963 to 1976, it has been much less dramatic than in the US. The Caesarean section rate has increased from 3·1% in 1963 to 6·5% in 1976.

More detailed evidence comes from the records of one London teaching hospital serving a population of 160,000 including a large number of poor immigrants, with an above average rate of unemployment and below average living conditions. The Caesarean section rate rose from 6·9% in 1973 to 10·8% in 1978 with little perceptible effect on either the perinatal or neonatal mortality rates (Table 3), which are of the same order as those in the US and Long Island.

The obstetric department of the London Hospital comprises two units delivering approximately equal numbers of women at Whitechapel and Mile End. The obstetric unit at Whitechapel is associated with a neonatal intensive care unit for the North-East Thames Regional Health Authority, and the reception of women

Table 2. Birth statistics, England and Wales, 1963–77

Year	Births No.	Births Rate*	Mortality rates Maternal†	Mortality rates Perinatal‡	% assisted births§ Forceps	% assisted births§ Caesarean section
1963	869,044	18·4	22	29·3	6·1	3·1
1964	890,518	18·8	20	28·2	NA	3·4
1965	876,566	18·4	19	26·9	6·1	3·5
1966	863,066	18·0	20	26·3	NA	3·5
1967	844,692	17·5	16	25·4	7·5	3·9
1968	831,120	17·0	18	24·7	NA	4·0
1969	808,192	16·5	15	23·4	7·7	4·4
1970	794,831	16·1	14	23·5	7·8	4·9
1971	793,054	16·0	13	22·3	NA	5·2
1972	734,029	14·8	12	21·7	NA	5·3
1973	645,234	13·7	10	21·0	11·9	5·2
1974	609,894	13·0	10	20·4	NA	NA
1975	574,819	12·2	11	19·3	NA	NA
1976	555,722	11·9	12	17·7	NA	6·5
1977	542,040	11·6	12	16·9	NA	NA

* Births per 1000 of the population.
† Maternal deaths per 100,000 total births.
‡ Stillbirths after 28 weeks plus first week neonatal deaths per 1000 total births.
§ Estimated from 10% sample of hospital activity analysis (Source: Annual Reports of the Hospital In-Patient Enquiry. DHSS/OPCS, HM Stationery Office).
NA = not available.

Table 3. Number of births and associated perinatal mortality rates, 1973–78, at the London Hospital (Whitechapel and Mile End)

Year	No. of births	% by Caesarean section	Mortality rates Perinatal	Mortality rates Neonatal
1973	2209	6·9	23	10·1
1974	2220	7·7	20·7	9·5
1975	2116	7·0	17·9	7·1
1976	2227	7·5	20·2	9·5
1977	2262	10·7	16·8	9·3
1978	2387	10·8	20·9	9·3

at higher risk than average accounts to some extent for the higher perinatal mortality rates. From February 1975 to July 1976 one of the authors (PJH) was jointly responsible with two other colleagues for maternity care at Whitechapel, then, from August 1976, transferred his obstetric responsibility to Mile End. A comparison of the practice in the two hospitals (Table 4) shows that the Caesarean section rate has increased at both hospitals with little effect on the perinatal mortality rate. A similar pattern applies to the incidence of assisted vaginal delivery at the two hospitals. The most marked recent change has been the reduction in the induction of labour. When the results are analysed according to the attitude of the obstetricians towards operative delivery (Table 5), it is apparent that more conservative policies are not associated with higher perinatal mortality rates.

At Mile End the Caesarean section rate increased with maternal age until 35 years (Table 6). The high Caesarean section rate in women with one child is accounted for by those having repeat Caesarean sections for disproportion. The Caesarean section rates were little different in the various racial groups, whilst the

Table 4. Operative delivery rates at the London Hospital, 1973–78: Whitechapel (W) and Mile End (ME)

Year	No. of deliveries		Perinatal mortality rate		% labour induced		% by Caesarean section		% assisted delivery*	
	W	ME	W	ME	W	ME	W	ME	W	ME
1973	932	1277	29·7	17·9	49	26	9·0	5·5	14·8	11·6
1974	912	1308	23·4	18·2	40	40	10·1	5·2	17·3	11·6
1975	991	1118	19·8	16·0	35	30	9·0	5·2	14·6	11·4
1976	1048	1179	22·7	17·7	29	20	8·4	6·7	13·4	12·2
1977	1096	1166	17·0	16·0	29	16	11·9	9·7	13·6	11·0
1978	1193	1195	24·8	16·7	19	13	13·2	8·5	11·9	8·2

* Includes all operative vaginal deliveries.

Table 5. Perinatal mortality rates (PNM) at the London Hospital (Whitechapel and Mile End) 1975–78, by rates of operative intervention and attitudes of the obstetricians

Year	Type of obstetric management	Total deliveries		Labour induced			Caesarean sections			Operative vaginal deliveries		
		No.	PNM	No.	%	PNM	No.	%	PNM	No.	%	PNM
1975	Active	1249	19·2	442	35	15·8	95	8	10·5	167	13	65·8
	Conservative	884	15·4	244	28	12·2	55	6	54·5	101	11	29·7
1976	Active	1374	20·3	399	29	10·0	119	9	16·8	159	12	37·7
	Conservative	869	19·3	144	17	33·5	56	6	nil	108	12	46·3
1977	Active	1573	19·7	429	27	9·3	188	12	15·9	242	15	45·5
	Conservative	726	9·6	82	11	12·2	71	10	28·2	113	16	17·6
1978	Active	1596	21·9	312	20	22·4	187	12	42·7	179	11	55·9
	Conservative	839	16·6	75	9	53·3	76	9	52·6	94	11	42·5

---

358   *C. Francome and P. J. Huntingford*

perinatal mortality rates from 1976 to 1978 were 14·2 per 1000 for whites, 26·2 per 1000 for blacks and 13·3 per 1000 for those of Asian origin. The high rate amongst black women is accounted for by the fact that more of them were young, unsupported, nulliparous women, whereas all of the Asian women were married, supported and of higher parity.

Table 6. Caesarean sections at the London Hospital (White-chapel and Mile End), by age and parity in 1978, and by ethnic origin, 1976–78

	No. of births	Caesarian sections No.	%	Perinatal mortality/1000 births
Age of mother (1978)				
20 or under	288	14	4·9	
21–30	710	58	8·2	
31–35	135	22	16·3	
35+	74	8	10·8	
Parity (1978)				
0	303	24	7·9	
1	104	16	15·4	
2–4	737	58	7·9	
5+	63	4	6·3	
Race (1976–78)				
White	2473	178	7·2	14·2
Black	650	58	8·9	26·2
Asian	225	21	9·3	13·3

A comparison of these data from the US and Britain shows that in recent years in both countries obstetric practice has become more aggressive, particularly in respect of the use of Caesarean section in the US. Although perinatal mortality rates are declining there is no good evidence to suggest that this is the result of an increase in obstetric intervention, since equally good results are obtained in the US and Britain, and by conservative obstetricians, as by those who intervene more readily during labour and births.

Medical factors

Medical reasons used to justify the increase in births by Caesarean section

If the increase in the use of Caesarean section, and indeed any obstetric operation, is soundly based then the literature should contain the results of controlled studies showing the benefits of the increased rate for either the mother, the baby, or both (Chalmers & Richards, 1977). Hospitals with high rates should show improved maternal and perinatal mortality rates, and fewer babies with

146

breathing difficulties at birth, compared with those hospitals having lower Caesarean section rates for a similar population. As the increase in the use of Caesarean section has been less in Britain than the US there should be some evidence that the health of British mothers and their babies is inferior. There is no such evidence available (Baskett, 1978). It is usually assumed in the medical literature that improving maternal and perinatal mortality rates are the result of changes in obstetric practice. But, the hypothesis that the improvements are the results of socioeconomic progress is equally valid and better supported by the data that do exist (Baird, 1960; Huntingford, 1978, 1979).

The safety of Caesarean section for the mothers

There is no doubt that Caesarean section as a method of giving birth has become much safer. Antibiotics, improvements in anaesthesia and the increased skill of obstetricians who perform more operations have all combined to reduce the maternal death rate. Nevertheless, so far as maternal health is concerned the evidence is clear that Caesarean section is more dangerous than vaginal delivery (Caire, 1978). In three surveys carried out in the US in the past 5 years the average mortality rate associated with Caesarean section was 1 per 1000 operations. In the most recent of these studies (Evrard & Gold, 1977) based on 160,000 births the maternal mortality rate was 2·7 per 100,000 vaginal deliveries compared with 69·95 per 100,000 Caesarean sections. The comparative risks are precisely similar in Britain (Department of Health and Social Security, 1979). The death rate in England and Wales for Caesarean section between 1973 and 1975 was 0·8 per 1000 operations. The proportion of those deaths in which there was an avoidable factor was 60·5%, which was the highest since 1952. Some of the deaths from Caesarean section are of course the result of the complications that necessitated the operation rather than of the operation itself. However, there can be no doubt that resort to delivery by an excessive number of Caesarean sections will increase maternal mortality and morbidity.

The use of fetal monitors

A major development in recent years has been the introduction of controlled labour surveyed by electronic fetal monitors. Fetal monitors were welcomed with some reservations; appropriately used they should not lead to an increase in the Caesarean section rate, but inappropriately used they would (Jones, 1976). There were also fears that the monitors themselves might cause problems, such as adverse effects from prolonged exposure to ultrasound, and the trauma and infection caused by the attachment of electrodes to the babies' scalp. In 1978 the Food and Drug Administration Commissioner told a Senate Health Committee that research does not support the assertion of physicians and the manufacturers that monitoring devices are entirely without danger.

In a community hospital with 17,000 births and a Caesarean section rate of 8%, fetal monitors probably prevented 28 operations, whilst they provided the indication for Caesarean section in 26 women (Kelly & Kulkarni, 1973). Although the introduction of fetal monitors to one hospital in Britain at first led to an increase in the Caesarean section rate, it fell from 9·7% in 1973 to 5·8% in 1974, whilst the perinatal mortality rate fell from 15·8 to 11·7 per 1000 births (Edington, Sibanda & Beard, 1975). Beard (1978, personal communication) observed that the major effect of fetal monitors should not be to increase the Caesarean section rate, but to identify more clearly those women in whom it might be necessary. He believes that fetal heart rate monitoring is a relatively imprecise method of diagnosing fetal asphyxia, but it is a good screening system giving warning of danger.

The results from nine studies carried out under controlled conditions show that there need be only a small increase in the Caesarean section rate when fetal monitors are used (Hughey *et al.*, 1977). However, in practice, with indiscriminate and unthinking use, they do increase the rate, if only because of the difficulty in detection and interpreting technical artefacts. There is evidence that nearly three times as many women who are monitored electronically in labour in the US have Caesarean sections compared with those who are not (Stein, 1978). The number of fetal monitors in use in the US increased rapidly after a marketing company took over another one manufacturing them (Cole, 1978) and one wonders how many obstetricians attended courses on their use and the interpretation of the results.

Caesarean section and perinatal mortality

An increase in the use of Caesarean section is claimed to be to the benefit of the babies by reducing the incidence of brain damage and perinatal deaths. The claim that as the Caesarean section rate goes up so the perinatal mortality rate falls (Cole, 1978) has been used to justify an increase in the rate from 4–5% up to about 10%. However, the data presented here show that this is not true. Jones (1976) has also criticized this attitude, because of evidence that an increase in the Caesarean section rate above 8–9% leads to little, if any, further reduction in perinatal mortality and morbidity. Furthermore, it may be questioned whether even this increase in the Caesarean section rate improves the health of babies. During the time when the Caesarean section rate has been rising there has been a decline in the birth rate largely due to the reduction in the number of births to women at high risk (Hughey *et al.*, 1977). This, together with advances in neonatal care, could well account for the observed improvements in perinatal mortality and morbidity (Hibbard, 1976). Indeed in some places the Caesarean section rate has been reduced at the same time that the health of the babies born has improved (Edington *et al.*, 1975). Our data confirm this experience. Further, an increase in the Caesarean section rate may actually cause other problems, such as an increase in the number of infants surviving with congenital defects, and in those born prematurely and/or with breathing difficulties (Editorial, 1976). More subtle is the destructive influence that operative delivery has on the development of parental relationships with the newborn baby (Coleman, 1978).

The optimal Caesarean section rate

The optimal Caesarean section rate in the best interests of mothers and babies is difficult to determine and must vary to some extent with the characteristics of the population. Haddad & Lundy (1978) suggested a primary Caesarean section rate of 9–11%, the indications being fetal distress in 1–1·5%, all breech deliveries amounting to 3%, cephalo-pelvic disproportion and/or abnormalities in labour

3–5%, and a variety of other indications in 2%. This figure is high, especially as it does not include repeat operations, but it is now well below that for many hospitals in the US. It is questionable whether all breeches should be delivered by Caesarean section. The allowance for fetal distress almost certainly reflects the lack of precision in diagnosis rather than its true incidence. If time were not a constraint in labour rooms, the need for Caesarean section for abnormalities in labour could probably be reduced by half. It is also not necessary for Caesarean section to be repeated in those women in whom the indication for the primary operation does not persist (Merrill & Gibbs, 1978). We believe that the case has yet to be made on medical grounds for a Caesarean section rate much in excess of 6% of total deliveries. Rates in excess of this figure must be shown to be in the best interests of the mothers and their babies.

Conclusion

The rise in the number of babies born by Caesarean section in the US and following obstetric intervention in general in Britain does not seem to be based on accurate evidence that it is in the best interests of either the women or their babies. Innovations in medical technology are used indiscriminately without proper evaluation so that instead of increasing diagnostic accuracy they lead to more surgical intervention.

A relative lack of pressure against the increase of surgical intervention in birth does not mean that the individual woman given the choice would wish to have her baby in this way. The press, medical literature and advice given to women in prenatal classes encourage them to accept medical opinions without question, at a time when they are most vulnerable and carrying responsibility for the unborn child. It is an unusual woman who in the middle of labour can challenge medical advice, especially when it is apparently based on objective evidence and accurate electronic observations.

We believe that the increase in surgical intervention in labour can be accounted for by non-medical factors that protect the interests and authority of the medical profession over women. Women who have Caesarean sections are more likely to have problems in later pregnancies, and many restrict the number of children that they have as a consequence. Following Caesarean section women take a longer time to recover from childbirth, and some will die unnecessarily, often without benefit to the health of their babies. We believe that this is an intolerable and unacceptable situation that calls for public audit of medical practices in childbirth.

Finally, the increase in the number of Caesarean sections in women who are becoming increasingly healthy raises questions related to sexist issues, particularly as the majority of obstetricians are male (Ehrenreich & English, 1978). How much of the increase is due to a need for male obstetricians to retain control of a process in which they cannot otherwise participate so that they remain dominant will be argued. But, we consider that it is a hypothesis for serious consideration and not one that can be dismissed by paternalistic and authoritarian responses that allow no challenge.

Acknowledgments

We would like to thank the following who helped us in our analysis: Dr R. Weiss of Nassau County Medical Center, Dr D. J. Pennington of Nassau Hospital at Mineola, J. Cuneo of Nassau County Department of Health, J. J. Tarney and G. Therriault of the State of New York Department of Health, and Marlene Mascarenhas for typing assistance. Colin Francome would also like to thank the Social Science Research Council for their financial help.

References

BAIRD, D. (1960) The evolution of modern obstetrics. *Lancet*, ii, 557, 609.

BASKETT, T.F. (1978) Cesarean section: what is an acceptable rate? *Can. med. Ass. J.* **118**, 1019.

BUNKER, J. (1970) Surgical manpower: a comparison of operations and surgeons in the United States and in England and Wales. *New Engl. J. Med.* **283**, 135.

BUREMETTA, E. (1974) *Trends in Cesarean section 1963–1972*. Department of Health, State of New York.

CAIRE, J.B. (1978) Are current rates of Cesarean section justified? *South. med. J.* **71**, 571.

CHALMERS, I. & RICHARDS, M. (1977) Intervention and causal inference in obstetric practice. In: *Benefits and Hazards of the New Obstetrics*, p. 34, Edited by T. Chard and M. P. M. Richards. Clinics in Developmental Medicine No. 64. Spastics International/Heinemann Medical, London.

COLE, K.C. (1978) Cesarean sections. *Newsday*, 18 September, 8A–9A.

COLEMAN, W.S. (1978) Mother–newborn relationship following Cesarean section. *J. Pediat.* **92**, 163.

DEPARTMENT OF HEALTH AND SOCIAL SECURITY (1979) *Report on Confidential Enquiries into Maternal Deaths in England and Wales 1973–1975*. HM Stationery Office, London.

EDINGTON, P.T., SIBANDA, J. & BEARD, R.W. (1975) Influence on clinical practice of routine intrapartum fetal monitoring. *Br. med. J.* **3**, 341.

EDITORIAL (1976) Caesarean section and respiratory distress syndrome. *Br. med. J.* **1**, 978.

EHRENREICH, B. & ENGLISH, D. (1978) *For Her Own Good: 150 Years of the Experts' Advice to Women*. Pluto Press, London.

EVRARD, J.R. & GOLD, E.M. (1977) Cesarean section and maternal mortality in Rhode Island. *Obstet. Gynec. N.Y.* **50**, 594.

HADDAD, H. & LUNDY, L. (1978) Changing indications for Cesarean section. *Obstet. Gynec. N.Y.* **51**, 133.

HIBBARD, L.T. (1976) Changing trends in Cesarean section. *Am. J. Obstet. Gynec.* **125**, 798.

HUGHEY, M.J., LAPATA, R.E., MCELIN, T.W. & LUSSKY, R.L. (1977) The effect of fetal monitoring on the incidence of Cesarean section. *Obstet. Gynec. N.Y.* **49**, 513.

HUNTINGFORD, P.J. (1978) Obstetrics: past, present and future. In: *The Place of Birth*. Edited by S. Kitzinger and J. A. Davis. Oxford University Press, Oxford.

HUNTINGFORD, P.J. (1979) Obstetric practice—whose baby? *Update*, **18**, 1529.

JONES, O.H. (1976) Cesarean section in present day obstetrics. *Am. J. Obstet. Gynec.* **126**, 521.

KELLY, V.C. & KULKARNI, D. (1973) Experience with fetal monitoring in a community hospital *Obstet. Gynec. N.Y.* **41**, 818.

MERRILL, R.S. & GIBBS, C.E. (1978) Planned vaginal delivery following Cesarean section. *Obstet. Gynec. N.Y.* **52**, 50.

OFFICE OF POPULATION CENSUSES AND SURVEYS (1979) *Infant and Perinatal Mortality*. DH1 79/1. HM Stationery Office, London.

STEIN, J.J. (1978) *Making Medical Choices*, p. 103. Houghton-Mifflin, Boston.

Received 6th September 1979

Copyright ©1977 Birth and the Family Journal

Having a Section is Having a Baby

Murray W. Enkin, M.D., FRCS(C)

Cesarean section was not always having a baby. For that matter, it was not always having a mother, either. The operation has been done even before the time of the Romans, but got its name not from Julius Caesar, who was not born by cesarean section, but from the Latin *caedere*—"to cut." Gnaeus Pompeius decreed that the baby be removed from the mother by an abdominal incision after the mother had died, so that they could be buried separately.[1] The first recorded performance of a cesarean on a living woman took place in 1500, not by a doctor or a midwife, but by a sow gelder named Jacob Nuffer, who knew nothing about midwifery. When his wife could not give birth, and the midwives and surgeons gave her up for lost, he did the obvious thing. She lived to the age of 77, but we have no record of what happened to the baby.[1]

From the beginning of the 17th Century, the operation was tried several times as a last resort, but the results were not always as good as Nuffer's. In 1784 Aitken wrote, after a good description of the technique, "This formidable operation, intended to save mother and child, has been performed during many centuries with various success. In Britain, it has never fully had the desired effect, all the mothers having died."[2]

Murray W. Enkin *is an Associate Professor of Obstetrics and Gynecology at McMaster University Medical School, Hamilton, Ontario. He is a board member of I.C.E.A., and vice president of the North American Society of Psychosomatic Obstetrics and Gynecology. This paper was presented at the La Leche League International meeting in Toronto, Canada, on July 15, 1977.*

BIRTH AND THE FAMILY JOURNAL VOL. 4:3 FALL 1977

This may give a little background to the concepts we have about this operation, and the fears engendered by the very name today. And yet recently, we have seen an incredible change in the attitude of obstetricians to cesareans, to the extent that while as recently as 10 years ago, we obstetricians had the difficult job of explaining to our peers why a cesarean was done, today we have the even more difficult job, often, of explaining why a cesarean was not done. Depending on the hospital, from 10-15% or more of births are by cesarean today. Whether or not this is justified is another concern. The fact is that today, not only is having a section having a baby, but often, having a baby is having a section.

Technically, a cesarean birth is simple and safe. Modern anesthesia has improved to the point where anesthetic risks are virtually nil. The risks of hemorrhage have been reduced with improved surgical techniques and blood transfusion. The fears of infection have been counterbalanced by proper attention to asepsis, and to the antibiotics we have available. The classical operation, with its dangerous and weak incision into the upper segment of the uterus, has almost completely disappeared. It has been replaced with an incision into the lower uterine segment, which is strong and virtually without risk of rupturing in a subsequent pregnancy.

So we may properly ask "Why avoid a cesarean—if it is safe for mother and baby, painless, risk free, and avoids the hazards, mess and discomforts of labor?"

99

151

We could just as easily make this argument for the other end of pregnancy, and start them all with artificial insemination, which is safe, painless, risk-free, and avoids all the problems of an ill-timed, unplanned and unwanted pregnancy. It allows exact knowledge of fetal maturity. Above all, we can avoid the fuss and mess and uncontrolled behaviour of sexual intercourse. Somehow, I don't think it will sell. There are satisfactions at both ends of pregnancy, when done in the old fashioned way, and some people feel that they are important.

The decision to do a cesarean is one which the doctor can make. The decision to have a cesarean birth is one which the parents should make. Parents must be given the information to make an informed decision, including what the operation entails, the indications, the risks, the benefits, the short and long term effects, what effects it may have on the baby and on the parent-child bond, on lactation and breastfeeding, and on subsequent pregnancies. Beyond the decision as to whether or not to have a cesarean, parents have the right to decide, within the limits of medical safety, how the operation is to be performed— electively, or after labor starts, with the mother asleep or awake, what medications are to be used, whether or not her partner should be with her, what happens to the baby after the delivery, and other decisions. These are questions which every woman who may have a cesarean—which means all who are pregnant—should ask.

There are times when a cesarean is unquestionably advisable, and lifesaving for mother or child or both, including severe cephalopelvic disproportion, hemorrhage which is life threatening, and a central placenta previa. Most of the time, however, the indications for the operation are less definite, and depend largely on a judgement call. How long is prolonged labor? At what point should it be terminated by cesarean? How great is the risk of a breech birth to the baby? Is the change in the baby's heart rate on a fetal monitor a real distress which demands that the baby be delivered immediately, or is it just the response of the baby to

the normal stress of labor? There is no easy answer to these questions. Despite a great deal of research, there is a lot of opinion and little fact. Feelings are important, and the obstetrician's feelings have to be considered, too. The decision as to whether or not to have a cesarean should be a carefully shared one between parents and doctor, although the ultimate decision is with the parents.

For the surgeon a cesarean operation is usually a simple one. After the usual prep and catheterization, the patient is anesthetized. An incision is made into the abdominal cavity, cutting through the skin, fascia and peritoneum. The bladder is then separated from the lower segment of the uterus and pushed down out of the way, and an incision is made into the lower segment of the uterus. The baby is removed, handed to someone else to look after, and the incision in the uterus is sutured. The bladder is stitched back into place. The abdominal incision is closed, and the surgeon goes about his or her business. The mother is usually seen once a day for 6 or 7 days in the hospital, and for one postpartum visit.

For the mother, and for her partner, and perhaps for the baby, it is not quite so simple to undergo a cesarean birth. If the cesarean has been planned, she has had a long period of fear and apprehension awaiting the surgery. If it is a sudden decision, she often feels cheated, and even devastated. If she has had prepared childbirth classes, she has usually been prepared only for a normal birth. She has heard of cesareans, but she feels sure that they happen to someone else. Then a number of small, but uncomfortable procedures follow. She is shaved, even in those hospitals enlightened enough not to shave the pubic hair for a normal birth. She has an intravenous. She is catheterized. She then has an epidural anesthetic, or she has a general anesthetic. She is probably separated from her partner throughout all these unpleasant procedures.

While the surgeon is working, the mother is unconscious or ignored by the nurses and doctors who are too busy to bother with her. If she had a regional

100

anesthetic, she is often given a narcotic or major tranquilizer as soon as the baby is delivered. This makes her too sleepy to relate to the baby. It may not matter, because the baby is probably taken to a special care nursery for 24 hours or more of observation. The mother will recover from the anesthetic with a sore abdomen. She will move stiffly and with difficulty, and will have need of assistance in looking after herself and her baby for the first few days. She is left with a scarred belly, a scarred uterus, and often a scarred mind. She is faced with the prospect of a repeat cesarean in subsequent pregnancies, although this is a questionable matter at the present time.[3]

And yet, we know that a cesarean is sometimes necessary, and must be done. What can be done to take advantage of the benefits of a needed cesarean, and yet minimize the damage? I would like to make 10 suggestions, which have come from practices which work at McMaster University:

1. Every pregnant parent should be aware of what a cesarean is, the fact that she may have one, and know enough about the operation to help in the decision. If the reasons for doing a cesarean are valid, she will be able to keep her self-esteem despite the fact that she can not give birth in the usual manner. If the mother knows what procedures will occur, and how they feel, and why they are done, then she will be able to cope with them, whether they are preps, enema, catheter, and whatever else is necessary.

2. The mother and her partner should have a choice in the timing of birth. Tests for fetal maturity are used to confirm the physical examination finding and parent's dates. These tests include ultrasound scans of the fetal biparametal diameter and general size at about 20 weeks gestation and also amniocentesis: withdrawing amniotic fluid, which is examined for lecithin sphyngomyelin. With fetal maturity, lecithin increases. While these tests and measurements give a good idea of whether the baby is ready to be born, the baby often decides the question.[4] Also, there is good evidence that even a little labor is good for the baby.[5] It may be best under some circum-

stances to wait for labor to begin and then have a cesarean.

3. The woman should have a choice of anesthesia. Some may prefer to be unconscious, while others prefer to be awake. There are advantages to each. Sometimes medical factors dictate which is best, but most often, the decision is not a medical one on the part of the doctor, but one of habit or convenience.

4. The mother should have the right to have her partner with her at this important time in her life. It is true that a cesarean is a surgical procedure, and rigid aseptic technique in the operating room is required. But there is no reason why any intelligent man cannot be shown how to put on proper operating room attire, wear a cap and mask, and keep away from the sterile field.

5. The feelings of the baby should be considered. Obviously there must be enough light for the surgeon to see, and for the baby to be examined. But there is no reason for the whole room to be brightly lit, or for there to be loud noises to disturb the baby. Also, there is no reason for the cord to be clamped until physiological adjustments have occurred, and the baby's breathing is regular. Finally, there is no reason why the baby cannot be cuddled by the father, unless the child needs medical attention.

6. The father's feelings should be considered as well. Parent-child bonding is as important to fathers as it is to mothers. The opportunity to hold and fondle and care for his new baby is his right and his responsibility. There is a beautiful term for the relation of a father to his new baby—engrossment—to make larger. Fathers who have early contact with their babies show an enthusiastic and intense involvement. They become aware early of the individuality of their infant and they experience elation and an increased sense of self-esteem.[6] This experience should not be denied the father, whatever the method by which his baby arrives.

7. While it is important that mother and baby both be carefully observed after a cesarean birth, there is no reason why they sould not be observed together. A recovery room bed is big enough to hold

a mother and baby, and one nurse can watch over both. In this way the important first hour after birth is spent developing what many consider to be a lifelong, unique bond of love.

8. Just as soon as she feels able, the mother should be allowed to start rooming in, and the baby should be with her in the hospital room. There should be no rigid feeding schedules, supplemental feedings, or other unnecessary intervention to interfere with normal and natural lactation.

9. Excessive narcotics, sedatives, analgesics, and other drugs which pass into the breast milk can be avoided. There are many ways besides drugs to make a woman comfortable after a cesarean. Adequate rest, hot water bottles, careful arrangement of position and pillows, reassurance and support, encouragement all help, and lessen reliance on drugs, which may be harmful to the baby.

10. Finally, after it is all over, the parents should have the opportunity for a full discussion with the doctor of why the cesarean was necessary, their feelings about it, and the prospects for future pregnancies. So often, this is left up in the air, and the repressed feelings and lack of understanding can cause untold fears, frustrations, uncertainties and anxieties.

Many hospitals are now incorporating many or all of these procedures. McMaster University Medical Centre has instituted these practices, with relative ease and to the increased satisfaction of parents and doctors.

REFERENCES

1. Graham, Harvey: *Eternal Eve* Doubleday, 1951.

2. Aitken, John: *Principles of Midwifery* Edinburgh, 1784.

3. Sloan, D.: Inconclusive conclusion. Am J. Obstet Gynecol 101:133, 1 May 1968.

5. Leggins, G.C. et al: Control of parturition in man. Biol Reprod 16:39, 1977.

6. Hibbard, L.T.: Changing trends in cesarean section. Am J Obstet Gynecol 125:798, 15 Jul 1976.

7. Greenberg, M. and Morris, N.: Engrossment: the newborn's impact upon the father. Am J Orthopsychiat 44:520, Jul 1976.

20th-Century Natural Childbirth

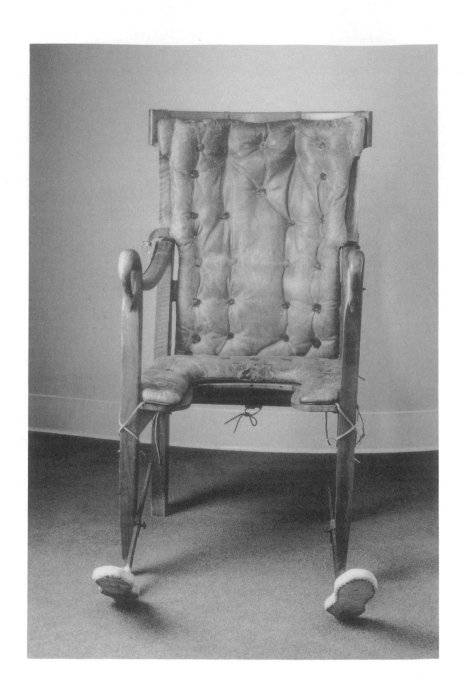

Is Natural Childbirth Natural?

ARTHUR J. MANDY, M.D.; THEODORE E. MANDY, M.D.; ROBERT FARKAS, M.D.;
and ERNEST SCHER, M.D.

FOR OVER one hundred years, since James Simpson first introduced anesthesia as an integral part of obstetrical practice, research has been directed toward making childbirth a more comfortable and happy event. Now the fashion in obstetrics is changing and a new philosophy threatens to undermine that progress. It is no longer considered smart talk at the bridge table to discuss twilight sleep or painless labor. The woman of the day is one who can vividly describe every last detail of her delivery, including the ecstasy of the unassisted expulsion of the placenta.

Doctors and patients alike are once more engaged in a debate over the following issues: Is pain in childbirth a culturally induced phenomenon? Must patients actively participate in the delivery? Are expectant mothers entitled to the benefits of modern analgesia and anesthesia? And is it psychologically damaging to either the mother or the child to be delivered in a state of unconsciousness?

For the past 3 years we have been engaged in a study of the natural childbirth program. During this period we have not only investigated the dynamics of the procedure in our own clinic, but we have also observed it in practically every community where the program has been in operation. Some of the conclusions we have reached from this study are

not entirely in keeping with those reported by the more enthusiastic advocates of natural childbirth, since, as we have stated elsewhere, the program may act not so much to develop a more mature expectant mother, as to encourage her dependence upon an important, authoritative figure supported by formal, complex, ritualistic routines (6).

This impression has been strengthened recently, as a result of a careful follow-up on 3 women, each of whom was successfully delivered by natural childbirth during the past year. The first patient attempted suicide with an overdose of barbiturates, 9 months after the delivery of her infant. She is now under active psychiatric treatment. The second, 7 months postpartum, is being threatened by her husband with divorce because of a serious conflict over the problem of frigidity for which she, too, is receiving psychotherapy. The third patient developed, shortly after childbirth, an intractable, widespread neurodermatitis which has been treated by several psychiatrists and at least four dermatologists, with only modest improvement. An interesting sidelight regarding this last patient came to our attention in conversation with Dr. Jacob Conn, her psychiatrist. While describing her to him as one of the most successful candidates we had ever conducted through natural childbirth (without an analgesia or anesthesia), he interrupted by stating, "That's interesting, because she has always been my best hypnotic subject."

Many interested individuals are disturbed today by what appears to be an organized confusion of thought on this subject. Even clinicians who have labored long to perfect a safe and effective agent for pain relief in labor are now asking themselves, "was it all in vain?" Ironically, the progressive obstetrician has believed, all this time, that he was

From the Obstetrical and Gynecological Psychosomatic Clinic, Sinai Hospital, Baltimore, Md.

Presented at the Annual Meeting of the American Psychosomatic Society, Atlantic City, New Jersey, April 28, 1951.

We are indebted to Dr. Alan F. Guttmacher for his interest and cooperation in the work of our psychosomatic clinic and to Mrs. Doris Morrow Dunlap for her able assistance in the preparation of this manuscript.

Received for publication April 26, 1951.

rendering a distinct service to the mother by sparing her the psychic trauma of a physically painful experience—one which has been repeatedly cited throughout medical literature as a precipitating mechanism for many of the functional gynecologic disorders. Instead he is now being accused of having denied the mother that vital experience necessary to provide for a healthy emotional relationship with her child. This is not an easy pill to swallow—nor is it a very convincing one, especially when thousands of women, awakening from their delivery have remarked, "This was wonderful—how soon can I have another baby?" In fact, it is no secret that some of the largest obstetrical practices in America have been built upon the obstetrician's reputation for "knocking his patients out cold."

It would be pointless in this paper to debate the relative merits of natural childbirth and the more orthodox procedures from the standpoint of the physical aspects of the delivery. Anesthesia at least permits unhurried, meticulous care at the delivery table, which no other technique can equal, and which not even the most ardent proponents of natural childbirth would deny. But thus far they have advanced no objective data in defense of their methods, nor are they likely to in the near future.

The principal benefits which have been claimed for natural childbirth are psychological. Grantly Dick Read has only recently written, "children who have been born according to the laws of nature will be evidence of its psychological value as they grow to maturity. It will be easy to recognize those who were born with instinctive maternal guidance in the first few moments of their lives" (1). If true, it would perhaps justify widespread extention of his methods, but this is a statement which few qualified psychiatrists feel prepared to support at the present time.

We should like at the very beginning to specifically emphasize one point. It is not our purpose to either condemn Grantly Dick Read or to denounce his doctrines. By so dramatically calling attention to the emotional needs of the expectant mother, Read has made a

lasting contribution to the practice of obstetrics. He is a physician of great dignity and personal charm, through which qualities he is capable of favorably influencing the course of his patients' pregnancies. His motives in developing the program of natural childbirth were unquestionably humanitarian. He is, moreover, a courageous pioneer with a missionary-like spirit. But his work, nevertheless, is not entirely free of criticism. In his enthusiasm for the project, Read has both exaggerated its applicability and confused its dynamics. He has, furthermore, permitted personal convictions to obscure the objectiveness of his observations, as a consequence of which it is often difficult to distinguish between fact and fantasy in his writings.

In order to understand more fully the genesis and meaning of Read's work, one must remember that his program was originally patterned for the needs of his own locale. Only later was it translated into concepts which have been modified for application to other parts of the world. During the past quarter century obstetrics in England has been vastly different from that which we have known in this country. Whereas in America, research in obstetrical anesthesia and analgesia had achieved a high degree of pain relief without appreciably increasing the risk to mother or child, no comparable progress was witnessed in England.

Last year the editors of the *British Medical Journal* published some very revealing statistics regarding current analgesic practices in England (1). No more than 5 per cent of all mothers confined at home were given any pain relief in labor. And while 48 per cent of mothers confined in the hospital were offered relief of pain, a large proportion of them considered it altogether inadequate relief. The majority of all deliveries were at that time being conducted by midwives and probably still are. When pain-relieving drugs were employed, they consisted chiefly of chloral, potassium bromide, tincture of opium, morphine, chloroform, and ether. In safe dosage, most of these drugs were unsatisfactory; in effective doses they were not without danger. Under the existing conditions it is quite understandable why Read should have felt compelled to make dramatic changes, and anyone who has observed his great personal charm can readily understand why the technique he chose was for him the most appropriate. That Read has been able to effectively utilize these qualities of his personality to enhance the conduct of his patients' labors has never for a moment been doubted.

Read's basic concept, that fear of childbirth increases the patient's tension state and thereby produces pain in labor, is sufficiently broad for general acceptance. There is little doubt that anxiety and fear of the unknown can magnify discomfort into alarming proportions, by both distorting perception of pain and by increasing the intensity of pain through disturbed uterine physiology. But this does not imply that labor is ordinarily altogether free of discomfort. His statement that "pain is an emotional anomaly" (12) is based upon anthropologic data of debatable validity (13). To be sure, certain investigators have reported that women in primitive tribes appear to have painless labor, but there have been no reports which describe how these observations were evaluated. Simply because a woman fails to scream aloud during childbirth, we cannot interpret it as evidence that she has endured no discomfort. We know that, in a large measure, cultural patterns determine the outward response of a patient to painful stimuli.

Although no completely satisfactory method of measuring visceral pain has yet been devised, the dolorimeter of Javert and Hardy offers a fairly objective approach to the study. In a careful report on the measurement of pain intensity in labor they recently had this to say, "The regimen known as natural childbirth has little if any effect on the pain intensity in labor. However, it does produce a satisfactory reaction pattern in the patient comparable to that obtained with moderate doses of heroin, morphine and demerol." But they also made the following statement, "most of the patients (delivered by natural childbirth) expressed themselves as having been deceived as to the amount and intensity of pain to expect in labor" (4).

Significantly, these investigators did observe a surprising degree of equanimity among patients prepared by natural childbirth indoctrination, despite the fact that many of these women interpreted the pain of labor at 10½ dols, which is the peak level of pain perception. Because of similar observations, Galloway has described natural childbirth as "Pain Without Fear" (2). It is interesting, nevertheless, to speculate upon how preparation for natural childbirth accomplishes this psychological lobotomy.

Read's program of natural childbirth has been developed around four major issues— diet, education, exercise, and relaxation (9). The first three phases can be dismissed with just a few words of comment. As far as we can determine, diet plays a negligible role upon the course of labor except perhaps under conditions of extreme deprivation. Education is of value only in the desensitization of some of the common taboos surrounding pregnancy and the childbirth process. Those who have attempted too intensive a program of education in anatomy and physiology are aware that such a procedure can arouse as much anxiety as it allays. The role of exercises is also a questionable one, since they are not only a nuisance to the patient, but they are impossible to evaluate objectively due to the difficulty in determining which patients have faithfully followed the prescribed routines and which have not. In Rodway's study of 340 exercise-participating patients and a similar group of controls, she was unable to demonstrate any advantage for the exercise group regarding the length of labor, pain in labor, postpartum hemorrhage, or fetal morbidity (14). Perhaps the greatest practical benefit from all three steps is the increased personal attention extended to the patient, and her exposure to group participation and group competition.

Relaxation techniques, on the other hand, form the cornerstone of every natural childbirth program. From the patient's proficiency in this single phase of the indoctrination, one can predict with a reasonable degree of accuracy how successfully she will complete her labor. Fearing that the stigma of hypnosis would discredit his program, Read unfortunately has gone to almost absurd lengths to distinguish relaxation from hypnotic techniques. Let us review for a moment his own description of patients who have been successfully indoctrinated. He writes, "Those who have learned relaxation not infrequently lay as if in a trance throughout the first stage, and throughout the second stage their receptivity to stimuli was lowered to such an extent that many were unconscious of incidents that occurred and words that were spoken during that time" (10). We submit, from this description, that the state of relaxation in these women is indistinguishable from a hypnotic trance.

In the labor room we have frequently demonstrated that anesthesia can be induced through the use of nothing more than the simple relaxation techniques which Read describes. In fact, by employing the very same approach, Dr. Theodore Mandy performed a classical cesarean section last year on a severely toxemic patient in whom practically all anesthesia was contraindicated. Prior to making the initial incision, the skin alone was infiltrated with procaine, and this was done to avoid further shocking of the patient in the event that the procedure was inadequate to the patient's needs. The technique was, however, eminently successful.

That relaxation and hypnosis are interrelated phenomena is further supported by Pascal, who drew the following conclusion from his investigations. "Simple relaxation seems to be sufficiently far along on the hypnotic continuum to facilitate recall and to increase the suggestibility of the patient" (8). We have been informed, furthermore, by Rosen, that Abramson and others who have had a wide experience with hypnotic techniques in obstetrical practice, are convinced of the relationship which exists between hypnosis and the relaxation techniques employed in the natural childbirth programs (15).

Anyone familiar with the induction of a light hypnotic trance state knows that the program of training is almost identical with that employed for relaxation. In both, the patient must have not only a need for, but also an abiding faith in the program, the therapist, or in the particular institution which she has selected. Moreover, from available statistics on natural childbirth, it is obvious that the number of patients who can be delivered without the aid of analgesic drugs, is not significantly different from the relative hypnotizability of the public at large. By supplementing natural childbirth with barbiturates, demerol, or other analgesic agents, the program can be adapted to a much larger segment of the obstetrical population. But it is also true that through the use of the same drugs a larger number of patients can be hypnotized than is otherwise possible.

In this light a new sense of understanding is given to the meaning of Read's work, for as soon as we can appreciate the medical application of hypnotic techniques, scientific reason will replace the speculations and hypotheses which have contributed to only further veil the program in an atmosphere of mystery. Unfortunately, hypnosis has been almost exclusively identified, in the public mind, with the somnambulistic states induced in especially suitable candidates for stage demonstrations. Wolberg and others have shown, however, that depending upon its depth, the range of hypnosis may extend from simple increase suggestibility and relaxation to total body anesthesia and amnesia (16).

Thus we are in a better position to evaluate the merits of the respective portions of the natural childbirth program. As it is now being carried out in Thoms' Clinic at the Yale University Hospital, it fully utilizes every device to establish and maintain a good patient-doctor, and patient-hospital relationship. Maximum effort is exerted to spare the expectant mother from the customary traumatic experiences of labor, and orientation in this direction has penetrated every level of the hospital personnel from the senior house resident to the obstetrical floor maid. There is no harsh treatment or discipline to which either the patient or her husband are exposed. There are no frustrated or sadistic delivery room nursing supervisors. Not only have the attendants attitudes been revised, but their language as well. Patients are spoken to warmly and sympathetically, and terms such as "uterine contractions" have been substituted for "labor pains." They have made capital of group competitive spirit and one gets the feeling that the majority of patients are anxious to "get into the game."

In short, a genuine attempt has been made by Thoms to replace the negative conditioning in pregnancy with a positive one. Yet even under such an ideally controlled environment the program must be supplemented in a large number of patients by substantial amounts of analgesia and anesthesia. The total amount of drugs administered to any patient is determined by the individual's needs and is limited only by the restriction that she must be kept conscious during her labor.

One might reasonably ask why is it, if childbirth is a natural physiologic process, that more women do not complete their delivery without the assistance of pain-relieving drugs? There are two principal reasons. In the first place, childbirth is seldom naturally free of discomfort. And secondly, this discomfort is accentuated by unconscious emotional conflicts which are not easily accessible to the peripheral approach of the natural childbirth program, but which are, nevertheless, capable of inducing disturbed uterine physiology.

While every expectant mother would undoubtedly benefit from a wider application of anxiety-alleviating techniques, we must recognize that anxiety in pregnancy is not the result of a single emotion of fear of childbirth on an otherwise normal psyche. It is rather a reflection of the patient's entire personality in relation to that specific event. Long before the onset of labor, in fact even prior to the pregnancy, a woman's emotional behavior is decisively influenced by the level of her psychosexual maturity and is evidenced by the kind of relationships she has established with mother, father, siblings, husband and colleagues.

The patient may have numerous fears, unrelated to the actual childbirth, such as the fear of increased responsibility, loss of personal freedom and companionship, economic deprivation, and inadequate housing. Occasionally she may also be disturbed with anxiety that the fetus will disfigure or permanently damage her body. For any or all of these reasons she may be overwhelmed with hostility and guilt toward both her husband and offspring. But while such anxieties are almost uniformly present in the expectant mother, we have found, as did Klein and Potter (5), that they are rarely presented as a spontaneous complaint.

In a recent publication we described how an emotional conflict produced a problem of uterine inertia during labor and how, under narcoanalysis, it was uncovered and corrected (7). The patient revealed, in an emotional outburst after receiving the drug intravenously, that, prior to meeting her husband, she had been criminally aborted. To this event she had attributed, on the basis of guilt, the deformed child which was born subsequent to her marriage, and for the same reason she feared that another imperfect child would result from the current pregnancy. The patient was reassured during the same interview that her delivery would proceed uneventfully, following which she immediately fell into active labor and delivered a healthy infant in one hour and thirty-five minutes.

Goodrich, who has been one of the pioneer contributors to the American literature on natural childbirth, made the following comment to us regarding this case: (3) "I was very glad that you made the point about the natural childbirth preparation program not being effective in allaying the anxieties concerning other things than labor pains. I have felt for some time that the most such a program can hope to do is to attack the superficial and mostly conscious anxieties concerning pregnancy and labor themselves. I also have observed that patients who have deeper anxieties are often classified as 'failures' by their attendants, who seem to feel that the program has failed in some way with these patients."

Discussion

As in demand-schedule breast feeding and the rooming-in plan, the benefits claimed for natural childbirth are primarily psychologic. Our methods for evaluating such data are far from perfect at present and care must be exercised to minimize errors in observation and interpretation. To determine the real worth of the program will require many more years of careful study, but even now certain conclusions are valid.

In the first place, natural childbirth is not a panacea for the emotional problems which beset the expectant mother or her offspring. For those women to whom the increased personal attention and moral support are important, the program serves an extremely useful purpose. There are, on the other hand, many women, more seriously disturbed, for whom such a program is evidently inadequate.

Secondly, the benefits which result from the complex procedure of indoctrination are

soever. Hingson, in a research study of conduction anesthesia jointly carried out at the Johns Hopkins and the Sinai Hospitals, in collaboration with Drs. Eastman and Guttmacher, has demonstrated that under suitable conditions a patient may have all of the advantages of natural childbirth with none of its discomforts.

On the other hand, active participation can be carried to absurd lengths as is evident when Read speaks of the ecstasy of unassisted expulsion of the placenta. Carrying this just one step further, we can conceive of a new cult arising which would advocate that only the mother could be permitted to sever the umbilical cord. Certainly such a philosophy

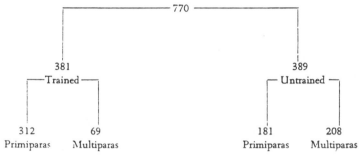

FIG. 1. Comparison of trained and untrained mothers during first seven months of 1950. Figures 1–3, from data of University College Hospital and Medical School, London, England.

not attributable to any specific portion of it. Instead, its success depends principally upon the value of the total program in developing a closer relationship between the patient and her doctor (or clinic). The faith of the patient in, and her need for, such a program regulate the degree to which the procedure can be applied, inasmuch as these factors influence the suggestibility and hypnotizability of the patient. For these reasons widespread application of the program is impossible without broad supplementation with analgesia and anesthesia.

Finally it remains to be proved what advantages accrue from active participation of the patient in childbirth. If it were really essential that the patient remain consciously alert during the delivery, this could be accomplished by caudal anesthesia with no discomfort what-

would not lack for proponents on the basis that this act is perhaps the most psychologically significant of all.

Since the completion of this manuscript we have had an opportunity to discuss the subject, during his visit to America this year, with C. W. C. Nixon, Professor of Obstetrics, University College Hospital and Medical School, London. Professor Nixon has been regarded as the best authority on natural childbirth in England since Read's departure, and for that reason we consider the unpublished statistics which he consented to leave with us very significant.

In a series of 770 cases collected during the first seven months of 1950, 381 patients were trained in natural childbirth, and 389 were untrained (Fig. 1). In Figs. 2 and 3 it will be observed that there was no significant dif-

PSYCHOSOMATIC MEDICINE

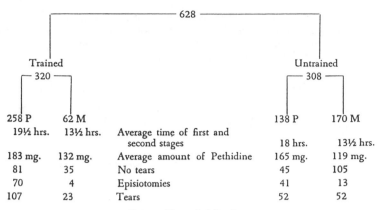

```
                                    ┌──────── 628 ────────┐
                                    │                     │

              Trained                            Untrained
           ┌─── 320 ───┐                       ┌─── 308 ───┐
           │           │                       │           │

        258 P        62 M                    138 P       170 M
        19½ hrs.    13½ hrs.    Average time of first and
                                    second stages          18 hrs.    13½ hrs.
        183 mg.     132 mg.     Average amount of Pethidine   165 mg.   119 mg.
         81          35         No tears                    45          105
         70           4         Episiotomies                41          13
        107          23         Tears                       52          52
```

FIG. 2. Normal deliveries.

```
  ┌─ Trained ─┐                                                    ┌─Untrained─┐
  │           │                                                    │           │

312 P        69 M                                               181 P       208 M
 11           1     Cesarian section                              8          18
 24           1     Forceps deliveries excluding twins or breech presentations   20    3
 14           6     Postpartum hemorrhage retained placenta      17           6
  9           0     Premature deliveries excluding twins and breech presen-
                       tations                                    6           9
 10           5     Others                                        9          10
```

FIG. 3. Complications.

ference in the length of labor, the amount of analgesia, or in the number of complications between the two groups studied by Nixon. Neither was there any significant difference observed in the attitude of the two groups of women regarding their childbirth experiences (Table 1). Indeed we were surprised to note that less than 50 per cent of either group had, at the end of six months, a pleasant recollection of the delivery. We are, at present, compiling our own data and although these statistics are not yet ready for publication, we can safely report that they will reveal a higher incidence of pleasant responses.

A word of caution must be introduced in regard to the methods of collection and interpretation of data concerning the patients' attitudes. One fact is certain. We cannot rely on the routine questionnaire for accurate evaluation of the program. While visiting one of

the clinics we had a unique experience in privately interviewing a patient who had just delivered and reported that she, too, was delighted with natural childbirth. Later, however, and only after learning that we were

TABLE 1. MOTHERS RECOLLECTION OF LABOR AFTER SIX MONTHS

Recollection	Trained (N = 396)		Untrained (N = 457)	
	No.	%	No.	%
Pleasant	180	45.5	168	36.8
Unpleasant	151	38.1	213	46.6
Other	65	16.4	76	16.6

from another city and not associated with the hospital in which she delivered, would the patient talk freely. She then told us that the delivery was more painful than she had anticipated or felt was necessary. The worst part was the tearing sensation just as the baby was being born, but she couldn't admit it to the house staff for fear of disappointing them.

Conclusions

1. Natural childbirth, as it is being interpreted and applied today, bears little resemblance to the procedure under which name it masquerades.

2. When adapted to the needs of the individual patient, however, it can serve as a useful obstetrical adjunct, but it cannot be expected to bring about, through regimentation, universally successful reforms.

3. With increased emotional support to the patient, the analgesic drug requirements can be reduced to levels of greater safety to the mother and infant; that is the principal advantage offered by the program. On the other hand, one can dispense with the complex preliminary routines and still accomplish the same end.

4. Perhaps the most objectionable feature of the program is in its emphasis that any *normal* woman can be delivered by natural childbirth. It is a condemnable act that attempts to stigmatize all those who fail to participate, especially when the benefits of full participation are far from established.

5. As an unfortunate consequence of the unbridled publicity currently attending these programs, potentially useful disciplines of therapy are in danger of being entirely discredited through gross exaggeration.

References

1. Editorial, *British Med. J.*, Feb. 26, 1949, p. 356.
2. GALLOWAY, C. E. *The Mother* 11:7, 1949.
3. GOODRICH, F. W., JR. Personal communication.
4. JAVERT, C. T., and HARDY, J. D. *Am. J. Obst. & Gynec.* 60:552, 1950.
5. KLEIN, H.; POTTER, H.; and DYK, R. *Anxiety in Pregnancy and Childbirth.* New York, Hoeber, 1950.
6. MANDY, A. J.; MANDY, T. E.; FARKAS, R.; and SCHER, E. *The Natural Childbirth Illusion,* in publication, *J. South. Med. A.*
7. MANDY, A. J.; MANDY, T. E.; FARKAS, R.; SCHER, E., and KAISER, I. *Am. J. Obst. & Gynec.* 60:605, 1950.
8. PASCAL, G. R. *J. Abnorm. & Soc. Psychol.* 42:226-242, 1947.
9. READ, G. D. *Childbirth Without Fear.* New York, Harper & Brothers, 1944, p. 82.
10. READ, G. D. *Childbirth Without Fear.* New York, Harper & Brothers, 1944, p. 115.
11. READ, G. D. *Brit. M. J.,* April 16, 1949.
12. READ, G. D. *Lancet* 1: April 30, 1949.
13. REID, D. E., and COHEN, M. E. *J.A.M.A.* 142:615, 1950.
14. RODWAY, H. E. *J. Obst. & Gynaec. Brit. Emp.* 54:77, 1947.
15. ROSEN, H. Personal communication.
16. WOLBERG, L. *Medical Hypnosis.* New York, Grune and Stratton, 1948.

The Western Journal of Surgery, Obstetrics and Gynecology

VOL. 62   DECEMBER, 1954   NO. 12

The Relief of Pain in Labour

GRANTLY DICK READ, M.A., M.D., CANTAB.

PETERSFIELD, HANTS, ENGLAND

THE PROBLEM OF PAIN

ABSTRACT

This contribution describes the procedures that avert severe pain in labour and relieve discomfort with the minimum of risk to both mind and body of mother and child.

The diagnosis of pain is discussed briefly and the cause of distress in normal labour. The syndrome of fear, tension and pain is explained and the psychosomatic processes by which it is established, and the manner in which its intensity disrupts normal physiological function alluded to.

The means of forestalling and breaking down the fear-tension-pain syndrome are commented upon. Fear and its profound influence upon childbirth and the neonate calls for logical indoctrination of confidence by education, which is one of the most important tenets of the author.

Antenatal education, the educators, and the labour ward staff are discussed as well as the obstetrician's role in pain-relief. The subject is reviewed at a high sociological level and the treatise is concluded by a synoptic summary.

Reproduction is the origin of a new life; the maternal invironment influences intrauterine growth, the manner of birth, and neonatal development. This may be observed throughout the whole realm of animal life, but never more clearly than in the human species.

The problem of pain in childbirth will not be solved by discussions upon drugs, analgesics and anaesthetics. The relative merits of different reagents and their mode of application has, for many years, occupied volumes of medical literature. The method of administration, the persons qualified or licensed to use the apparatus of election, and the organization of services for distribution and employment of pain-relieving measures, constitute a new dialectic branch of medical science.

These observations are not relevant to physical obstetric abnormalities, which occur probably in less than five per cent of all labours. These are pathological states which are painful and must be treated as such by the immediate employment of measures for relief. But 95 per cent, possibly even more, of all labours are normal in every way, except

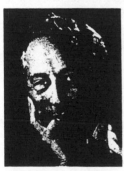

Born at Beccles, Suffolk, England, January 26, 1890. From boyhood was keen on natural history, entomology and zoology, and at an early age questioned why women had pain in childbirth while the animals seemed happy and proud to have their young. Educated at Bishop's Stortford College, and St. John's College, Cambridge. Honours Degree in Natural Science, and later Master of Arts and Doctor of Medicine from Cambridge University. In 1914, was called into service with the Army, landed at Gallipoli; in 1917, Medical Staff Officer, Indian Cavalry Corps, France, where first introduced to relaxation by Subahdar Major. Released from army to become demonstrator in Pathology, Cambridge University. Appointed Resident Accoucheur, London Hospital in 1920; continued research into the physiology of childbirth. In 1921, evolved theory of Natural Childbirth; book written in 1929, published in 1933, by Heinemann's, London. In 1935, contributed to Prof. F. J. Browne's textbook, Antenatal and Postnatal Care (Influence of the Emotions on Pregnancy and Parturition). Further publications followed. Invited to lecture in America in 1947, under the sponsorship of the Maternity Center Association of New York. Lectured in France, South Africa, Ireland and the Scottish, Welsh and English universities, 1947-1948. Practised in South Africa during the period, 1949-1953. By 1954, Natural Childbirth principles were accepted in all countries and the books have been translated in ten languages.

for the presence of unbearable pain. There is no physiological provision for this pain upon which its use or purpose can be sustained.

Certain aspects of the pain of labour and the rationale of its relief may have escaped the notice of those who have applied themselves only recently to the unravelling of its mysteries.

All essential physiological functions, whether concerned with maintenance or reproduction, when implemented within the normal mean are discharged without involving the protective mechanism of pain. This is equally true of breathing, eating, defaecation, micturation, copulation and parturition. These activities, necessary for the survival of the individual and the species, are pleasurable and become painful only when some disruption of the natural processes occurs. Pain arises from injury and initiates protective motor activity for the purpose of escape or mitigation, only when physiological integrity is subjected to assault.

THE DIAGNOSIS OF PAIN

The diagnosis of the cause of pain is one of the fundamental principles of clinical medicine and those who obliterate it before its origin is determined, as accurately as possible, may court disaster. This axiom is applicable to childbirth. For generations pain has been accepted as a normal manifestation of parturition—women have been told they must suffer because it is natural and unavoidable—and they have suffered. But the cause of their distress is not generally understood either by the attendants at labour or by the women themselves. Anaesthesia has been used as the easiest method of alleviating pain, the origin of which remains undiagnosed. With the possible exception of psychoanalytical procedures, this is the only example of empirical narcosis in general use.

Before legislation or organization to prevent or overcome the discomforts of labour is decided upon, the most frequent cause of dystocia should be examined.

PAIN AND FEAR

The human race has developed two protective faculties, both closely associated inasmuch as they are activated by motor responses to stimulus. They are *pain* and *fear*. As the mechanism of *pain* has been evolved in order to fortify reaction to injury, so the mechanism of *fear*, which is phylogenetic injury,

intensifies the alertness to the presence of danger and reinforces the powers of combat or escape. Similar neuromuscular and chemical changes occur in the presence of (pain) or the threat of (fear) injury, and if either condition persists in an intensified form, a state of shock supervenes involving exhaustion of nerve cells by depleting them of substances necessary for their efficiency. Thus shock may damage, beyond repair, the nervous mechanism of the higher centres of the brain. The integrity of interpretation of sensory impulses from the periphery may be disturbed permanently by pain and fear resulting in diminished or exaggerated motor responses. The mind does not escape trauma. The vivid memory of painful or terrifying labour is reinforced by fear of its recurrence and intensified by the conflicting desire for more children.

It has been said that over 60 per cent of women in institutions for treatment of psychopathies in the United States are suffering from the experience of, or the fear of childbirth. In mothers, whose reactions to mental and physical suffering are less severe, the conflict between mother-love and resentment has produced marked changes in behaviour, often at the expense of harmony in the family unit.

THE PHYSIOLOGY OF UTERINE PAIN

Since we are considering the relief of pain in childbirth, the neuromuscular mechanism of its origin must be explained.

There are sense organs in the body for recording painful stimuli, which were designated by Sherrington—"nociceptors." Their distribution is purposeful, for areas and parts exposed to primitive injury are more liberally supplied with nociceptors than parts of the body structurally protected from physical assault. Each of these sense organs has a specific function—some record touch, others temperature and others pressure, some laceration and others tissue tension, and so forth. The uterus is furnished with only two types of nociceptors and they are activated by laceration and excessive tension. Since there does not appear to be any necessity or provision for laceration of tissues within the uterus in normal birth, we are left with the conclusion that the pain of labour is almost entirely due to excessive tension. The *cause of pain*, therefore, is tension greater than that which is within the normal physiological mean, which will vary as the threshold of pain varies in the individual.

It has been shown that, under the influence of fear, the muscles supplied by the sympathetic nervous system contract. The only muscles in the uterus with this nerve supply are circular fibres mainly disposed in the lower uterine segment and sometimes the cervix. In a state of contraction they are inhibitory to the dilatation of the lower segment and the outlet of the uterus. Resistance to the efforts of the longitudinal muscles to dilate the cervix about the presenting part increases muscular tension. When two groups of muscles act simultaneously in opposition to each other, tension, pain and exhaustion result. This absence of neuromuscular harmony or polarity in uterine action produces painful sensations. When there is no fear stimulus, the circular fibres are relaxed and do not resist the expulsive effort, but with the earliest discomfort of increased tension a woman's apprehension is intensified and strengthens, through her protective neuromuscular mechanism, the contractions of the inhibitory muscle fibres.

Thus, *the pain of labour is due to tension caused by fear*. The pain intensifies the fear which in turn increases the tension by resistance. At length the vicious circle of these three evils destroys all confidence and self-control—then fear is magnified to terror; pain becomes the agony of torture; and tension, the Gargantuan grip of paralysing rigidity from which there is no escape. The almost maniacal screams and pitiful prayers to be freed from the torment of fear and pain portray the psychopathy of childbirth in its most hideous manifestations. At some time or other, in our obstetric careers, most of us have witnessed and been called upon to give immediate relief to women in this sorry state.

If this syndrome is established, it must be broken down as quickly as possible, for its ultimate development usually results in the necessity for instrumental interference with labour, a risk of serious shock and permanent injury to the mind of the mother. Effective anaesthesia must be administered without delay for, in such cases, unconsciousness is the lesser evil.

At first sight, this appears to be a satisfactory solution to the problem, but although inhalation anaesthesia induces unconsciousness, the influence of fear continues in that part of the brain which remains active beneath the consciousness. The processes of shock and brain cell exhaustion are not arrested by analgesics although pain sensations are obliterated.

FEAR IN CHILDBIRTH

Fear is, therefore, the great enemy of parturient women. It is largely responsible for the development of pain, and its harmful effects are not dissipated in unconsciousness induced by inhalant analgesics.

Women who have been numb or insensible during labour frequently describe dramatically the horrors of childbirth. Their memory is of distracting and unbearable suffering, but we know, from the depth of their narcosis, that they were unaware of pain sensations; only fear, imprinted in ghastly endogenous images upon the mind, was recalled with the return of consciousness and recounted as reality.

The pain of normal childbirth is almost negligible in the absence of fear. Relief from the discomforts of labour is found in the mind of the woman herself, not in the phials and philtres of the physician.

In this campaign against the suffering of women, fear, the arch enemy, must be allayed. As an adjuvant in this assault, introduce the art of controlled respiration, and relaxation to combat excessive tension. If, in spite of careful antenatal preparation, fear, tension and pain supervene, narcotics and analgesia should be available for immediate use, and must be employed to bring relief before the vicious circle of this syndrome is established.

1. *The first principle* of the relief of pain in childbirth is progressive education of the young. By this means only can the ignorance and fear of childbirth be forestalled and replaced by confidence and understanding.

In order to do this, changes must be brought about in the attitude of men, women and children alike toward childbirth. The most wonderful and satisfying of all human experiences should be placed in its correct perspective in the upbringing of children and in the education of young girls.

The laws of nature will be taught in schools; simple botany and biology for the juniors; elementary human physiology in the senior classes. A girl of 15 or 16 years of age is physiologically mature, and her mind is attuned to the reception of instruction in mother-craft and baby care. If it is important in this modern age to teach young women how to be self-supporting, it is, as a corollary,

167

far more important to instruct them in the science of marriage, reproduction and motherhood.

The fear of childbirth persists because adequate knowledge of the subject is systematically withheld from the young. Their information is often gleaned from the whisperings of those who have heard whisperings. With minds warped by misunderstandings and filled with apprehension born of ignorance, they marry and become pregnant. Then the full force of fear is brought to bear upon them by the ill-judged sympathy of friends and affectionate relatives who have suffered the same indignity of culture. This series of events, with minor variations, is remarkably constant. Young women are prepared for every calling in life except that which the majority of them will embark upon in the full joy and blindness of youth and love.

2. *Education of the Pregnant Woman.* Throughout the antenatal months, women must be instructed in matters concerning pregnancy and be made familiar with the changes within and about her.

In the third trimester, they learn of labour and by demonstrations from diagrams and in discussion are led to understand how to help, and how to avoid hindering, the uterus as parturition proceeds. They become aware of themselves as an integral part of the event and find fear-destroyed confidence in the knowledge that they can assist and protect the child during its birth.

This prenatal instruction is invaluable for the relief of pain; it is reinforced by advice upon personal hygiene and physical fitness. The control of respiration is practiced and its value during labour explained. Relaxation of the body as an adjuvant to overcome general muscular tension, and its use in pregnancy and labour is described and the methods of acquiring efficiency in the art are taught.

One of the most pleasing observations upon antenatal teaching is the ability of pregnant women of all social grades to understand and become interested in this subject. Rich, poor, illiterate and scholars react alike to the solution of the problems that have weighed heavily and fearfully upon their minds.

3. *The Education of those Giving Antenatal Instruction.* These people have a grave responsibility for, with much greater power than is realized, they wield a strong weapon in this fight against the pain of childbirth.

They must be enthusiasts with a balanced outlook, for the exaggeration of any branch of the teaching at the expense of an essential part, may easily prove disappointing in the test of labour. There are many who believe in the alleviation of fear and pain in childbirth, but whose pupils do not reach a high standard of success. This frequently occurs in antenatal schools where physical fitness is made the predominant feature. Exercises, relaxation and breathing are excellent accessories to pain relief, but the ambitious and sincere physiotherapist, however highly qualified, who has little knowledge of the phenomena of parturition and no practical experience of obstetric procedures, is too often disconcerted by the behaviour of her patients in labour.

It must not be overlooked that there are many women who, for some reason or other, have been unable to take part in physical exercises, yet they have studied books upon the natural processes of childbirth and have born their children with the utmost ease and the minimum of discomfort.

Those who conduct antenatal classes of instruction need to follow only one education curriculum to enable them to obtain maximum success—they need not be nurses, midwives, physiotherapists or doctors but they must have applied themselves to the study of antenatal education and preparation and all it entails. It is a highly specialized subject requiring a wide knowledge of many aspects of childbirth. The ideal teacher is one who has experienced a natural birth of her own offspring. She must be able to impart, with the aid of diagrams, the elementary anatomy and physiology of reproduction, and explain in simple words how the baby is nourished in the womb. An outline of the processes of birth is given and the reasons why patience is required during the long first stage and hard work in the second stage of labour. The exhortation to confidence and self-control, based on understanding of the changing phases of labour, has a salutory influence in avoiding self-inflicted discomfort.

The teacher must be familiar with the theory and practice of Natural or Physiological Childbirth so that each progressive step, throughout the psychological and physical education, may be clearly understood. To ask pregnant women to carry out a procedure and not be able to answer the question

168

"Why?" introduces an element of empirical suggestion which is not always acceptable to intelligent pupils.

The instructress, to be competent to discuss all branches of the subject, must have labour-ward experience. It is the only way in which she can appreciate the significance of her ex-positions and learn, by observation, the art of helping parturient women to implement the antenatal teaching they have received.

And now come our greatest problems.

4. *The Labour-Ward Staff.* Frequently the nurses in attendance upon women during the course of labour unwittingly disturb the par-turient and foil her efforts and good inten-tions. A firm but kindly sympathy must be sustained by an accurate knowledge of the mental as well as the physical phenomena of childbirth.The labour-ward sister must be a bulwark against the onslaughts of fear and a tower of strength in time of doubt, weakness or wavering self-control. Her attentions should be personal and her visits frequent. Assistant nurses should be instructed in the causes of alarm and studiously avoid them. No sensory system is so receptive as that of a woman in labour; a sharp voice or a careless movement may agitate a tranquil mind. The sight or clang of instruments will cause dis-tressing apprehension followed by painful contractions of the uterus. The sister in charge should use her position of responsibili-ty and authority to appease the frightened, not to admonish the weakling who has no courage to persist. The more alarmed the woman, so much the more companionship and help she requires, for her physical suffer-ing is commensurate with her fear. Such pa-tients should never be left alone "because they have hours of labour ahead of them," nor should they be told "to get on with it and not make a noise for they will receive attention when necessary." This attitude still exists in some maternity hospitals which are overcrowded and understaffed. The intensity of discomfort often varies with the skill and understanding of the labour-ward sister. Those who combine the virtue of imparting confidence with a kindly understanding of a woman's fears and feelings will prevent more pain than the ultra-efficient organiser who practices impersonally an academic rule of thumb.

5. *The Obstetrician's Role in Pain Relief.* Every day hundreds of labours are made painful because of the firmly rooted belief that drugs and anaesthetics are the only means by which a woman can be relieved of pain in childbirth.

There are two types of doctor: the one who understands the phenomena and psychoso-matic manifestations of parturition, and the one who does not. The former observes in each successive phase the significance of the *fear-tension-pain syndrome.* The latter believes that childbirth is a painful illness and should be treated as such. He sees no influence of the woman's mind upon her uterus and the sooner she is unconscious, the better for her—and the more quickly he can finish the labour. He may show little consideration for his patient's wishes, and even less for the ultimate well-being of her neonate. It is easier, possibly more profitable, to be brilliantly active in the pres-ence of an unconscious woman than it is to resist the urge to interfere whilst a conscious woman, confident in the presence and advice of the doctor, gives birth to her child with neither alarm nor discomfort.

Professionally and academically the teach-ers of obstetrics have it in their power to revolutionise childbirth. By sending out into the world doctors equipped with the knowl-edge of the mental as well as the physical phenomena of labour, they will change the approach of the obstetrician to the woman bearing a child. These men would be familiar with the psychosomatic manifestations—the harmony or discord between the mind and the body which are interdependent compon-ents of the mechanism of parturition. The fear of childbirth would be recognised as an unusual and pathological state within two or three generations and the suffering of women avoided without the necessity for applied medicinal relief, to the extent of incurring many of the disadvantages of its use.

Such obstetricians would approach preg-nancy and parturition in a new light. Attend-ance at labour may require time, concentra-tion and personal skill, but is it not a wom-an's right to expect such care? The doctor will no longer be called to "confinements" but to women who desire his understanding and his protection whilst they give birth to their children with conscious pride and dig-nity. It is an occasion when a little time is well spent in order to ensure the happy and comparatively painless outcome of parturi-tion which is incontrovertably more important and far reaching in its benefits than many hysterectomies. Childbirth is the greatest achievement and the most satisfying experience of a woman's life—it is the culmination of the most beautiful and delectable emotions. It is the ultimate accomplishment of the design of God or Nature, according to personal belief, for the procreation of the race. It is not only the arrival of a new being with all its potentialities, but also the making or marring of a woman's life as a mother, wife and influential member of society. This rich reward of perfection in the physical and spiritual purpose of human love has no biological justification for pain. The pathological labour is painful, and the mind fraught with excessive fear is pathological.

A SOCIAL RESPONSIBILITY

The relief from fear and pain of childbirth is not only a medical problem. It is a necessity for the survival of the cultural standards of the race, as surely as strength of arms is necessary for the survival of a nation.

The administration of this momentous task must be the responsibility of the rulers of the people, guided and instructed by those whose special calling endows them with the knowledge to advise. The obstetric physician of the new school will have the courage to protect women of our time from the well-intentioned but misguided orthodoxy of an obstetric era now ripe to be reformed. Relief from pain, and the fear of pain in childbirth is the most important service that can be rendered to humanity, and should take priority over other branches of medical science.

The medical obstetrician will not only be competent to meet all emergencies of childbirth, but will have specialised training in the psychology, neurology, biochemistry and endocrinology of pregnancy and parturition. The physiology and pathology of the reproductive function in all its aspects, will be the foundation of his clinical experience. His ambition will be to perfect motherhood, his responsibility, the birth of a new generation, uninjured by interference with the natural or physiological mechanism.

He will bring a vast fund of modern science to reinforce the humanitarian but half forgotten art of the great clinicians of the past. The significance of fear both in childbirth and disease was observed and recorded by the ancient physicians over two thousand years ago. In this there is nothing new, but the manner in which the mind influences childbirth has been demonstrated only in recent years. The *fear-tension-pain syndrome* has been proved by observers in many countries to hold the key to the relief from pain in labour.

One of the greatest barriers to the acceptance of a new concept in the science of healing is the conservative attitude of the teachers and senior members of the medical profession. This was understandable over 20 years ago when my first book Natural Childbirth* was published. Since then many teaching centres and maternity hospitals all over the world have applied this method and made observations with controls. They are unanimous in declaring that the removal of fear is the best approach to the relief from pain. It has become difficult to appreciate the adverse criticism of those who have made no effort to employ these procedures for the alleviating of discomfort in childbirth.

An even stronger argument in favour of natural methods is that the accurate implementation of the tenets of this teaching gives the practical clinical result which is claimed for it. This minimizes the importance of the academic and theoretical objections to the method raised by those who have no experience of its application. It is incomprehensible that doctors who are ostensibly concerned with the means of relieving human suffering should seek recognition by condemning procedures of proved value without subjecting them to trial.

In the early days this method of pain relief appeared at first sight to be so revolutionary that we could sympathise with those who were unwilling to believe, but today the truth of its contentions is emphasised in obstetric text books and journals. The subject is read and followed in practically every civilised nation, having been translated into the languages of the people. The publication of records from different countries and many maternity hospitals show a striking similarity; 90 to 95† per cent of normal births are conducted with the women in a state of full consciousness, so little distressed by discomfort

*Read, Grantly Dick: Natural Childbirth, William Heinenann, Ltd., London, 1933.

†In my recent travels through Africa, and The Belgian Congo, this figure was 95 to 98 per cent amongst over 200 tribes and sub-tribes from whom I obtained information about primitive childbirth.

that they refuse to accept the analgesia which is offered to them. With few exceptions, these women speak with enthusiasm of the achievement and wonder of childbirth, and many desire to repeat the experience not only because they want more children, but because it has brought them a happiness incomparably greater than any other moment of their lives.

SUMMARY AND CONCLUSIONS

1. The vicious circle of the *fear-tension-pain syndrome* is responsible for the pain of labour. In 90 to 95 per cent of cases, severe pain can be avoided or overcome by the elimination of fear and tension. This minimises but does not preclude the use of drugs and analgesics, but decreases the risks incurred by both mother and child in deep or prolonged narcosis.

2. The assets of fearless normal labour outweigh the liabilities of labour with fear and pain covered by analgesics.

3. The approach to and conduct of natural childbirth is no longer experimental or theoretical. Ample evidence, with and without controls, proves its claims to be understated rather than exaggerated.

4. Education* and antenatal instruction are

*Read, Grantly Dick: Childbirth Without Fear, Harper & Brothers, New York, 1944.

important factors in the relief of pain in childbirth.

5. Those who attend women in labour must be familiar with the emotional as well as the physical phenomena of parturition.

6. The quality of obstetrics and the care of mothers and newborn babies indicate the cultural standard of a community. This highly specialised and comprehensive subject concerns not only the present but the future of the human race. The fear of childbirth and its accompaniment of pain is one of the most insidious social evils of our time.

7. The fear and pain of childbirth is the province of the obstetric physician whose specialised education and intellectual bent facilitate the understanding of emotional states and sensory disturbances. To be successful he employs mental attributes different from those of the specialised gynaecological surgeon. The incompatibility of these two authoritative vocations makes unanimity difficult upon the subject of pain relief in labour.

8. The teachers of obstetrics have it in their power to revolutionise childbirth by introducing rational and harmless pain relieving measures. The physiology of the majority of childbearing women must receive attention at least equal to the pathology of the few.

Grantley Dick Read and Sheila Kitzinger: Towards a Woman-Centred Story of Childbirth?

TESS COSSLETT

The aim of this paper is to look back at part of the history of the natural childbirth movement in Britain, by concentrating on what I see as two key texts: Grantley Dick Read's *Natural Childbirth* (1933) and Sheila Kitzinger's *The Experience of Childbirth* (1962). The question I want to ask is what happens when a concept that was very male-centred in its original formulation,[1] is appropriated by a woman for a woman-centred approach. In looking at these two texts I am particularly interested in what might be called 'literary' concerns: the language they use, their point-of-view, their implied audience, and above all the *stories* they tell about birth, the way they dramatise and illustrate their ideas with anecdotes or ideal narratives about how 'primitive' women, or typical women, or 'trained' women give birth. I see all these 'literary' features as carrying important *ideological* implications about woman's role and woman's nature; for instance, the appeal to the example of the 'primitive woman' carries implications about women as 'natural' mothers, as of course does the very term *'natural'* childbirth.

The natural childbirth movement has been the main opponent of what has been called the 'medical model' of birth (Rothman, 1982: 23-4). The way in which male medical 'experts' have written about childbirth has been much analysed and attacked by feminists (Oakley, 1984; Martin, 1987; Rich, 1977; Rothman, 1982). The experts' mechanical language takes institutional shape in the rigid routines of hospitalised birth. But sometimes a simple opposition is assumed, between male experts and hospitals on the one hand, and women and the natural childbirth movement on the other (Martin, 1987: 139-165; Rothman, 1982; Arms, 1977). Such a model ignores the extent to which 'natural childbirth' is itself a cultural product, and in fact a male-authored one; it also ignores the way some women have seen the natural childbirth movement as potentially oppressive (Oakley, 1980: 2, 64; Rich, 1977: 173). Some writers have noted how the natural childbirth movement has been co-opted by the medical institution (Karmel, 1959: 129-40; Oakley, 1980: 36-7; Rich, 1977: 176; Wertz and Wertz, 1979: 192-5), but to understand its inherent contradictions, and

29

the ways it can serve both to liberate and oppress women, it is necessary to go back to the work of its founding 'father', Grantley Dick Read.

On first reading Dick Read, I was surprised by the *tone* of his book, and its implied reader. The modern birth books I had read were all clearly written for the information of a pregnant woman reader, even if she was not directly addressed (e.g. Bourne, 1975). Read's book, however, is addressed over her head to other medical experts. Not only is the language extremely technical, but Read tells jocular stories about the 'types' of women who consult him, as if to fellow practitioners who might come across similar specimens. In addition, his theory assigns a totally passive and dependent role to the woman patient, and an all-powerful one to the male obstetrician, who is thus the person to be convinced. Later, Read claimed that the book *was* addressed to and written for women, and signs of this change of heart appear in later editions. Failing in his attempt to gain recognition from the medical establishment, Read found his ideas being taken up by women who were perhaps already opposed to the standard forms of medical control of childbirth. Here he found a secondary source of support, on which he tried to build. But his theory has many problems for a woman-centred approach.

Read's theory of childbirth depends on a simplistic opposition of nature and culture, the primitive and the civilised, in which the natural and primitive is valued above the cultured and civilised. Women of 'primitive races', he alleges, give birth without intervention and without pain.[2] Using a pseudo-evolutionary model, he sees such women not as the product of *different* cultures, but as those 'whose natural development has not attained a state of civilisation', 'women without culture' (1933: 22). Pain in childbirth is only produced by fear, which is created by the false beliefs and practices of 'civilisation'. This idealisation of the 'natural' woman has some very questionable implications. Motherhood is seen as women's essential role, obscured by the distortions of civilisation. Thus 'among the primitive races a girl is brought up from the point of view of survival. Sexual life and the reproduction of her kind are the fulfilment of her highest ideals' (1933: 42). Attempting to revive this primitive attitude, Read starts his book with the premise that 'childbirth is the perfection of womanhood' (1933: ix). And yet Read's idealisation of motherhood has some very 'civilised' ends in view:

> A healthy and happy parturition ... is the making of a mother who will in every way be fitted to carry out the duties of motherhood, which is not only to bear children, but to be the corner-stone of the temple of Home, without which no home can produce a family of worthy citizens ...

30

Children born in pain, born of fear ... cannot ... be expected to produce a high level of national efficiency. (1933: 99)

Thus a particular ideology about women as domestic angels contributing to the strength of the nation-state is being promoted under the label 'nature'.

Read is only participating here in a prevailing ideology of his time: the campaign to produce a better imperial race by improving childbirth education and facilities (Lewis, 1980). Woman at home giving birth is analogous to man abroad fighting for his country, and at times Read deserts his 'primitive' imagery for a contrasting set of *military* images - civilised woman's extreme terror at childbirth is compared to the extreme terror Dick Read has witnessed and experienced in the First World War. The alleviation of this terror is like a military campaign:

The work of readjusting the minds of women occupied in the primitive functions of childbirth requires as much skill, precision and foresight on the part of those who are concerned with it as the counter-measures against bombs from aeroplanes, gas attacks, magnetic and acoustic mines, submarines and all the improvements of modern warfare demand from those whose business it is to understand these things. (1933: 51)

Interestingly, the intelligent military strategist becomes *not* the woman herself, but the male medical expert, 'whose business it is to understand such things'. This appropriation by the obstetrician of the active role in childbirth is essential to Read's approach.

We have seen that Read's 'natural' woman is a cultural construct, with anti-feminist implications. Who exactly are the 'primitive' women that Read lauds and wishes his patients to emulate? A central scene is one where Read watches a 'primitive' woman leaving her work to give birth painlessly in a thicket by herself. This 'primitive' woman, often identified as 'African', still regularly pops up, as an instantly recognisable stereotype, in ante-natal books and talks. Read, in his seminal account, puts in details that suggest the scene is taking place in Africa, or at least somewhere very remote, so that the woman can represent to his readers a genuinely primitive person: 'a *sub-tropical* sun was beating down: the temperature was nearing 100 ... I was known by the *natives* as "the doctor"'; the woman's contractions appeared much more violent than 'those of the *average European woman*' (1933: 40-1, my italics). All this suggests an incident taking

31

place in some far-distant tribe, but if we read Read's official biography we find out that the description is based on an incident in *Belgium*, behind the lines, during the First World War (Thomas, 1957: 56). The woman is a Belgian peasant, upon whom Read projects his stereotype of the primitive woman. He only went to Africa much later in his career. His main experiences of seemingly painless and fearless childbirths were among the working-class women of the East End of London, and he argues that the working classes are more 'primitive' in their mental development than the middle classes: 'The practice of repression is not found here - there is little "personality pride" and no suppression of instinctive urge in the face of social convention' (1933: 44).

So Read is concerned with a relatively small group of upper- and middle-class women, whom he wishes to save from the fears induced by their false cultivation, and to return to a state of natural motherhood. But while his accounts of the Belgian woman, and of his lower-class patients, seem to emphasise the women's independence and control over the process of birth, this is not what he seeks to restore to his middle-class patients. Paradoxically, it is only the highly-trained, male obstetrician who can counter the women's 'civilised' fears, and restore them to their 'natural' state. To do this, he makes use of another 'natural' quality of women, their essential 'dependency':

> In spite of the emancipation of woman, in spite of her having attained equality in many paths of life, in her normal state she is found subconsciously to look upon man as the protective sex of the genus. She appreciates his aggression and defence; she is activated almost entirely by motives of dependence upon man. Some psychologists go so far as to say that the seeds of resentment in women can sometimes be traced to the sense of something lacking in them that man possesses. (1933: 102)

The reactionary, anti-feminist, pseudo-Freudian basis of Read's project is here made quite clear.

This belief in female dependency is used to support a vision of the obstetrician as ideal male protector. Some very romantic language is used to create this picture: 'a knight, a valiant protector from all harm, on whose knowledge and power she can depend with unwavering faith' (1933: 65). Thus it is not surprising that Read addresses his book over the heads of his patients, to his fellow obstetricians, attempting to awaken them to their high calling. This is especially evident in Chapter III, in which he tells the stories of various 'types' of women

32

who have consulted him: 'from the earliest meeting with these patients who request that *we* should attend them at their confinements, it is necessary to create the atmosphere that can give confidence in *our* teaching and that can allow *us* the influence essential for the control of their emotions' (1933:26, my italics). 'Control' is an interesting word here - just as in the medical model the doctor tries to 'control' the woman's body, so here he tries to 'control' her emotions: 'natural' is a paradoxical word to use for this process. Read's subsequent descriptions of the different types of women, 'as they enter your consulting room' (1933: 27), also strive for control by categorisation, putting women into the old-fashioned categories of choleric, sanguine, phlegmatic and melancholic. He then proceeds to tell two exemplary stories, contrasting the choleric and the phlegmatic.

Having set up this sort of category, Read can describe the women's characters by means of their outward appearances - but a sexual appraisal is also going on, the male 'gaze' evaluating their femininity. Thus the choleric woman, who turns out to be a model patient, is described like this: 'A tall, fair girl, with large blue eyes, a thin, sensitive mouth, slightly tapering chin beneath her oval face, came into my consulting room. She was beautifully dressed in such a way that her excellent proportions were adequately demonstrated to the world' (1933: 29). By contrast, the phlegmatic woman, a hopeless patient, is described as sexually unattractive, 'Large, red and plainly dressed' (1933: 30). Sexual attractiveness equals true womanhood and results in natural childbirth, via dependence on men. This last point is made clear by the other major difference between the two women: in the first story, the only other character is a dashing, military husband; in the second, it is a dominant and fear-inspiring mother. The first woman responds with a kind of military courage when Read uses the words 'confidence' and 'guts' to her. After the birth, 'Six foot four of magnificent manhood pushed me out of the way. He had just returned from manoevres ... He had only one thought and one expression on his face - adoration' (1933. 31). This adoration is not interpreted as any tribute to his *wife's* courage - rather, it reveals to the doctor that this husband was responsible for his wife's success: 'I felt that I had succeeded, until her husband came in, and then I knew that the success was his' (1933: 31-2).

By contrast, the other woman's husband is not in evidence: 'I did not see her husband; he was something in the city' (1933: 31). He has left her to the baneful influence of her mother, who accompanies her to the consulting room: 'a large, severe lady with an aquiline nose and a firm mouth above an almost masculine chin brought her daughter in' (1933: 30). Notice again that her femininity is being impugned. A similar story is told later in the book, and again the mother's lack of

33

femininity is stressed: 'Her mother was a lady whose experience of life had somewhat destroyed her confidence in men, and not without reason. She herself was suffering from rather pronounced climacteric symptoms' (1933: 67). In both cases, the mothers fill the daughters with fears about the pains of childbirth, and by their presence prevent the male obstetrician from exercising his charismatic effect. In the first case, 'the influence of the physician was neither allowed nor expected' (1933: 31); in the second, the mother finally yields when 'I pointed out to her that so long as she was in the room I could do nothing' (1933: 68), and an easy birth ensues once she has left.

In these stories, the mother is clearly set up as the enemy of the male obstetrician, and the husband as his ally. The mothers' attempts to exercise control are dismissed as unfeminine. Natural childbirth, for Read, is an essentially male-dominated activity. The mothers' bad effect is especially via the *stories* they have told their daughters: 'She had told her of the trials of childbirth ... this girl had been introduced to all that was terrifying in parturition' (1933: 30). Mothers' oral stories about birth have always constituted an alternative tradition to the written versions of medical experts, and male experts have often been hostile to the 'old wives' tales' of this oral tradition (Cosslett, forthcoming). This opposition could be seen as part of a whole history of gradual male domination of childbirth, including also the take-over by male doctors from female midwives (Donnison, 1977; Towler and Bramall, 1986). Midwives hardly feature in this first edition of Read's book, and when they do, they are put firmly in their place:

> ... an accurate knowledge of the limits of safety is of much greater importance than an academic knowledge of those things which belong to the sphere of the qualified medical man. A knowledge of human nature, and an instinctive faculty for human kindness are the greatest assets that a good midwife can possess. (1933: 117)

The duty of a midwife is not to criticise the doctor, but to 'place him on a pedestal' (1933: 120).

Nevertheless, Read got nowhere with his attempt to persuade the medical establishment of the value of his ideas, while midwives and birthing women did begin to take them up. His biographer comments again and again on the professional jealousy that hampered his career (Thomas, 1957: 65, 71, 84, 98, 107, 112, 133), and also reveals that the most favourable reviews of his book were in *Nursing Notes* and *Nursing Times*, contrasting with 'the cautious, if not puzzled, attitude of the reviewers who wrote in journals usually taken to be the voices of medical authority' (1957: 107). Midwives had, to some extent, already

34

anticipated some of Read's ideas, as he concedes in *Natural Childbirth* (1933: 78). And of course Read's original inspiration is supposed to have come from those 'primitive' women of the lower class, who knew instinctively about natural childbirth. Women reading the book may have seen a way to greater control of the birthing process themselves. Be that as it may, it was among women, as midwives and patients, that Read found his greatest support. The second edition of his book, *Revelation of Childbirth* (1942), takes some account of this. Dick Read explains how women educated in natural childbirth ideas 'became interested in the performance of their own parturition ... They were able to criticise their own sensations during labour, and to differentiate between hard work and pain' (1942: 94). A more active participation by women themselves is being recognised. He still claims to be writing for his professional peers (1942: 225), but at the same time he appeals for more first-hand accounts from *women*, in order to persuade other *women* (1942: 226).

The third edition, *Childbirth Without Fear* (1954), goes even further in the direction of addressing itself to women. It claims to be written 'for the mothers of the rising and succeeding generations' (1954: v). Read writes of the thousands of letters he has received from mothers, confirming his theories, and he presents his philosophy of natural childbirth as originating from the *voice* of a woman in Whitechapel, who said, after giving birth, 'It didn't hurt. It wasn't meant to, was it, doctor?' (1954: 6, 10). The book is presented as both written for and originating from women. Read's increasing reliance on women's support is reflected in his biography (1957), where history is revised and he is presented as having addressed himself to women from the start. Thus, in *Natural Childbirth*, 'Scorning the style which would be acceptable to the academic mind, he wrote in a form that he thought might appeal to women, and thereby brought down on himself, later on, much bitter and cynical criticism' (Thomas, 1957: 95); and again, in the second edition, 'he decided to write for the womenfolk. The academics could take it or leave it, just as they chose' (1957: 115). These claims are patently untrue, given the tone and style of the first two editions, and must reflect the way Read was projecting himself as a champion of women in the 50s, as well as his resentment at his neglect by the medical establishment.

The contradictions in Read's books show how on the one hand the philosophy of 'natural childbirth', while claiming to rest on an innate power and competence in women, was nevertheless founded on anti-feminist and male-centred ideologies. On the other hand, the instability of the contradictions, and the changes in later editions, also reveal how the philosophy could be taken over by women, as a basis for a female-centred, female-empowering account of childbirth. This has

35

been achieved most successfully by the influential childbirth writer, Sheila Kitzinger.

Kitzinger's tone, and her implied readers, are both quite different from Read's. The Foreword, by a highly qualified male obstetrician, describes the book as 'written by a layman *(sic)* for laymen *(sic)*', but also stresses Kitzinger's 'authority' and her 'wide knowledge' (1962: 11-12). In the Author's Note, Kitzinger describes herself as someone who has been preparing mothers for childbirth, and who has had four babies herself. Her role thus transgressively combines several sometimes contradictory functions: the expert, the teacher and confidante of birthing women, the woman who has given birth herself. Women's experience lies behind her claim to authority, but she also lays claim to 'male' medical knowledge and terminology, which she wishes to make accessible to other women. Kitzinger's multiple, shifting role is reflected in the shifting point of view and addressee of her writing: sometimes, it is the experiences of a generic 'woman' that are being described, sometimes 'the woman' shifts into 'one', which includes the author as a possible participant in the experiences (e.g. 1962: 22-3). In the section describing exercises, a 'you' is suddenly introduced as addressee, as direct instructions are given to the reader as pregnant woman (1962: 71). Very occasionally, the author appears in the first person: 'I have noticed that among women attending my classes', or, after a description of birth, 'I have tried to describe my personal sensations' (1962: 60, 130). While the second quotation here is, necessarily, totally unlike anything in Read, the first might remind us of Dick Read observing his typical patients - but Kitzinger is in a much more reciprocal relationship with hers: 'I used to tell mothers that they would feel "a splitting, burning sensation", until one newly delivered mother wrote to tell me that she had not felt anything like this and that it had been pleasant' (1962: 150, footnote). As Kitzinger writes in the Author's Note, 'The descriptions of phases of labour which preface certain of the chapters come from the accounts of these newly delivered women' (1962: 13). The book thus gives the impression of a co-operative effort, written for women, with help from women, by a woman who has herself undergone the same experiences.

One central feature of the natural childbirth model is that it draws attention to the subjective experience of the birthing woman, not just to her objectified body, as in the medical or 'mechanical' model. Her state of mind is the key to a successful birth. As we saw, Read took the consequence to be that the male obstetrician must *control* that state of mind. Kitzinger, on the other hand, seeks to give control to the woman herself: 'She is no longer a passive, suffering instrument. She no longer hands over her body to doctor and nurses to deal with as they think best. She retains the power of self-direction, of self-control, of

36

choice, and of voluntary decision' (1962: 20). This empowering of the woman leads to a rather less glamorous view of the obstetrician than Dick Read gives us. Kitzinger discredits the idea that 'natural childbirth implies a sort of hypnotic relationship between the doctor and patient', and insists that a woman can put the method into practice 'even if the obstetrician or midwife knows nothing about it at all' (1962: 24). Women who are over-dependent on their doctors are seen as immature types looking for father-figures (1962: 108). We are treated to a woman patient's view of famous men:

> Obstetricians and nurses need to be far more aware of the impression they create upon their patients. Many would be appalled if they realized what they thought about them. I know that one obstetrician who prides himself upon his sympathy is described by more than one patient as 'unapproachable' and 'always so rushed'. (1962: 59)

This extends into a revolutionary attack on the social status of doctors,

> ... a tradition that there must exist a social distance between doctor and patient which serves to maintain his dignity and status *vis-à-vis* the layman and to make his pronouncements worthy of respect. The 'bedside manner' disappeared with the doctor who acted the part of kindly father confessor and avuncular adviser - a role which itself served to maintain this distance by its assumption of implicit authority and superior status - and in his place has come the clinician, the foreman and manager of the baby factory who treats the women lying on the examination tables as if they were so many fish on a slab. (1962: 59)

Here, both the Read type father-figure, and the unsympathetic proponent of the mechanical model are attacked as remote and authoritarian. It is refreshing to read this typology of unsatisfactory doctors, after Read's typology of unsatisfactory patients.

So far, in my argument, it may have seemed as if Kitzinger has dispensed with 'nature' altogether; the emphasis on the conscious, informed, active woman is similar to that of the Lamaze method, which presents itself as *better* than nature (Karmel, 1959: 42). The Lamaze method involves learning specific breathing techniques, and is based on a Pavlovian model of conditioning the body to ignore pain (Lamaze, 1958). Kitzinger claims to be adapting her ideas from both Read and Lamaze (1962: 13). Lamaze dispensed with Read's 'mystical' ideas on motherhood, and offered instead an image of the mother as highly

37

181

trained athlete, not as 'primitive woman' (Karmel, 1959: 22, 49, 67, 92, 140). We often find Kitzinger too using this kind of image: she advises that a birthing woman should take no drugs 'that a car driver would not take before setting out on a night journey in fog, or an athlete before taking part in a race' (1962: 121). She also tells us,

> I know one woman who drove to hospital on the back of a motorbike, relaxing well whilst using a sufficient degree of muscular tension to sit firmly on the machine and not fall off. One mother who came to my classes was an aeroplane pilot, and flew up till the date of her delivery; she practised relaxation in the small space afforded in the cockpit, just in case she should start labour when in the air. (1962: 75)

The introduction of cars, motorbikes and aeroplanes here takes us even further from the primitive woman: these women are successful achievers, in control of machines and bodies. Yet, despite her own use of these images, Kitzinger feels she has to attack both the emphasis on 'athletic skill' in the Lamaze model, and its 'mechanistic' aspect, and reinstate Read's 'spiritual' dimension (1962: 21, 23, 141, 144). She sees the Lamaze approach as too dangerously like the 'fish on the slab' mechanical model, and the way in which Lamaze breathing techniques have been easily co-opted into the dehumanising routines of American hospitals may prove her right (Rothman, 1982: 92, 177; Wertz and Wertz, 1979: 193-4). But while Kitzinger's insistence on the 'spiritual' dimension of birth can be seen as a defence against its mechanisation, it does also carry along with it the anti-feminist traditionalism of Read, as we will see.

In attempting to restore the 'spiritual' dimension to birth, Kitzinger makes use of two methods: the use of religious imagery, and a pseudo-Freudian account of the unconscious and its primitive urges. The religious imagery is relatively empowering: '... as the baby develops and can be felt moving inside, to some women annunciation, incarnation, seem to become facts of their own existence' (1962: 22). The appropriation of Marian imagery here is transgressive in that it attributes to *all* women what should be the experience of only one perfect woman, though it also carries all the reactionary implications of that imagery - motherhood as central to woman's being, passive mother subordinated to divine baby, etc. (Warner, 1976). A later use of religious imagery is even more transgressive, as Kitzinger attributes creative power to women: 'One can only be in awe and deliver oneself over, in faith, to this wonderful thing - one's own body at the work of creation' (1962: 132). Read too, occasionally uses religious imagery. There is one particularly telling passage, when he ends *Natural*

38

Childbirth with an image of doctor and midwife standing on the shore, encouraging the frail bark of the baby through the waves of labour. Lest this image seem to put the doctor into too marginal a position, Read adds a final image implicitly likening him to Christ walking on the water (1933: 123; see also Cosslett, 1989: 276). The religious imagery aggrandises the male obstetrician, not, as in Kitzinger's case, the birthing woman.

A large part of Kitzinger's book is devoted to what she calls the 'psychology of pregnancy'. As we saw, she gives primacy to a woman's state of mind, and she presents herself as able to let us into the secrets of pregnant women's psychological state (1962: 53): she has the authority of experience. But what we get is a very oppressive pseudo-Freudian account based on the idea of 'adjustment' - the woman's adjustment (or failure to adjust) to her roles both as mother and wife. Well-adjusted women give birth easily; poorly-adjusted women have difficulty. Giving birth naturally is depicted as an adjustment to heterosexual sexuality. A woman stuck in a long labour is 'not able to *give* birth', 'for some reason which may have its origins in her own childhood and which is probably linked to the quality of her marriage relationship' (1962: 105-6). Just as in Read sexual attractiveness to men went along with the ability to give birth naturally, so here sexual adjustment to men has the same effect. Later, in another context, Kitzinger insists that a long labour can be pleasurable, to a well-prepared woman (1962: 119); here the model is of the woman in control, making what she wants out of her experience. But in the psychological section, Kitzinger is carried away by the logic of her model of the inhibited woman unable to adjust to her primitive sexual urges. The model inevitably leads to the language of blaming and of prescription; thus the deep-seated guilt of a woman afraid of bearing a mal-formed baby is 'unmasked' when her first question is 'Is it all right?' (1962: 62); and the hope that a woman 'should long to savour the experience of birth to the full, not wanting to hold back or to give only half of herself' (1962: 103), starts to sound like a prescription which we may fail to live up to. The many exhortations that a woman 'need not feel she has "failed" if ...' (1962: 136, 147) only increase this reader's sense of anxiety, by introducing the notion of 'failure' in some test of essential womanhood.

This prescriptive tone is most strongly felt in a birth-story that Kitzinger tells in the present tense, recounting the experiences of 'the woman' - a character who is both typical and ideal:

> The woman feels as if her whole body is becoming a
> gateway into the world for her child ... [the baby]
> suddenly turns red and the mother gasps with pleasure at

39

183

this ... She wants to take him into her arms immediately ... she realises that this child is exactly what she desired ... the mother ... is radiant and transfigured now ... [the husband and wife] have experienced together something incomprehensibly wonderful - a peak of joy in their married life ... (1962: 152-5)

The present tense encourages the reader to build up the fantasy along with the writer, to see it as if unfolding before her. At the same time, read differently, the present tense can introduce a prescriptive tone - this is how it *is*, not how some particular birth *was*: but what if the woman doesn't feel and act as she is meant to? In a more subtle way than Read's portraits of his patients, Kitzinger's birth-story also implies a sheep-and-goats division of women into ideal or unsatisfactory types, on very traditional lines.

Central to Kitzinger's ideal of well-adjusted womanhood is, as in Read, the notion that women are essentially *mothers*: 'The experience of bearing a child is central to a woman's life' (1962: 17); 'A woman expresses herself in childbearing. Without this experience she feels that she has missed something, that she is incomplete, in some way, wasted' (1962: 68). Moreover, motherhood is seen in the context of a traditional marriage relationship: birth is essentially 'part of a marriage, and can enrich or deprive it according to how the experience is lived through by both man and woman' (1962: 192). As we have seen, the quality of the marriage relation is alleged to affect the woman's ability to give birth; and the husband's participation and presence throughout is insisted on. Kitzinger is a little more aware than Read of the culturally conditioned aspect of the mother and wife role she holds up as 'natural'; she discusses the difficulties of sustaining these roles in the face of 'the general lack of clarity in masculine and feminine roles within our society at this time ... a general lack of acceptance of the roles of wife and mother as they have been known for centuries in Western society' (1962: 55). This suggests a nostalgic harking back to times when roles were clearer - but a later section points out that different difficulties arose under the old system, when an over-devoted mother could stunt her children's psychological growth (1962: 191). As in the discrepancy about long labours, we have the impression of Kitzinger pulled in different directions by the different models she is using.

But notice that her objection to the traditional mothering role is one that *blames* the woman again - in many ways the book is not as woman-centred as it purports to be. In particular, the emphasis on husbands as ideal birth-partners is very male-centred; the husband takes over the Dick Read role, 'her guide and counsellor, who will

40

gently and firmly correct her faults, encourage her when she begins to lose confidence, and let her know by his pride in her that she is doing well' (1962: 99). Like Read, Kitzinger is suspicious and dismissive of the female oral tradition of birth-stories and advice: 'the dread and horror that is associated with most "old wives tales"' (1962: 18). It is the husband who protects his wife from these, *and* from the soulless medical 'experts': he is to 'stand between his wife and the sceptics, the bearers of old wives tales and those who see birth as a sort of major surgical operation' (1962: 199).

In later editions, Kitzinger revises 'marriage' to 'relationship' and 'husband' to 'partner'; on the other hand, she also adds a much more searing attack on dominant mothers as a pernicious influence on daughters (1984: 50, 80-4). The seeds of this are evident in the 1962 edition, not only in the attack on dominant traditional mothers, but also in a passage discussing the woman who *is* dependent on her birth attendants: the woman dependent on a male doctor gets off lightly; she needs 'a father figure who must care for her and let her come to no harm - who will be firm, authoritarian and kind, like a loving father'. But the woman who needs a mother figure is criticised for 'girlhood dependence', especially if she is the daughter of a 'mother-dominated home' (1962: 108). A portrait is provided of an 'over-motherly midwife' who may 'use her kindness in order to get power over her patient', exercising 'a will of iron' (1962: 109). 'Wilful' midwives here come in for criticism that 'authoritarian' doctors escape - despite Kitzinger's earlier criticism of doctors' remoteness. Read's stereotype of the dominant mother, interfering in childbirth, is alive and well. Thus Kitzinger's insistence on the husband's participation involves a denigration of mothers and other women helpers. In fact, the natural childbirth movement's emphasis on the birth as the couple's experience fitted in very well with the culture of the 50s, with its emphasis on marriage and the 'feminine mystique' (Wertz and Wertz, 1979: 181-9). Kitzinger's 1962 book retains a lot of this 50s ideology, as well as anticipating the sexual 'liberation' of the 60s in its frank discussion of sexual relations and impulses. As we have seen, this also leads to a very traditional model of women's role.

I do not want to give the impression in my analysis that Kitzinger is any more contradictory than Read, who often reads as a strange amalgam of 18th century Natural Theology, 19th century evolutionism and imperialism and 20th century Freudianism, plus vague spiritual references. But all these discourses are pulling *together* for Read, towards his ideal of dominant male obstetricians and subservient natural mothers. On the other hand, they also leave loopholes for an *active* female appropriation, by his female followers, by Kitzinger, and by Read himself, as he changed the direction of his

41

message. In Kitzinger's book, there is more a sense of different discourses and models pulling in different directions as she opens up those loopholes and inserts herself as an active, disruptive woman into discourses that imply her passivity. As Rothman points out, the contemporary home birth movement in America rests on a sometimes uneasy alliance between feminists, with a highly developed critique of patriarchal institutions, and traditional women, seeking to return to family-centred values (Rothman, 1982: 24, 32, 49, 94, 97, 109). *Both* these impulses can be seen in embryo in Kitzinger's book, and any woman taking up her approach must chart a wary course between them: it is not so easy, I would suggest, to pry them apart and come up with a 'correct' feminist approach to childbirth.

Notes

1. Read was in fact indebted to some female predecessors (see Kitzinger, 1962: 18, 42, 80); but he got into print first, and his is the name which became attached to the idea of natural childbirth.

2. For a critique of this notion see Freedman and Ferguson, 1950 and Macintyre, 1977.

Bibliography

Arms, S. 1977, *Immaculate Deception*, Boston: Houghton Mifflin.

Bourne, G. 1975, *Pregnancy*, London: Pan.

Cosslett, T. 1989, 'Childbirth from the Woman's Point of View in British Women's Fiction: Enid Bagnold's *The Squire* and A. S. Byatt's *Still Life*', *Tulsa Studies in Women's Literature* vol. 8, no. 2 (Fall 1989), 263-86.

Cosslett, T. (forthcoming), 'Questioning the Definition of Literature: Fictional and Non-fictional Accounts of Childbirth'. In J. Aaron and S. Walby (eds.), *Out of the Margins: Women's Studies in the Nineties*, Basingstoke: Falmer Press.

Donnison, J. 1977, *Midwives and Medical Men: A History of Inter-Professional Rivalry and Women's Rights*, London: Heinemann.

Freedman, L. and Ferguson, V. M. 1950, 'The Question of "Painless Childbirth" in Primitive Cultures', *American Journal of Orthopsychiatry* 20 (1950), 363-72.

42

Karmel, M. 1959, *Babies Without Tears: A Mother's Experience of the Lamaze Method of Painless Childbirth*, London: Secker and Warburg.

Kitzinger, S. 1962, *The Experience of Childbirth*, London: Gollancz.

Kitzinger, S. 1984, *The Experience of Childbirth*, 5th ed., Harmondsworth: Penguin.

Lamaze, F. 1958, *Painless Childbirth*, London: Burke.

Lewis, J. 1980, *The Politics of Motherhood: Child and Maternal Welfare in England 1900-1939*, London: Croom Helm.

Macintyre, S. 1977, 'Childbirth: the Myth of the Golden Age', *World Medicine* vol. 12, no. 18 (1977), 17-22.

Martin, E. 1987, *The Woman in the Body: a Cultural Analysis of Reproduction*, Boston: Beacon Press.

Oakley, A. 1980, *Women Confined: Towards a Sociology of Childbirth*, Oxford: Martin Robertson.

Oakley, A. 1984, *The Captured Womb: A History of the Medical Care of Pregnant Women*, Oxford: Blackwell.

Read, G. D. 1933, *Natural Childbirth*, London: Heinemann.

Read, G. D. 1942, *Revelation of Childbirth*, London: Heinemann.

Read, G. D. 1954, *Childbirth Without Fear*, London: Heinemann.

Rich, A., 1977, *Of Woman Born: Motherhood as Experience and Institution*, London: Virago.

Rothman, B. K. 1982, *In Labor: Women and Power in the Birthplace*, New York and London: Norton.

Thomas, A. N. 1957, *Dr. Courageous: The Story of Dr. Grantley Dick Read*, London: Heinemann.

Towler, J. and Bramall, J. 1986, *Midwives in History and Society*, London: Croom Helm.

Warner, M. 1976, *Alone of All Her Sex*, London: Weidenfeld.

43

Copyright © 1978 Birth and the Family Journal

Lamaze Childbirth Training and Changes in Belief about Personal Control

Gary S. Felton, Ph.D.

Florrie B. Segelman, R.N.

ABSTRACT: *This study explored changes in parents' beliefs about the origin of control for behavior and its consequences after completion of Lamaze classes, Red Cross classes, and no classes. Results indicate that Lamaze training for women, led to a significant increase in new mothers seeing themselves as origins of control (as against seeing others or chance as agents of control). Other modes showed no significant change for women. No significant postpartum findings emerged for men under any condition. These findings are discussed and suggestions are made for modification of Lamaze training to improve it and to better meet the immediate needs of expectant and new parents. (Birth Family J 5:3, Fall 1978)*

Introduction

The purpose of this study was to learn and measure the degree to which beliefs about the origin of control for behavior and its consequences might change on the part of men and women who complete Lamaze childbirth training classes. Such beliefs relate to the concept known as internalization/externalization[10] —the degree to which an individual perceives the origin of control to reside within or outside himself or herself. Specifically, internality relates to the belief that the person is directly responsible for behavior and its consequences and can have effect and impact on the environment. Externality relates to the belief that behavior and its consequences are regulated by fate, luck, chance, or other exterior dimensions.

Among many areas where this concept has been studied, research on the psychotherapeutic process has shown an important, direct relationship between the degree to which clients see themselves as the origin of control and rated favorable outcome.[5,6,8] These findings suggest that learning to perceive an internal origin for responsibility helps people to implement new and effective behaviors. In addition, research has shown that such an orientation can be taught systematically to clients in individual psychotherapy[9] and in group psychotherapy.[3,4] Since this

Gary S. Felton, Ph.D. *is a clinical psychologist teaching at Los Angeles City College in the Human Services Curriculum, Department of Psychology, is author of the book* Up from Underachievement, *and is Director, Center for Interpersonal Studies, Suite 22, 11941 Wilshire Boulevard, Los Angeles, California 90025.*

Florrie B. Segelman, R.N. *is a practicing childbirth educator in the Los Angeles area for over seven years, and has trained several thousand couples in the Lamaze method of childbirth preparation and lectures frequently in the Los Angeles area about childbirth preparation. She is a member of the American Society of Psychoprophylaxis in Obstetrics. She was the technical advisor for the ABC Television Network "Movie of the Week"* Having Babies *(1976).*

perception correlates positively with favorable outcome in psychotherapy,[5,6,8] enhancing it in training Lamaze couples could facilitate their immediate pre- and post-natal adjustment. The first step in considering such an approach is to measure the pre-existing degree to which such persons see themselves as the origin of control and the degree to which such a view emerges among Lamaze-trained couples, purely as a function of Lamaze training.

Major goals of Lamaze training are to help expectant women and men recognize their fears and deal with them, to describe the process of labor and delivery, to teach techniques of breathing, relaxation, and concentration, to develop a physical and emotional support system (coach and other class members), to offer a way to experience birth with dignity and awareness, actively and with control. In addition, Lamaze training helps participants learn which questions to ask and actively pursue and how to recognize one's body signals and respond appropriately to them. Furthermore, instructors of Lamaze classes hope to aid in the creation of better consumers and to teach about alternatives available within various class participants' areas, both for health care and for community resources.[1,2,7]

Although the purpose of this study was not to compare different childbirth methods, we included for control purposes participants in the American National Red Cross Preparation for Parenthood classes. These classes focus on teaching aspects of anatomy, physiology, pregnancy, and the birth process. In addition, participants are taught about the importance of nutrition prenatally as well as postnatally and are familiarized with such parent/infant experiences as preparing the layette, bathing and holding the infant. Further features of this training include viewing films about giving birth and breast feeding and learning about feeding approaches, growth and development, and parenting. Red Cross

Preparation classes bring to the general community some valuable information regarding health care. Because charges are minimal or non-existent, and Red Cross Centers are widespread, this training is available to a wider segment of the community than are many private or hospital classes.

Due to the differences in classes and populations served, we hypothesized that women's belief about the origin of control would shift significantly toward seeing themselves as the origin of control, over the course of Lamaze training, and would shift in a similar direction but not as significantly for Red Cross participants. For men, we theorized that two experiences would occur. First, men independently would respond to childbirth preparation in ways similar to women's responses. Second, these response patterns would be reinforced through transfer of training and learning from women to their male partners. Thus, we theorized that men also would show a shift toward seeing themselves as the origin of control. As with women, we predicted that Lamaze-trained men would shift significantly toward seeing themselves as the agent of control, whereas Red Cross-trained men would shift in a similar direction but not as significantly. To our knowledge, among Lamaze-trained couples or among Red Cross-trained couples there are no reported studies of internal-external belief systems.

Method

Participants in the study consisted of three groups of men and women. One group was comprised of 26 male and 33 female members of six different Lamaze childbirth training classes conducted by one of us (Segelman). These classes consisted of six weekly two-hour meetings. Each class was composed of six couples. The participants in this study primarily were Caucasian, middle-class residents of the western Los Angeles area. Most people had completed college and they ranged

142

in age from 22 to 35, with the average age approximately 28 years. Of these 59 participants, 81.4% were preparing for their first child, 13.6% were preparing for their second child, and 5.0% were preparing for their third child. Of those preparing for a second or third child, 54.6% (n=6) had been trained in the Lamaze technique for their previous deliveries.

A second group was comprised of 21 male and 21 female members of four different American National Red Cross Preparation for Parenthood classes. These classes consisted of six weekly two-hour meetings. Each class was composed of 16 couples. The participants from these classes were matched as closely as possible demographically to members of the Lamaze classes. They primarily were Caucasian, middle-class residents of the western Los Angeles area. Most of them were college graduates and they ranged in age from 21 to 39, with the average age approximately 26 years. Of these 42 participants, 81.0% were preparing for their first child, 9.5% were preparing for their second child, 4.8% were preparing for their third child, and 4.8% were preparing for their fourth child. Of those getting ready for second, third, or fourth children, 62.5% (n=5) had received Red Cross training for previous deliveries.

A third group of expectant parents consisted of 18 women and 12 men who underwent no formal training prior to the births of their babies. Although a little more difficult to control for identical personal parameters, these participants were Caucasian, middle-class college graduates who resided in western and central Los Angeles. Their age range was 24 to 37 with an average age approximately 29 years. Twenty-eight members (14 couples) of this group were preparing for their first child and had had no previous childbirth training.

These groups were chosen to allow us more accurately to know how much our findings truly are a function of La-

maze training, how much they are a function of training per se, and how much they are a function of the experience of giving birth.

Instrument

The instrument used was the Rotter Internal-External [I-E] Scale.[10] This 29-item, forced-choice scale assesses the degree to which a person believes the origin of control to be internal or external to himself or herself. Each item consists of two statements from which the individual respondent must choose one as best typifying his or her belief about the specific content in those two statements. For example, one question from the scale reads as follows:

a) When I make plans, I am almost certain that I can make them work.

b) It is not always wise to plan too far ahead because many things turn out to be a matter of good or bad fortune anyhow.

Statement *a* is scored as *internal;* statement *b* is scored as *external.* The scale takes 10-15 minutes to complete and has a score of 0 (maximally internal) to 23 (maximally external). Six items are filler items which are not scored.

Procedure

Over a seven-month period, the I-E Scale was administered to 66 members of six different Lamaze classes six to eight weeks prior to the births of their full-term babies. All but six participants in the classes volunteered to take part. The pretest was administered in the first class of the series to all 66 participants. The posttest was completed by 33 of the participants (16 men and 17 women) in the sixth class, and by 26 of the participants (10 men and 16 women) at home after delivery of the baby.

Over a six-month period, the I-E Scale also was administered to 49 members of four different Red Cross classes six to eight weeks prior to the births of their full-term babies. All but nine participants in these classes volunteered to take part. The pretest was administered in the first class of the series to all 49 participants. The posttest was completed by 22 of the participants (11 men and 11 women) in the sixth class, and 20 of the participants (10 men and 10 women) at home after delivery of the baby.

Over a four-month period, the I-E Scale also was given to 16 married couples who were undergoing no formalized training prior to childbirth. The pretest was administered at a time designated by each individual couple as six to eight weeks prior to expected delivery. The posttest was completed by 16 of the participants (8 men and 8 women) at a time designated by each couple as one to two weeks prior to delivery, and by 14 of the participants (4 men and 10 women) at home after delivery of the baby.

Participants in the three groups returned their answer sheets by mail immediately after completing them. The above particular research design was selected because of the possible habituation effects which probably would occur were we to administer the scale more than twice in a ten-week period; i.e., class No. 1, class No. 6, *and* after delivery.

Assignment to each of the groups was random (using the table of random numbers). Participants were neither assigned to nor informed of their posttest grouping until the sixth class or its time equivalent. Sixteen persons of the 147 participants in the entire study declined to return the posttest information. Feedback about performance score was available to any participant who requested it.

Results

In all statistical comparisons, *t* tests were performed to assess the significance of the differences between average scores (means). The mean pretest scores of the

144

male and female participants were evaluated statistically for all possible comparisons. There were no significant differences in these scores and these pretest scores did not differ significantly from norm scores of the general population. These findings suggest that we are dealing with a representative sample of the general population and that men compared with women. Also, participants who tested for a second time in class No. 6 were compared with participants who were tested for a second time after delivery. All started with equal degrees to which they see themselves as the origin of control. Score changes with a negative sign are in the direction of *greater* belief in oneself as the origin of control; those with a positive sign are the converse.

As a group, the Lamaze participants who were given the second test in class No. 6 showed a non-significant change toward seeing themselves as the origin of control (mean change, −0.46 points). Similarly, as a group, the Lamaze participants who were given the second test after delivery showed a non-significant change toward seeing themselves as the agent of control (mean change, −1.38 points.) At the same time, however, men who completed the second test in class No. 6 and women who completed the second test after delivery both showed significant changes in the direction of viewing themselves as the origin of control (men: mean change, −2.43 points, t=1.64, p<.06, women: mean change, −3.06 points, t= 3.55, p<.005). Women who completed the second test in class No. 6 and men who completed the second test after delivery both showed non-significant changes in the direction of seeing outside factors as controlling (men: mean change, +1.30 points; women: mean change, +1.41 points).

As a group, the Lamaze participants who completed the second test after delivery showed a greater but non-significant change toward seeing themselves as agent of control than did the participants who completed the second test in class

192

No. 6 (mean change, −1.38 points as compared with −0.46 points). Women who completed the second test after delivery changed significantly more toward seeing themselves as control agent than did their female counterparts in class No. 6 (mean change, −3.06 points, as compared with mean change +1.41 points, $t=4.34$, $p<.0005$). Men who completed the second test in class No. 6 changed significantly more toward viewing themselves as the origin of control than did their male counterparts completing the test after delivery (mean change, −2.43 points, as compared with mean change, +1.30 points, $t=4.07$, $p<.0005$).

As a group, Red Cross participants who completed the second test in class No. 6 showed a slightly greater and non-significant change toward seeing outside factors as controlling than did the participants who were tested after delivery (mean change, +1.14 points, as compared with +1.10 points). Men who completed the second test after delivery changed non-significantly more toward seeing external factors as controlling than did their male counterparts who completed the second test in class No. 6 (mean change, +1.90 points, as compared with mean change, +0.46 points). Women who completed the second test in class No. 6 changed non-significantly more toward seeing outside factors as controlling than did their female counterparts completing the test after delivery (mean change, +1.81 points, as compared with mean change, + 0.30 points).

As a group, those persons who underwent no training for childbirth showed non-significant change in score toward seeing external factors as control agent, both at a time equivalent to class No. 6 (mean change, +1.24 points) and at a time equivalent to being tested after delivery (mean change, +0.50 points). Women who were tested at a time equivalent to class No. 6 changed non-significantly toward seeing external factors as controlling (mean change, +1.74 points) as did their counterparts who were tested at a time equivalent to being tested after delivery (mean change, +0.50 points). Men who received the second test at a time equivalent to class No. 6 changed non-significantly toward seeing outside factors as controlling (mean change, +0.74 points) as did their counterparts who were given the second test at a time equivalent to after delivery (mean change, +0.50 points). Chi square analyses allowed us to learn whether our significant changes are attributable to several large score changes intermixed with changes which are minimal, or are a function of consistent, sizeable score changes throughout the distribution. The results of these analyses show that where we found significant changes in score from pre- to posttest, in all conditions tested, the changes are attributable to consistent, sizeable score differences throughout each distribution.

To understand the trend of score changes for all participants in the study, we looked at the sequential scoring from class No. 1, to class No. 6, to after delivery for the Lamaze and Red Cross participants and the sequential scoring from time period 1, to time period 2, to after delivery for the non-trained participants. These directional patterns for the first two groups are displayed in Figures 1 and 2.

Additionally, it occurred to us that since 18.6% of the Lamaze participants and 19.0% of the Red Cross participants already had experienced childbirth training prior to this study, there might be differences in the results accounted for by this fact. No pretest differences existed in the scores of these participants compared with those of their childbirth training counterparts. In addition, the change scores of such participants did not differ significantly from the change scores of participants who had had no previous childbirth training.

Finally, two other comparisons were

made: 1) score changes of Lamaze men tested in class No. 6 versus those of Red Cross men tested in class No. 6; 2) score changes of Lamaze women tested after delivery versus those of Red Cross women tested after delivery. The results of these comparisons show that Lamaze men tested in class No. 6 changed significantly more toward seeing themselves as control agent than did Red Cross men tested at the same time (mean change, −2.43 points, as compared with +0.46 points, t=2.75, p<.01). Lamaze women tested at home after delivery changed significantly more toward seeing themselves as control agent than did Red Cross women under the same testing conditions (mean change, −3.06 points, as compared with +0.30 points, t=3.61, p<.0025).

Since in each case the difference between mean score change of Lamaze men tested in class No. 6 and non-trained men tested in class No. 6, and between mean score change of Lamaze women and non-trained women both tested at home after delivery is greater than the difference between these same Lamaze participants and their Red Cross counterparts, these former differences also are significant.

Discussion

Often it has been true that Lamaze classes have been situated in geographic areas serving upper-economic sectors of the population whereas Red Cross classes have been situated in lower-economic sectors. Where these differences have been

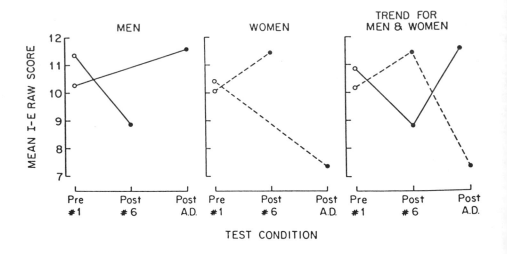

Figure 1. Graphic display of pre- (class No. 1) and posttest (class No. 6 and after delivery) mean I-E raw scores for men alone, for women alone, and for the integration of all scores to depict trend among persons who complete Lamaze training.

146

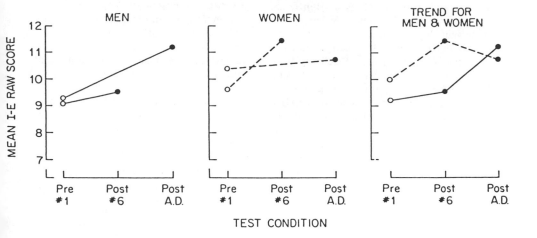

Figure 2. Graphic display of pre- (class No. 1) and posttest (class No. 6 and after delivery) mean I-E raw scores for men alone, for women alone, and for the integration of all scores to depict trend among persons who complete Red Cross training.

operating, we might reasonably expect that Lamaze participants would inherently more likely view themselves as the agent of control and that Red Cross participants would more likely see the external world as a determinant of their experience. In fact this often is the case and thus we might find such differences complicating any comparison of these two teaching methods. It is possible that some of these differences were operating in the present study despite all efforts to prevent such happening by working with Red Cross and Lamaze participants who were balanced regarding economic background, education level, geographic residence, etc. In reading and interpreting Figures 1 and 2, it is important for the reader to understand that the findings depicted therein are illustrative and descriptive in nature and are not quantitative.

After Training

Our results show that the experience of Lamaze training and childbirth has a significant impact on the participants' belief systems as to where personal control lies. We originally hypothesized that *both* men and women would change significantly toward seeing themselves as control agents by the end of training. This is not what we found. By the end of training only men saw themselves as control agents significantly more than before. Women more saw external factors as controlling. The differences between these opposite changes are significant, and since these findings are not what we predicted, they need analysis.

If the premises we outlined earlier regarding an internal view of control hold up, then it follows that men will become significantly more so because of the training. Statistically this is what we obtained, and oral as well as written feedback supports this finding. Much of the view men have of themselves as control agents derived from the feelings and beliefs that in the birth and delivery process they are essential to the full and healthy functioning of their women partners and their newborns. They see and believe themselves to have this great responsibility and believe that they are the origin of control for it. These beliefs are reflected in the self-as-control-agent scores they obtained by the end of training. This change toward seeing themselves as control agents was the finding which distinguished Lamaze-trained men from Red Cross-trained men and from men who did not attend any preparation for childbirth classes.

Unexpectedly, women more viewed outside factors as controlling by the end of training. Based on formal written and oral reports and on anecdotal sharing by participants, we found that these scores obtained by women reflect three main areas of concern for women in the latter stages of pregnancy and of Lamaze training. Women focus on what their control over their bodies will be like during labor and delivery, on whether they will be able to complete the experience without unexpected difficulty, and on the survival of their newborns. If we break down these dimensions, we can begin to understand the results obtained for women.

First, we found that Lamaze-trained women consistently feel and express, at the end of training, general overall confidence in their ability to maintain control over their body throughout the labor and delivery experience. We have not found this to be true for women who underwent no training. Second, in the latter stages of Lamaze training, women also begin to believe that, although most likely they will retain control in the childbirth process, there may be some difficulty in giving birth which is unanticipated and unrelated to their control. Third, women fear that something may be wrong developmentally with the neo-

148

nate or that the neonate may be stillborn, another factor women believe to be fully out of their control.

Essentially we found, through written evaluations and discussion sessions, that women believe strongly that with regard to labor and delivery, they are in control, and with regard to unexpected happenings and health of the newborn, they are not. The focus appears to be much more on fear about the latter two issues and much less on their belief in themselves as control agents over their bodies during labor and delivery. To a large extent, for this reason women score more in the direction of seeing outside factors as control agent than expected. Women in all three groups were more in this direction after training or its equivalent in time; none of these changes was significant in this direction.

After Delivery

Originally we hypothesized that both men and women would change significantly toward seeing themselves as control agent by the time following delivery. Also, we hypothesized that both men and women would feel themselves significantly more as origins of control after birth of the baby than they would at the end of the Lamaze classes. We found these hypotheses to be borne out partially. After the births of the babies, Lamaze women scored significantly more toward seeing themselves as control agents than they did after training. However, after the birth, Lamaze men scored significantly more in the direction of seeing outside factors as controlling than they did after training. For women, this highly significant change from initial scores and the difference between these scores and class No. 6 posttest scores is what we predicted. It appears that once women experience the actual labor, childbirth, and early postpartum activities, as well as feel their Lamaze training work in all of these areas, feel their belief about origin of control substantiated, find their fears about ill health of the neonate abated, and know that few unexpected or difficult events occurred, they relax and incorporate an even greater belief in themselves as origin of control. This change is clearly reflected in greater scores of seeing oneself as control agent and is talked about by women in discussion sessions. This finding distinguished Lamaze-trained women from Red Cross participants and from women who had no formal classes.

The after-delivery change scores obtained by men are opposite to what we predicted. They were significantly more in the direction of external factors as controlling after birth of the baby than after training. In talking with men and in evaluating their written reports, it appears that one major factor operating here is that prior to the birth men believe themselves to be responsible for the welfare of their partner and they concentrate most of their focus and energy on these issues. After birth, it seems that they begin to realize the full impact of their new, day-to-day practical responsibilities, e.g., being a parent, being a father, having to provide for another person, having a great amount of practical responsibility for the new baby's life, having a family to support and relate to, and feelings of displacement. At this juncture, men experience some feelings similar to those of culture shock. They express feelings of not being prepared (both out of societal tradition and from their own experience) for these new demands and realities, and the fears and inadequacies they feel are reflected in their change scores.

With regard to the above findings, it is conceivable that Lamaze-trained women might have experienced less medication during the delivery process than women in either of the other two groups and therefore might feel much more in control during delivery by virtue of this discrepancy. Our records show that no significant differences occurred between groups in the amount, frequency, or incidence of medication during labor and delivery.

Trend

The analyses of the proportion of scores which changed in the same direction as the mean score, for each of the comparisons made, show that a significantly greater number of scores changed in the direction of the mean rather than away from it, for all four Lamaze conditions (men tested in class No. 6, women tested in class No. 6, men tested after delivery, women tested after delivery), confirming that we are dealing with a consistent finding. Our learning about this pattern is important because it shows that a significant number of people respond similarly rather than having a few large scores which offset a number of small ones. For Red Cross participants the only two conditions where significance of this nature was found were women tested in class No. 6 and men tested after delivery, indicating that such changes were less consistent for this group.

Conclusion

The findings from this study open the way for better understanding of the emotional responses and belief systems which such men and women experience in the latter stages of Lamaze training, just prior to delivery. Such awareness on our part allows us to design more effective Lamaze training sequences and elements of teaching and counseling, which are critical ingredients of this childbirth approach. Such new directions include a greater focus during training on 1) women's feelings about unexpected elements in the childbirth process and the neonate's health; 2) the postnatal responsibilities men will encounter; 3) change in the family structure with the addition of a baby; and 4) the commonness of these feelings and experiences among other people.

REFERENCES

1. Bean, C.A. *Methods of childbirth: A complete guide to childbirth classes and the new maternity care.* Garden City, Doubleday & Co., 1974.
2. Bing, E. and Karmel, M. *A practical training course for the psychoprophylactic method of childbirth (Lamaze technique).* New York, The American Society for Psychoprophylaxis in Obstetrics, Inc., 1965.
3. Felton, G.S. and Biggs, B.E. Psychotherapy and responsibility. *Small Group Behavior, 4,* 147-155, (May) 1973.
4. Felton, G.S. and Biggs, B.E. Teaching internalization behavior to collegiate low achievers in group psychotherapy. *Psychotherapy: Theory, Research, and Practice, 9,* 281-283, (Fall) 1972.
5. Gillis, J.S. and Jessor, R. Effects of brief psychotherapy on belief in internal control: An exploratory study. *Psychotherapy: Theory, Research, and Practice, 7,* 135-136, (Fall) 1970.
6. Kirtner, W.L. and Cartwright, D.S. Success and failure in client-centered therapy as a function of initial in-therapy behavior. *Journal of Consulting Psychology, 22,* 329-335, 1958.
7. MacFarlane, A. The psychology of childbirth. Cambridge, Harvard University Press, 1977.
8. Perry, C. Client internalizing and/or client externalizing consistency or change: Its effect on therapeutic process and outcome. Unpublished doctoral dissertation, Michigan State University, 1969.
9. Pierce, R.M., Schauble, P.G., and Farkas, A. Teaching internalization behavior to clients. *Psychotherapy: Theory, Research, and Practice, 7,* 217-220, (Winter) 1970.
10. Rotter, J.B. Generalized expectancies for internal versus external control of reinforcement. *Psychological Monograph, 80* (Whole No. 609), 1-28, 1966.

Copyright © 1977 Birth and the Family Journal

The Transition from Home to Hospital Birth in the United States, 1930-1960

Neal Devitt

During the period from 1930 to 1960 the proportion of births in hospitals increased from 36.9 percent (1935) to 88 percent (1950) to 96 percent (1960), as shown in Table 7. Nationwide statistics on the place of birth were not available until 1935. During this period the campaign to hospitalize birth achieved support from obstetricians, public health officials, upper class women and insurance companies.[41] Also, in 1946, the Hill-Burton Act provided funds for the construction of hospitals in rural areas, creating the possibility of hospital birth for populations which previously had no choice but to give birth in the home.

Many proponents of hospital birth attribute the reduction in obstetric mortality over the past sixty years to the advances in medical care in hospitals. Pearse[54] wrote in 1976:

In 1940 half the deliveries in the United States were carried out at home, and the maternal mortality was 60 per 10,000 live births. In 1975, with over 99 percent of deliveries in hospitals, maternal mortality is less than 3 per 10,000 live births. This is not purely a coincidence.

Neal Devitt *received an A.B. in Biology from Harvard University in 1977. He will begin medical school this September at Rush Medical College in Chicago. He is a member of* Birth Day, *a Boston-based home birth organization, and is the father of two children, the second one born at home.*

A few obstetricians who were familiar with the statistical studies evaluating hospital birth opposed the trend. George Kosmak, editor of the *American Journal of Obstetrics and Gynecology*, wrote in 1938:

. . . during the last 25 years . . . the hospital has been substituted for the home in from 75 to 80 percent of all cases . . . This undoubtedly has contributed to the ease and comfort of patients, although not necessarily to their safety. The more frequent resort to hospitals has provided a temptation for operative interference, with ultimate results that are often deplorable.[34]

Lay opposition to the hospitalization of birth began in the 1950's with the publication of Ashley Montagu's article "Babies Should be Born at Home" in the *Ladies' Home Journal*.[48] However, vocal, organized lay opposition to hospitalization of normal birth did not appear until the late 1960's. There are now six nationally known organizations of lay and professional people who support home birth.[57] David Stewart of the National Association of Parents and Professionals for Safe Alternatives in Childbirth (NAPSAC) sums up the disenchantment with hospital birth, "Hospitals have never been proven to be the safest place for most mothers to give birth."[13]

In order to address this controversy, we reviewed the historical basis for the hospitalization of birth in the United

47

199

States, surveying the medical and popular literature from 1930 to 1960 with the following questions in mind: What was the historical basis for the shift to the hospital? How did the home confinement of the past compare to that advocated today? What was the relative safety of birth at home compared to birth in the hospital?

Historical Attitudes toward Home and Hospital Birth

Several changes before 1930 influenced the attitudes of many regarding childbirth. Infant mortality had risen precipitously in the mid-1800's as a result of the related pressures of industrialization and urbanization, which pauperized the working class. In the latter 1800's, in response to the urban reform movement and the growing influence of the infectious theory of disease, infant mortality began a decline which has continued to the present. By 1910, New York City had again attained its infant mortality rate of 1810.[3] Massachusetts in 1910 had just fallen below its infant mortality rate of 1855-59.[26] Thus the decline in obstetric mortality from 1930 to 1960 cannot be understood solely as the result of changes occurring during that period, but must be seen as part of a process that began in the 1870's.

Also prior to 1930, the midwife was virtually eliminated. Midwife-attended births dropped from about 40 percent in 1915 to 10.7 percent in 1935.[32] The remaining practice of midwifery was concentrated largely in the rural South. In 1935 midwives attended only 4.5 percent of all Caucasian births, but 54% of all nonwhite births.[32] As a result, in contrast to Europe, the United States had no class of accoucheurs expertly trained in domiciliary obstetrics.

Between 1920 and 1930 there was a heated controversy between "radical" operative and "conservative" obstetrics. In 1920 De Lee introduced his famous "prophylactic forceps" operation.[11] Others advocated that all babies be delivered by cesarean section to "preserve in its original state the genital tract . . . conducive to a happier marital state."[5] In

1937 Irving[31] wrote in the *New England Journal of Medicine:*

> We have prophylactic forceps, prophylactic version, and even prophylactic rupture of membranes. It is not evident against what the prophylaxis is directed, unless it be against normal childbirth.

Of 223 United States Hospitals surveyed in 1932, 37 percent reported their incidence of forceps deliveries to be 20 percent or higher, ranging up to 81 percent.[68] Due to this rise in forceps deliveries, and other interventions in birth, from 1918 to 1925, infant deaths from birth injuries rose 5 percent per year, an increase of 44 percent for the entire period.[18] Rudolph Holmes, the obstetrician who introduced scopolamine to United States obstetrics, later said, "I wish to God I hadn't done it."[9] He concluded:

> The basic error has crept into the obstetric field that pregnancy and labor are pathologic entities, that childbearing is a disease, a surgical malady which must be terminated by some spectacular procedure. There is too insistent preachment by those who are defending a reign of terror, of promiscuous operative furor, on the argument that women have so degenerated that childbearing is a phase of pathologic anatomy.[28]

Holmes realized that obstetric mortality could be reduced below the rates then obtained without recourse to surgical obstetrics. He cited studies from the eighteenth and nineteenth centuries to show that the best clinics in Europe and the United States had 100 years earlier achieved mortality rates comparable to the obstetric mortality of the United States in 1920.[28] This was also found by Peller[55] who studied obstetric mortality among 8,269 births to the European royal families from 1500 to 1930. For the 1600 births in the 1800's, neonatal mortality (under one month) was 32 per 1000 live births, a rate not equalled in the United States until 1937. For the 811 births from 1850 to 1899, the neo-

48

natal mortality rate of 17 per 1000 live births bettered the 1966 United States rate. However maternal mortality was unexceptional, largely due to lack of techniques to diagnose or manage placentae abruptio and previa, cephalopelvic disproportion, and hemorrhage

Despite the operative and anesthesia dangers of hospital obstetrics, during the 1930's women increasingly sought hospital births. The belief in a pathologic nature of pregnancy had spread from the medical to the popular consciousness. Science popularizer Paul de Kruif[35] wrote in 1936 that "human reproduction has become the same as a dangerous sickness." Physicians encouraged hospitalization for birth in part because the popular "operative interference" of hospital obstetrics decried by Kosmak was even more dangerous at home. Women who submitted to surgical obstetrics needed effective anesthetics. The popular press celebrated the development of each new childbirth anesthetic and procedure.[10,64] Women were warned that "New methods of painless childbirth can be used only in up-to-date hospitals."[67]

Obstetricians saw anesthetics and hospital based obstetrics as tools to slow what they thought was an alarming decline in the birth rate of the upper classes.[23,39,69] One enthusiastic father[44] wrote that widespread use of scopolamine-nembutal anesthesia would remove women's dread of labor so that more children would be "born in the white collar and professional groups where at present the low birth rate is causing grave alarm."

Physicians also sought to limit deliveries to the hospital to ease the demand of obstetrics on their time. Between 1900 and 1935 the elimination of the midwife, and the reduction in the number of physicians following the publication of the Flexner report on medical education in 1910, increased the obstetric case load of physicians. The draft of physicians into the military for World War Two, during a period of increasing birth rate, further strained the remaining civilian physicians, a group already complaining of exhaustion and fearing heart

attacks.[1] Since hospitalization of deliveries decreased the time spent by the physician on each case, Falls[16] concluded in 1943 that "It should be our aim . . . to encourage as far as possible the entry of obstetrical cases to the hospital services."

Paradoxically, in contrast to the popular demand for hospital care and anesthetic oblivion,[59] several recent studies have found that about 80 percent of women who gave birth both at home and in the hospital prefer birth at home.[22,37,53]

How did Home Confinement of the Past Compare to that of Today?

From 1930 to 1960 children were born at home usually because the parents were too poor to afford a hospital birth, according to Olson,[52] O'Brien[51] and the New York Academy of Medicine,[50] or because they lived in an area where there was no hospital. Many of these poor women were ill-nourished. "Poor nutrition [had] been a problem from the beginning" of the New York Maternity Center Association Clinic.[36] The women often were in poor health or had a bad obstetric history. Kooser[33] described the population served by the Frontier Nursing Service of Kentucky:

The majority have parasitic infestation [such as] ascariasis and *Nectar americanus.* Most of them show varying degrees of endemic thyroid disease and low-grade dental infections. The incidence of gonorrhea and syphilis is very low . . .

He also reported that 16 percent of the women had secondary anemia with hemoglobins of 8 mg. or less. The normal is 14 mg. Steele[60] reported that 13 percent of the first 4000 women attended by the Frontier Nursing Service midwives exhibited symptoms of pre-eclampsia. 29 percent had had six or more children. Laird[36] reported that 36.4 percent of the clients attended at home by the Maternity Center Association in New York showed secondary anemia. In addition 5 percent of the mothers attended at home were in their tenth pregnancy and 6.3 percent tested positive for syphilis.

49

In addition to the poverty and pre-existing disease of the mothers, many of these women who gave birth at home between 1930 and 1960 were at risk for complications of birth. Miller[47] discovered that the midwives of the Catholic Maternity Institute in Santa Fe successfully attended 4 women at home after previous Cesarean sections. The Institute also reported that, of a series of 2303 home births, 24 percent of the mothers were grand multiparas, having had six or more children.[47] The New York Maternity Center reported that, in a series of 6000 births, 55 mothers with multiple pregnancies were delivered at home.[36]

The condition of the homes in which the children were born was often much worse than the health of the mothers. The midwives of the Catholic Maternity Institute, for example, often attended births in homes with no electricity or running water.[17] Byington[8] described the house of an immigrant steel worker in 1910, probably not different in degree from the tenements where the poor of the 1930's gave birth:

[The lodging house] consisted of two rooms, one above the other. . . . In the kitchen was the wife of the boarding boss getting dinner . . . In these two rooms besides the boarding boss . . . his wife and two babies, lived 20 men.

A 1942 survey of 15 medical schools which conducted home delivery services revealed that only 10 investigated the home beforehand "to determine its suitability as a place for delivery,"[40] perhaps because their clients could not have afforded any alternative. Buxbaum[6] described the birthplaces of Chicago's poor:

. . . the homes are usually of the worst type in which to do good aseptic obstetrics. Oftentimes our doctors are compelled to work without the aid of hot water, heat or even light, and the sanitary conditions are indescribable.

The physician who attended home births was often poorly trained in obstetrics, although the graduates of the Chicago Maternity Center Clinic were exceptionally well-trained. In 1931 the Council on Medical Education of the A.M.A. reported that of 1,491 interns in approved teaching hospitals, 334 graduated without having delivered any infants, and 235 had not even observed deliveries; more than 200 had attended fewer than 10 deliveries and only 70 had attended 50 or more.[4]

The survey of home delivery services of 15 medical schools in 1941[40] revealed that at two schools medical students usually were not supervised even for their first delivery at home, while at 10 schools the student was supervised by an intern or resident for his or her first and perhaps second delivery. "The work of the students during the immediate puerperium was characterized in nearly every school by the casual care given the newborn . . ." The author concluded:

Students assigned to home delivery service are receiving their first practical obstetric training. For a school to have this take place under the worst possible circumstances, with a minimum of equipment, inadequate facilities for efficiently carrying out good aseptic technique, and little or no supervision at any time seems nothing short of criminal . . . Is it any wonder that almost all physicians have a false feeling of confidence that they are perfectly able to deliver almost any woman?

In spite of the frequent poor health and high risk conditions of women who delivered at home in the years between 1930 and 1960, and in spite of poor home conditions and lack of adequate training of doctors who did home deliveries, in many parts of the country birth attendants did not have access to a hospital for emergencies. The Chicago and New York Maternity Centers had very efficient emergency hospitalization procedures, however.[42] Elsewhere, lack of hospital back-up and the current popularity of operative obstetrics resulted in many operations and complicated deliveries carried out at home. Garrison in 1943 stated that he had done more than 2500 forceps deliveries and 1000 versions

50

at home.[20] In a review article on home obstetrics, Buxbaum of the Chicago Maternity Center advised:

> Forceps delivery, version, breech extraction, manual removal of the placenta, uterine tamponade and primary perineorrhaphy can readily and safely be performed in the home.[7]

Where a hospital was not available for emergencies, even cesarean sections were performed at home. Plass[56] reported in a study of 56,000 home births, that 111 cesarean sections and one craniotomy had been done at home births. Inhalation anesthesia was freely used at home births as well. In 6 of the 15 medical school home delivery services surveyed by Makepeace[40] in 1941, the medical student routinely gave inhalation anesthetics, while at another 6 schools, the student occasionally administered these anesthetics. One attendant[21] reported the use of open drop ether and scopolamine at home, and another,[46] chloroform. Buxbaum[7] advised that "local anesthesia is the anesthesia of choice, but ether can be employed using a tea strainer as a mask." Beard[2] found that his clients could not afford "to pay fees commensurate to having an anesthetist or nurse in attendance, so we depend upon members of the family . . . to drop chloroform."

Couples who have a home birth today choose it because they perceive it to have medical and/or socio-psychological advantages over hospital birth. The few studies of home birth populations[25,45] found the couples to be almost entirely white, middle class, well-nourished and often college educated. Also in contrast to home birth between 1930 and 1960, the attendants today, although composed not just of doctors and nurse-midwives, but mainly of lay midwives, carefully screen their clients to insure that only healthy women who are not likely to develop complications are followed during home birth.[13,14] Although it is often difficult for lay midwives to obtain, hospital back-up is almost uniformly arranged, in case of complications of home birth or early postpartum period. Except

for occasional episiotomies, no operations are now performed at home births. High risk conditions such as premature birth or low birth weight babies are carefully screened and not delivered at home. Low birth weight accounts for 66 percent of our perinatal mortality[30] and is largely associated with poverty and multiparity.[58] 75 percent of the recent reduction in neonatal mortality has been attributed to reduction of the incidence of low birth weight rate, and *not to changes in obstetric care.*[38] Diabetes, hypertension, toxemia, multiple gestation, and intercurrent illness indicate hospitalization for birth. Drugs used during home births today are limited to local anesthetics, oxytocin after the birth of the baby, vitamin K, silver nitrate, and antibiotics if needed.[13]

Safety of Home Birth Compared to Hospital Birth from 1930 to 1960

Because of the frequent poverty and resultant poor health of many women who gave birth at home between 1930 and 1960, and because of the poor condition of their homes, the poor training and "operative furor" of many of their attendants, and often the impossibility of hospital emergency care, one would expect that maternal and perinatal mortality would be high. This is not shown by the literature of the period.

A number of studies completed between 1930 and 1960 attempted to determine the relative safety of home and hospital birth. Each of the studies was either a crude comparison of the mortality rates of a local home birth population to the national rates or to a local hospital birth population. Since the mean socioeconomic status of the home birth population appears to have been below that of the hospital populations, and since socio-economic status is directly related to successful obstetric outcome,[56] the obstetric outcome for women who gave birth at home would have to have been matched to that of hospitalized parturients by economic status, and age, parity, and health status as well for an accurate comparison. Since this was not done, few

Table 1

Table 1
Maternal Mortality by Place of Birth—Minneapolis

	Live Births	Maternal Mortality/1000 live births Home			Maternal Mortality/1000 live births Hospital			
		Home %	Total	Sepsis	Hemorrhage	Hosp %	Total	Hosp Sepsis	Hemorrhage
1925	9423	28	3.1	1.9	0	72	3.5	0.3	0.4
1926	9192	25	3.0	0.9	0	75	5.6	1.4	0.4
1927	8620	23	2.5	2.0	0	77	2.5	0.7	0.6
1928	8348	21.5	5.0	3.4	0	78.5	3.8	0.4	0.9
Total	35583	24.2	3.4	2.0	0	75.8	3.9	0.74	0.59

From Holmes RW: Maternal Mortality. JAMA 93:1440-47, 1929.

solid conclusions can be based on the data presented.

Also, reliable statistics were not kept by individuals who attended home births, in contrast to the meticulous records of the 3 established midwifery services—Maternity Center Association, Frontier Nursing Service, Catholic Maternity Institute of Santa Fe—and the home birth services conducted by medical schools, such as the Chicago Maternity Center, and Boston Lying-In.

Holmes[29] presented data (Table 1) comparing home and hospital birth in Minneapolis from 1925 to 1928. The difference between home and hospital for the total maternal deaths in 1928 is not significant (p value = .48) nor is the difference in the total death rate for all four years significant (p value = .50). However the rate of puerperal sepsis following delivery in the hospital was significantly lower than at home (p value = .003). Thus in Minneapolis sepsis mortality was more prevalent at home and hemorrhage more frequent in the hospital so that the overall maternal death rate did not differ significantly between the two places of birth.

The most famous and controversial[43] comparison of the relative safety of home birth was the New York Academy of Medicine study of maternal mortality in New York City in the early 1930's (Table 2). The total maternal mortality rate, the rate of maternal mortality from puerperal septicemia, and the rate of mortality from hemorrhage were all significantly lower at home (all p values less than .0001).

Since "domiciliary obstetrical practice [was] largely confined to the foreign born and economically less fortunate,"[50] and since "the general puerperal death rate among foreign born women [was] considerably higher than that among the native born,"[50] the lower maternal mortality rate at home is surprising. The study committee cautioned that midwives and general practitioners, who attended the bulk of the home births, generally had less complicated cases than the obstetricians who confined their practice to the hospitals. But the committee thought it improbable that one-half of the obstetricians' cases were abnormal "as would be necessary if the rate were to be lowered to that of the general practitioners."[50] The committee concluded:

Table 2
Maternal Mortality in New York City 1930-1932

Place of birth	Total births	%	Maternal deaths	MMR/ 1,000	Sepsis deaths/ 1,000	Hemorrhage deaths/ 1,000
Home	102,105	29.3	189	1.9	0.9	0.26
Hospital	246,205	70.7	1,111	4.5	1.6	0.61
Total	348,310	100	1,300	3.7	1.5	0.51

MMR: maternal Mortality rate

from New York Academy of Medicine: *Maternal Mortality in New York City*. The Commonwealth Fund, New York, 1933.

Table 3
Iowa: Stillbirths by Place of Birth

Place of birth	Total births	%	Stillbirths %	Operative deliveries %	% Stillbirths Spontaneous births only
A. Communities greater than 10,000					
Home	11,858	39.2	2.7*	7.5	2.0†
Hospital	18,393	60.8	3.9*	23.1	2.5†
Total	30,251	100	3.4	17	2.3
B. Communities less than 10,000					
Home	49,542	80.6	2.7	8.1	2.0*
Hospital	11,945	19.4	2.7	14	1.2*
Total	61,487	100	2.7	9.3	1.6

*significant, p less than .0001
†significant, p = .009

from Plass ED, Alvis HJ: A Statistical Study of 129,539 Births in Iowa. Am J Ob Gyn 28:293-305, 1934.

. . . there can be little doubt that the ready facilities of a hospital tend to cause casual operative interference while conditions at home preclude operation unless there are urgent indications . . . [T]he patient who is delivered at home is subjected to fewer potential sources of danger . . . It would seem that the present attitude toward home confinements requires re-examination, and a program looking toward an increase in the practice of domiciliary obstetrics deserves careful investigation.

Plass and Alvis[56] studied the incidence of stillbirth among 129,500 births in Iowa (Table 3) and concluded that:

The significant increase in the stillbirth rate in urban hospitals over that of other groups is probably related to the increased incidence of operative delivery.

While, overall, the stillbirth rate was lower for home than for hospital, women who had a spontaneous hospital birth had a significantly lower stillbirth rate than their counterparts at home in the smaller communities. This relationship is reversed in the larger communities.

Hannah[24] reviewed 1809 home births compared to 436 hospital births on the Baylor Hospital charity service in 1939 (Table 4). The stillbirth rate was significantly lower at home (p value less than .0001) while the neonatal death rates did not differ significantly. Operative in-

terference in birth was much more common in the hospital. Hannah attributed the better results at home to the higher proportion of multiparas delivered there and the lesser degree of sedation used at home.

Stout,[61] of Johns Hopkins, studied the incidence of puerperal infection among women who had spontaneous multiparous births in the home and in the hospital charity service there. In his first series (819 deliveries) he found a maternal infection rate of 4.4% in the hospital and 0.8% at home. In the second series (875 births), when the temperature of the woman at home was taken in the afternoon in addition to a morning reading, the rate of infection was 4.9% at the hospital and 8.4% at home (significant, p value = .044). There was no difference in the severity of infection between the two groups. However the rate of mortality from puerperal infection was not different between home and hospital groups. Dowling,[12] in a survey of maternal mortality in Alabama, found no significant difference (p = .52) in the rate of death from puerperal sepsis: a mortality rate of 8.4/1000 live births for 16,633 home deliveries and 9.0 per 1000 for 22,728 hospital births.

Irving[31] examined maternal mortality in Massachusetts according to place of birth (Table 5). While the maternal death rate was significantly higher at home than in maternity hospitals or than in all hospitals, Irving attributed the poor record of home deliveries in Massachusetts

Table 4
Charity Service: Baylor Hospital

Place of birth	Total births	PMR/ 1000	Stillbirths/ 1000	NMR/ 1000	Maternal infection	Episiotomy	Forceps
Home	1809	38	2.8	23.8	5.2%	5.3%	10.3%
Hospital	436	78	27.5	22.9	4.8% *	74.3%	63.8%
Total	2245	46	7.6	23.6		18.7%	20.7%

PMR: Fetal, intrapartum, and neonatal deaths
NMR: Neonatal mortality rate
* Charity and private patients

from Hannah CR, et al: A Review of 4,000 Consecutive Deliveries in the Baylor Out-patient and Hospital Service. Tex St J Med 35:535-40, 1939.

to inadequate care delivered by physicians or to unnecessary intervention in labor. In contrast, the home delivery service of the Boston Lying-in Hospital, which was conducted by supervised fourth year medical students, had a mortality rate far below that of any class of hospital. This home delivery service found it necessary to transfer only 2.1% of its clients to the hospital.[31]

Tucker and Benarm[66] reported the results of 12,597 home deliveries attended by the physicians of Chicago's Maternity Center Clinic from 1932 to 1936. 15% of the women had not received prenatal care at the clinic and were seen for the first time in labor. 4.4% of the women were eventually hospitalized. 18 women died, 5 of whom were seen fo ꞏhe first time in labor. The maternal ꞏ ortality rate was 14.2 per 10,000 live bi ꞏhs at a time when the national rate wa: 59. If the 5 deaths from tuberculosis and the 2 from pneumonia were excluded, the corrected mortality rate would have been 9/10,000, a rate finally achieved by the United States as a whole in 1949—13 years later.

Laird[36] reported the results of 5,765 births attended by the nurse-midwives of the Maternity Center Clinic in New York from 1931 to 1951. 13.5% of the women were eventually transferred to the hospital. 5 maternal deaths gave the Center a maternal mortality rate of 8.8 per 10,000 live births (compared to a U.S. rate of 31.7 in 1941) and a neonatal death rate of 15 per 1000 live births. Laird emphasized that

In this group there was a high incidence of poor nutrition, poor home conditions, low income, unmarried mothers, and high parity. In spite of this, our neonatal death rate is much lower than the rate for the whole clinic area.

The final report of the Maternity Center home delivery service compared the record of the clinic to the mortality rates of the New York Hospital and concluded that the Maternity Center Association Clinic had achieved "results in maternal and perinatal mortality comparable to a fine teaching hospital."[15]

Table 5
Maternal Mortality in Massachusetts

Place of Birth	Live Births	Maternal Deaths/1000 Live Births	
Maternity Hospital	9,873	2.9	
General and Other	74,697	4.9	
All Hospitals	84,570	4.6	1934-1935
Home	42,191	5.5	
Boston Lying-In Total	10,590	3.5	
			1933-1935
Boston Lying-In Out-patient	3,301	0.3	

from Irving FC: Maternal Mortality at the Boston Lying-In Hospital in 1933, 1934, and 1935. N England J Med 217:693-95, 1937.

For the first 4,000 deliveries attended by the nurse-midwives of the Frontier Nursing Servcie from 1925 to 1940, Steele[60] reported a maternal mortality rate of 7.6/10,000 compared to a U.S. rate of 62/10,000 in 1933. The clients of the Frontier Nursing Service had a stillbirth rate of 30.2/1000 pregnancies and a neonatal mortality rate of 30.3/ 1000 live births compared to a U.S. rate of 34 at the midpoint year. 7.3% of the women required hospitalization. However the rate of hospitalization increased during the series to 12.3% in the fourth 1000 births. The episiotomy rate was 0.4%.

In contrast to the relatively favorable reports of homebirth presented above, Newberger[49] found that both the fetal and maternal death rates were significantly higher at home than in the hospital in downstate Illinois (Table 6). However the meaning of the difference in maternal mortality cannot be settled without knowing the place of occurrence of the 27 deaths due to criminal abortion and ectopic pregnancy since there were only 30 maternal deaths at home. With 94% of all births taking place in the hospital, the few women remaining at home were more likely to be poor, and in poor health. Record keeping by individuals doing home deliveries was also poor, compared to the careful statistics kept by the medical school home birth services and the 3 midwifery home birth services of the period.

normal labor. The recent claim that hospitalization, *per se,* is pathogenic in normal birth, cannot be evaluated from the information presented in these studies. However, Tew[63] has recently shown that in Britain the stillbirth rate is lower at home even for supposed high risk births. She concludes:

> The conventional apology for this wide disparity is that a far greater proportion of births at high risk, with inevitably high death rates, takes place in consultant hospitals than at home . . . [Even if one assumed] that 20 percent of hospital births had three or more high risk characteristics and had the very high average stillbirth rate of 50.0 per 1000, the stillbirth rate for the remaining 80 percent, with less than three high risk characteristics, would have been . . . one third higher than the home rate . . . [given the actual stillbirth rates of 14.8/1000 (hospital) and 4.5/1000 (home) in Britain for 1969-1973.]

Particularly at the New York Maternity Center and the Frontier Nursing Service, the relative safety of home birth should not be attributed solely to the poor quality of hospital obstetrics but also to the skill and dedication of nurse-midwives trained to understand normal childbirth and familiar with the home conditions of their clients.

Table 6
Maternal Mortality in Downstate Illinois

	Live births	% at home	Fetal deaths/1000 live births		Maternal deaths/10,000 live births	
			Home	Hospital	Home	Hospital
1948	103,777	6.9	38	16	17	8
1949	107,015	5.3	35	15	18	7
1950	107,464	4.2	37	14	18	6

from Newberger C: Maternal Mortality in Downstate Illinois. JAMA 149:328-30, 1952. Used with permission of the JAMA. "Copyright 1952, American Medical Association"

The above studies were so different in design and population and so limited in analysis that few generalizations can be made from them. It is evident that much of the poor record of hospital births was due to the greater tendency of hospital-based physicians to interfere in

Table 7 presents data on parallel declines in home birth and obstetric mortality from 1935 to 1961. In order to quantify any causal relationship between parallel declines, correlation coefficients are computed for annual percent changes in maternal mortality and hospitalization

55

207

Table 7

	MMR/ 10,000	% Decline	NMR/ 1,000	% Decline	Hospital Births %	% Increase
1935	58.2		32.4		36.9	
1936	56.8	2.4	32.6	+0.6	40.9	10.8
1937	48.9	13.9	31.3	4.0	44.8	9.5
1938	43.5	11.0	29.6	5.4	48.0	7.1
1939	40.4	7.1	29.3	1.0	51.1	6.5
1940	37.6	6.9	28.8	1.7	55.8	9.2
1941	31.7	15.7	27.7	3.8	61.2	9.7
1942	25.9	18.3	25.7	7.2	67.9	10.9
1943	24.5	5.4	24.7	3.9	72.1	6.2
1944	22.8	6.9	24.7	0	75.6	4.9
1945	20.7	9.2	24.3	1.6	78.8	4.2
1946	15.7	24.3	24.0	1.2	82.4	4.6
1947	13.5	14.0	22.8	5.0	84.8	2.9
1948	11.7	13.3	22.2	2.6	85.6	0.9
1949	9.03	22.8	- .	3.6	86.7	1.3
1950	8.33	7.8		4.2	88.0	1.5
1951	7.50	10.0		2.4	90.0	2.3
1952	6.78	9.6	21.3	1.0	91.7	0.8
1953	6.11	9.9	19.6	1.0	92.8	1.2
1954	5.24	14.2	19.1	2.6	93.6	0.9
1955	4.70	10.3	19.1	0	94.4	0.9
1956	4.09	13.0	18.9	1.0	95.1	0.7
1957	4.10	+0.2	19.0	+0.5	95.7	0.6
1958	3.76	8.3	19.5	+2.6	96.0	0.3
1959	3.74	0.5	19.0	2.6	96.4	0.4
1960	3.71	0.8	18.7	1.6	96.6	0.2
1961	3.69	0.5	18.4	1.6	96.9	0.3

MMR: maternal mortality rate
NMR: neonatal mortality rate

Maternal mortality rates from *Historical Statistics of the United States: Colonial Times to 1957.* GPO, Washington, D.C., 1960.

and Garfinkel J, et al: Infant, Maternal, and Childhood Mortality in the United States, 1968-1973. DHEW #75-5013, 1975.

All other data from Trends in Infant and Childhood Mortality, 1961. Children's Bureau Statistical Series #76. GPO, Washington, D.C., 1964.

of birth (R = -0.26, p = 0.2, not significant). The figures do not prove that hospitalization has no impact upon obstetric mortality, but simply that any causal relationship is not shown in the nationwide data for the years 1930 to 1960.

Those in medicine and public health have justified hospitalization and other medical intervention in childbirth by pointing to declines in perinatal mortality which were concurrent with increases in whatever surgical or technological practices were in vogue. However, perinatal mortality is largely dependent on social factors, especially nutrition and standard of living, rather than birth practices. Many social changes between 1930 and 1960 worked to reduce obstetric mortality. The New Dealers[62] emphasized that ". . . the decrease in both maternal and infant mortality rates have been greater during the 5 years of Federal and State cooperation under the Social

Security Act than during the 5 previous years." Another reason for the decline in obstetric mortality in the mid-thirties was the introduction of sulfanilamide to obstetrics in 1936.[31] The availability of penicillin for clinical practice in the early forties may have also contributed to the decline in obstetric mortality. In any period of very low birth rate, such as the 1930's and the 1970's, perinatal mortality can be expected to decline due to the reduction of multiparity and thus low birth weight babies. Both the low birth rate periods of the 1930's and the 1970's have been periods of rising obstetrical intervention, the early period being one of forceps and anesthesia, and the present period one of fetal monitoring and cesarean section. It is fascinating that in both cases, falling perinatal mortality due to lower birth rates, both stimulated increased obstetrical intervention, and was cited as its justification.

Conclusion

While the techniques of modern hospital obstetrics have saved the lives of many women and infants from genuine pathologies of birth, the literature of obstetrics in the United States from 1930 to 1960 does not show that healthy women with normal pregnancies benefitted from hospital obstetric care. Although statistically inconclusive, most of the comparative studies of home and hospital birth from the period, show that the incidence of birth injuries and obstetric mortality was greater in hospitals, probably due to interference in the normal birth process. These studies suggest that, despite the poverty, ill health and frequent high risk conditions of women who delivered at home, and despite the frequent poor training of attendants, and the operations and anesthesias used—often in crowded unsanitary settings—home birth was not less safe than hospital birth from 1930 to 1960.

REFERENCES

1. Bartholomew RA: Utopian Obstetrics. Am J Ob Gyn 44:553-58, 1942.
2. Beard HE: Home Obstetrics. W Virginia Med J 36:18-22, 1940.
3. Bolduan C, Weiner L: Infant Mortality in New York City One Hundred Years Ago. J of Pediatrics 7:55-9, 1935.
4. Boyd MS: Why Mothers Die. Nation 132: 293-5, 1931.
5. Brown WE: The Trend of Modern Obstetrics. J Iowa St Med Soc 20:550-3, 1930.
6. Buxbaum H: Out-patient Obstetrics: A Review of 6,863 Cases. Am J Ob Gyn 31: 409-19, 1936.
7. Buxbaum H: Obstetrics in the Home. Surg Clinics of N Am 23:45-58, Feb 1943.
8. Byington M: Homestead, the Households of a Mill Town. Russell Sage Foundation,1910, reprinted: University of Pittsburgh, 1974.
9. Childbirth: Nature vs. Drugs. Time 27:32-36, May 25, 1936.
10. Childbirth without Pain. Newsweek 21:65, Feb 1, 1943.
11. DeLee JB: The Prophylactic Forceps Operation. Trans Am Gyn Soc 45:66-83, 1920.
12. Dowling JD: Points of Interest in a Survey of Maternal Mortality—Alabama. Am J Public Health 27:803-08, 1937.
13. Epstein JL, et al: A Safe Homebirth Program that Works. in Stewart L, Stewart D (eds.): Safe Alternatives in Childbirth. NAPSAC, Chapel Hill, 1976.
14. Ettner FM: Study of Obstetrics. 1975. Ibid.
15. Faison JB: Report of the Maternity Center Association Clinic, 1952-1958. Am J Ob Gyn 81:395-402, 1961.
16. Falls FH: Effect of the War on the Maternal Welfare Program in Illinois. Ill J of Med 83:259-63, 1943.
17. Fell F: A Midwifery Delivery Service. Am J Nurs 45:220-22, 1945.
18. Frankel LK: The Present Status of Maternal and Infant Hygiene in the United States. Am J Public Health 17:1909-39, 1927.
19. Garfinkel J, et al: Infant, Maternal, and Childhood Mortality in the United States, 1968-1973. DHEW #75-5013, 1975.
20. Garrison JE: Delivering Babies at Home. J Med Assoc Alabama 12:228-31, 1943.
21. Giletto BJ: Management of Home Deliveries. Med Clinics of N Am 29:1525-37, 1945.
22. Goldthorp WO, Richman J: Maternal Attitudes to Unintended Home Confinement. The Practitioner 212:845-53, 1974.
23. Guttmacher AF: Obstetrics Today and Tomorrow. Bull NY Acad Med 19:555-62, 1943.
24. Hannah CR, et al: A Review of 4,000 Consecutive Deliveries in the Baylor Out-patient and Hospital Service. Tex St J Med 35: 535-40, 1939.

25. Hazell LD: Birth Goes Home. Catalyst Publishing Co., Seattle, 1974.

26. Historical Statistics of the United States: Colonial Times to 1957. GPO, Washington, D.C., 1960.

27. Holmes B: The Hospital Problem. JAMA 47:318-20, 1906.

28. Holmes RW: The Fads and Fancies of Obstetrics. Am J Ob Gyn 2:225-37, 1921.

29. Holmes RW: Maternal Mortality. JAMA 93:1440-47, 1929.

30. Hunter Jones O: Cesarean Section in Present Day Obstetrics. (Editor's note) Ob Gyn Survey 32:220-24, 1977.

31. Irving FC: Maternal Mortality at the Boston Lying-in Hospital in 1933, 1934, and 1935. N England J Med 217:693-95, 1937.

32. Jacobson PH: Hospital Care and the Vanishing Midwife. Millbank Memorial Fund Quarterly 34:253-61. 1956.

33. Kooser JH: Rural Obstetrics: A Report of the Work of the Frontier Nursing Service. Southern Med J 35:123-31, 1942.

34. Kosmak GW: The Favorable and Unfavorable Results from the Practice of Modern Obstetric Trends and Procedures. Mississippi Doctor 16:1-11, 1938.

35. de Kruif P: Why Should Mothers Die? Ladies' Home J 53:8+, Mar 1936.

36. Laird MD: Report of the Maternity Center Association Clinic, New York, 1931-1951. Am J Ob Gyn 69:178-84, 1955.

37. Lee F, Glasser J: The Role of Lay Midwifery in Maternity Care in a Large Urban Area. Public Health Rep 89:537-44, 1974.

38. Lee K, et al: Determinants of Neonatal Mortality. Ob Gyn Survey 32:153-55, 1977.

39. Letourneau CU: Hospitals and the Prevention of Neonatal Mortality. JAMA 153:476-79, 1953.

40. Makepeace AW: The Home Delivery Service. The Child 7:36-9, 1942.

41. Maternal Mortality Lowest where Hospital Confinement is most Frequent. Statistical Bull, Metro Life Ins Co 26:6-8, 1945.

42. Maternity Center Association—New York: Preparing for a Delivery in the Home. Am J Nursing 40:1323-27, 1940.

43. Maternity Death Rate. News Week 2:27, Nov 25, 1933.

44. McEvoy JP: Our Streamlined Baby. Readers' Digest 32:15-18, 1938.

45. Mehl LE, et al: Complications of Home Birth. Birth and the Family J 2:123-31, 1975.

46. Miller DG: Home Obstetrics. New Orleans Med and Surg J 101:167-71, 1949.

47. Miller E: Grand Multiparas. Ob Gyn 4:418-25, 1954.

48. Montagu MFA: Babies Should Be Born at Home. Ladies' Home J 72:52+, Sep 1955.

49. Newberger C: Maternal Mortality in Downstate Illinois. JAMA 149:328-30, 1952.

50. New York Academy of Medicine: *Maternal Mortality in New York City.* The Commonwealth Fund, New York, 1933.

51. O'Brien J: Factors in Obstetric Care. N Y St J of Med 43:236-44, 1943.

52. Olson RM: A Home Delivery Service. Am J Nursing 42:877-8, 1942.

53. Pathak UN: The Place for Confinement: Home or Hospital. Brit J Clinical Practice 14:111-14, 1960.

54. Pearse WH: The Image of the Obstetrician Gynecologist. Ob Gyn 48:611-12, 1976.

55. Peller S: Studies on Mortality Since the Renaissance. Bull Hist Med 13:427-61,1943.

56. Plass ED, Alvis HJ: A Statistical Study of 129,539 Births in Iowa. Am J Ob Gyn 28:293-305, 1934.

57. Proc of the 1975 Conference on Women and Health. (Chapter on Resources, p. 57) Boston Women's Health Collective, Box 192, W. Somerville, Ma. 02144.

58. Rider RV, et al: Associations between Premature Birth and Socio-economic Status. Am J Public Health 45:1022-28, 1955.

59. Smith HH: Back to the Midwife? New Republic 79:207, 1934.

60. Steele EJ: Report on the Fourth Thousand Confinements. Quart Bull Frontier Nurs Serv 16:4-13, 1941.

61. Stout ML: Incidence of Puerperal Infection. Am J Ob Gyn 29:588-90, 1935.

62. Tandy ED: Maternal and Infant Mortality in 1939. Child 5:189-96, 1941.

63. Tew M: Where to be Born. New Society 120-21, Jan 20, 1977.

64. Todd CL: Easier Motherhood. Ladies' Home J 47:9+, Mar 1930.

65. Trends in Infant and Childhood Mortality, 1961. Children's Bureau Statistical Series #76. GPO, 1964.

66. Tucker B, Benarm H: Maternal Mortality of the Chicago Maternity Center. Am J Public Health 27:33-36, 1937.

67. Vogue Answers Questions on Childbirth. Readers' Digest 43:33-35, Sep 1943.

68. White House Conference on Child Health Protection: Forceps and Cesarean Section. *Fetal, Newborn and Maternal Mortality.* D. Appleton-Century Co., New York, 1932.

69. The Week. New Republic 66:339-40, 1931.

58

PIONEERING IN FAMILY-CENTERED MATERNITY AND INFANT CARE: EDITH B. JACKSON AND THE YALE ROOMING-IN RESEARCH PROJECT*

Sara Lee Silberman

> It is too bad that good things that get started
> have to be stopped and forgotten; and then
> started as something new.
>
> —Edith B. Jackson, 23 August 1965[1]

Historians have recently chronicled dramatic changes that occurred during the first half of the twentieth century in three related areas of American medicine: (1) birthing procedures; (2) infant-feeding practices; and (3) the role of the hospital. In *Brought to Bed: Childbearing in America, 1750–1950*, Judith Walzer Leavitt details "the single most important transition in childbirth history," namely, the movement of parturition from "a natural home event" presided over by a woman's relatives and friends, to "a physician-directed medical and surgical event" that women experienced "alone among strangers" in the hospital.[2] Rima D. Apple's *Mothers and Medicine: A Social History of Infant Feeding, 1890–1950* addresses the "profound transformation of infant feeding and of mothers' nurturing role" that paralleled those changes in birthing. She points out that in 1900 "the overwhelming majority of infants received their nourishment at the breast" and "few physicians concerned themselves with infant feeding," whereas by 1950, "American women commonly bottle fed their infants" under the supervision of doctors who "stressed that they, as medical practitioners, were the experts who held knowledge unavailable to the laity."[3] Finally,

* This article is an expanded version of a talk presented at the sixtieth annual meeting of the American Association for the History of Medicine, Philadelphia, Pennsylvania, 2 May 1987. I am grateful to two anonymous *Bulletin* referees for very helpful comments on an earlier draft; to Garry M. Brodsky for careful readings of two drafts; to *Bulletin* copyeditor Miriam Kleiger; and to Connecticut College for a grant that facilitated final revisions.

[1] Edith B. Jackson to Morris [Wessel], 23 August 1965, Edith B. Jackson Papers, Schlesinger Library, Harvard University, Cambridge, Massachusetts.

[2] Judith Walzer Leavitt, *Brought to Bed: Childbearing in America, 1750–1950* (New York: Oxford University Press, 1986), pp. 195, 140, 171.

[3] Rima D. Apple, *Mothers and Medicine: A Social History of Infant Feeding, 1890–1950* (Madison: University of Wisconsin Press, 1987), pp. 3, 4, 94, 18. Apple acknowledges that many mothers between 1910 and 1920 "demanded that doctors supply them with formulas." She quotes a St. Louis practitioner who claimed that his colleagues "have to [prescribe formulas], for if we did not the other doctor across the street would." *Ibid.*, p. 75.

Charles E. Rosenberg, in *The Care of Strangers: The Rise of America's Hospital System,* notes a "transforming"[4] experience in American hospitals during that same period. Whereas in the eighteenth and nineteenth centuries the nation's few hospitals cared for the indigent and the homeless, Rosenberg shows that by the 1920s, when a hospital could offer antiseptic surgery, the X-ray, and the clinical laboratory, even the wealthiest Americans wanted their surgery, acute ailments, and parturitions attended to there.[5] Equally striking were simultaneous changes in hospital procedures and governance. The casual, paternalistic practices of the traditional institutions' lay founders were replaced by "an impersonal, intrusive, and highly structured routinism" that made it clear that doctors and such Progressive Era values as bureaucracy, efficiency, and medical professionalism had come to dominate twentieth-century American hospitals.[6]

Although the transformations in birthing, infant feeding and hospital care occurred independently of one another, they had characteristics in common. First, each represented a technological approach to one of the health and social problems that increasingly engaged Americans' attention early in the twentieth century: respectively, the maternal death rate in childbirth;[7] an alarming infant mortality rate that experts widely attributed to poor nutrition;[8] and the decreasing availability of female friends and relatives to help women through parturition.[9] In response to those circumstances, the modern, antiseptic hospital offered women both a supervised, safe, and even painless labor and delivery and the expertise of pediatric house officers who prescribed exactly when and what "scientific" formula infants should be fed.[10] For newborns, the hospital offered protection in an isolated, well-supervised nursery against disease from fellow patients, their own fathers, or other visitors.[11]

[4] Charles E. Rosenberg, *The Care of Strangers: The Rise of America's Hospital System* (New York: Basic Books, 1987), p. 341.

[5] *Ibid.,* chap. 10.

[6] Rosenberg, *Care of Strangers,* chaps. 11, 12. Quotation is on p. 290. For a characterization of Progressive Era values, see Robert Wiebe, *The Search for Order, 1877–1920* (New York: Hill & Wang, 1967).

[7] For a judicious treatment of what Leavitt calls the "almost impossible" task faced by historians who seek an accurate reading of the maternal mortality rate in childbirth in the nineteenth and early twentieth centuries, see Leavitt, *Brought to Bed,* pp. 23–28. Beyond dispute is the fact that women's fears of dying in childbirth remained intense into the 1920s; by then many had come to believe that hospital birthing might be safer than giving birth at home.

[8] Apple, *Mothers and Medicine,* p. 4.

[9] Leavitt, *Brought to Bed,* p. 194. In *The Care of Strangers,* Rosenberg makes it clear that the transformation in usage and governance of the American hospital had many more causes than the decreasing availability of a female support system for women in labor. I mention the last-named factor here because, starting in the 1920s, it was responsible for significantly increasing the desire of middle-class, married women to give birth in a hospital.

[10] "We pediatricians of that day did not allow our mothers to use their own judgment in feeding their babies," one of them later recalled. "They were taught that the feeding schedule should be rigidly followed" and "that the time to indicate [sic] regular habits began in early infancy." [Edith B. Jackson], "Evolution in the Psychological Care of Infants and Children," 1947, p. 3. (Typed manuscript in the private papers of William S. Jackson, Denver, Colorado.) I am deeply indebted to William S. Jackson, Edith Jackson's nephew, for access to this and many other papers that belonged to his aunt.

[11] At most famous European maternity hospitals, nurseries were unheard of in the first half of the twentieth century, and hospital nurseries did not become prevalent in the United States until the turn of the century.

Second, each transformation had these consequences: American women relied less on instinct and friends and more on science, medical professionals, and the hospital when they experienced childbirth and cared for their newborns; and they substantially benefited from the changes. By 1950, thanks to antibiotics, transfusions, and analgesics available only in hospitals, childbirth was both safer and less painful than ever before. In addition, mothers who bottle-fed their infants a physician-prescribed formula got relief not only from anxiety about whether their babies were getting adequate nutrition but also from the confinement that being their newborn's sole source of nourishment entailed. Finally, a ten-day postpartum stay in a clean, well-run hospital, with responsibility only for every-four-hour daytime feedings of their infants, allowed modern American mothers far more rest after their hospital deliveries than had been possible for their foremothers who gave birth at home. Not surprisingly, then, American women increasingly sought hospitalization for childbirth in the 1930s and 1940s and readily accepted physician-directed bottle feeding of their infants.[12]

In the late 1940s, however, a few women had begun to perceive and to deplore the costs, many of them psychological, of what they had gained in safety and convenience.[13] Unhappy with the impersonality and rigidity of hospital maternity and neonatal procedures that left them unconscious during delivery and largely separated from their infants during the lying-in period, they formed the small vanguard who adopted Grantly Dick-Read's natural childbirth techniques;[14] opted to "room-in" with their newborns in the few hospitals where that was possible at the time; and welcomed breast-feeding assistance when the La Leche League was formed in 1956. In each case, and with considerably more urgency and support from their peers by the 1960s and 1970s, American women sought, while retaining the gains, to recapture the human satisfactions and comforts of childbirth and breast-feeding that they had lost when "medicine intervened."[15]

This essay will describe an intervention by medical professionals in the 1930s and 1940s of a significantly different order. Intimately related to the

---

The New York Hospital, for example, had no nursery in 1896, and the Johns Hopkins Hospital was built without a nursery and had none until after 1890. Angus McBryde, "Compulsory rooming-in in the ward and private newborn service at Duke Hospital," *JAMA*, 1949, *145*: 627.

[12] Leavitt, *Brought to Bed*, chaps. 5, 7; Apple, *Mothers and Medicine*, chap. 9.

[13] Leavitt, *Brought to Bed*, p. 215; Apple, *Mothers and Medicine*, pp. 177–78. It should also be noted that some Progressive reformers, as early as the turn of the century, had rued the modern hospital's increasing concern with "diseases, not patients." In some localities, reformers managed to establish public health nursing and hospital social services that recognized "the need to follow the patient into his or her home." Rosenberg, *Care of Strangers*, pp. 152, 314. See also Charles E. Rosenberg, "Inward vision and outward glance: the shaping of the American hospital, 1880–1914," *Bull. Hist. Med.*, 1979, *53*: 349, 378.

[14] Grantly Dick-Read, *Childbirth without Fear: The Principles and Practice of Natural Childbirth* (New York: Harper & Row, 1944).

[15] Rosenberg, *Care of Strangers*, p. 347.

transformations in childbirth, infant feeding, and hospital care described by Leavitt, Apple, and Rosenberg, it nonetheless receives only passing mention in their books. I refer to the work of several small groups of psychologically oriented, hospital-based academic pediatricians, obstetricians, and child psychiatrists who shared neither the enthusiasm of their colleagues nor the optimism of their patients about the medical developments that were so rapidly and decisively changing the parturition and infant feeding experiences of American women.[16] Sooner than their patients, these physicians perceived what Rosenberg later explained so well: (1) the internal environment of the modern hospital, like that of "every other major institution in twentieth-century America," reflected the efforts of "increasingly self-conscious interest groups"—nurses, physicians, and administrators—"to find mutual adjustment" for their "competing needs;" and (2) because "no advocate of the patient's interest" had "figured in this evolution," the "patient's feelings" had played "no prominent role in the gradual definition of the hospital's internal environment."[17] In that context, these clinicians in effect *became* the advocates of the patient's interest in the impersonal, bureaucratic American hospital of the 1930s and 1940s. As such, their contribution to the history and practice of American medicine involved an effort to control, rather than advance, the processes whereby "the hospital had been medicalized" and "the medical profession had been hospitalized"[18] in the first half of the twentieth century.

To characterize and assess the contribution of these physicians, this essay will focus on the work of one of them, Edith Banfield Jackson (1895–1977).[19] A graduate of the Johns Hopkins University School of Medicine in 1921, an analysand of Sigmund Freud's from 1930 to 1936, and a clinical

---

[16] Two groups were especially notable and influential. The first included Erik H. Erikson, Benjamin Spock, Edith B. Jackson, and about a dozen other invited participants in the Conferences on Problems of Infancy and Childhood convened annually between 1947 and 1953 by the Josiah T. Macy, Jr., Foundation. These child psychiatrists, pediatricians, obstetricians, nurses, and nursery school educators, who regretted the thorough-going embrace by most doctors and their female patients of somatic, hospital-centered obstetrics and pediatrics, together hammered out arguments for a restoration of "family-centered" parturition and care of infants; the transactions of the Macy conferences, edited by Milton J. E. Senn, were published annually by the Josiah T. Macy, Jr., Foundation. A second interdisciplinary group equally committed to promoting family-centered maternity and infant care was based in Detroit and called itself the Cornelian Corner. *Newsweek*, reporting in 1949 on the origins of "what is regarded as one of the most revolutionary steps in pediatrics and obstetrics in the last 25 years," cited the seminal work of the Cornelian Corner, which advocated returning "to the practices of 50 years ago when babies were born at home, nursed by their mothers as often as they needed nourishment, and given unlimited 'mothering.'" Medicine, *Newsweek*, 21 March 1949, p. 52.

[17] Rosenberg, "Inward vision," p. 388.

[18] Rosenberg, *Care of Strangers*, p. 346.

[19] Edith Jackson was among the dozen regular participants at the Macy Conferences, and her views on breast-feeding and rooming-in clearly shaped the conferees' thinking; note that she and a nurse edited the conference's supplement on family-centered maternity and infant care. Edith B. Jackson and Genevieve Trainham, eds., *Family Centered Maternity and Infant Care: Report of the Committee on Rooming-in*, suppl. 1 to *Problems of Infancy and Childhood Transactions, Fourth Conference, 1950* (New York: Josiah Macy, Jr., Foundation, 1950). Note also that Benjamin Spock twice solicited Jackson's views on breast-feeding and rooming-in, once for an article he was writing for *Ladies' Home Journal* and once for a new edition of his celebrated *Baby and Child Care*. Ben [Spock] to Edie [Jackson], 16 September 1955, and Ben [Spock] to Edith [Jackson], 1 December 1955, Jackson Papers, Schlesinger Library. Jackson also corresponded regularly with members of the Cornelian Corner and on several occasions was an invited guest at their meetings in Detroit.

professor of pediatrics and psychiatry at the Yale School of Medicine for
more than two decades thereafter, Jackson directed an experimental
rooming-in project at the Grace–New Haven Community Hospital from
1946 to 1952. In that brief period, more than four hundred doctors, nurses,
and hospital administrators came from all over the world to observe the two
four-bed units in which mothers, attended by specially trained nurses and
pediatric fellows, roomed with their infants, calmly learning their babies'
needs and habits and nursing them at will.[20]

Historians of American medicine have variously forgotten, underesti-
mated, or misunderstood the significance of Jackson's work. In·1976 the
noted pediatrician Julius B. Richmond introduced a widely hailed book on
parent-infant "bonding" by his colleagues Marshall H. Klaus and John H.
Kennell as if their argument that hospital protocols should allow newborns
and their parents to be together after birth were original.[21] Richmond called
the authors "pioneers" in "reopening the nurseries ... to parents and their
families,"[22] even though every major idea in their book had been implemented in Jackson's Rooming-In Research Project thirty years earlier. More
recently, Rima Apple has acknowledged that rooming-in, for those few
women who experienced it in the 1940s and 1950s, effectively "eased the
tensions of new motherhood" by allowing the mother "to become familiar
with her infant before leaving the hospital." Apple misperceived the radical,
innovative character of the rooming-in concept, however, writing that
rooming-in ultimately "enhanced the medicalization of infant feeding by
promoting physicians and hospital personnel as the experts on child
care."[23] In fact, such was neither the intention nor the outcome of Jackson's
rooming-in project. Rooming-in was not one of the factors contributing to
the medicalization of parturition and infant care in the twentieth century.
Correctly understood, it stands—along with natural childbirth, a contempo-
raneous innovation—as a partially successful effort both to humanize birthing and feeding in a hospital setting and to re-empower the mother in those
crucial, natural, life experiences.

By describing Jackson's Rooming-In Research Project, it is possible both
to correct the historical record on rooming-in and to provide a case study
that makes concrete and particular several broader themes in twentieth-
century American medicine. First, in searching out the origins and purposes
of rooming-in, one can see that medical resistance to somatic, "hospitalized"
obstetrics and pediatrics in the United States has had virtually as long a

---

[20] "Guest Book of the Rooming-In Unit at Grace–New Haven Hospital," 9 April 1947 through 30 June 1952,
Edith B. Jackson Papers, Yale University Library, New Haven, Connecticut.

[21] The book, *Maternal-Infant Bonding: The Impact of Early Separation or Loss on Family Development*
(St. Louis: C. V. Mosby, 1976), is now in a revised, third, paperback edition: *Bonding: The Beginnings of
Parent-Infant Attachment* (St. Louis: C. V. Mosby; New York: New American Library, 1983).

[22] Julius H. Richmond, "Foreword," in Marshall H. Klaus and John H. Kennell, *Maternal-Infant Bonding*
(1976), p. x.

[23] Apple, *Mothers and Medicine*, pp. 178, 179.

history as has medical acceptance of this approach. Briefly stated, Jackson's program itself rested on ideas available decades earlier in the pediatric and psychoanalytic literature. Equally, though, the history of rooming-in at Grace–New Haven hospital reveals how thoroughly the developments noted by Leavitt, Apple, and Rosenberg had transformed American medicine by the middle of the twentieth century, because any account of Jackson's project must pay attention to the curious fact that rooming-in, although enormously satisfying for its participants and enthusiastically endorsed by physicians, nurses, and hospital administrators familiar with it, became the norm neither at Grace–New Haven nor at most other American hospitals after the project ended.[24] By detailing the medical establishment's resistance to "family-centered" infant and maternity care in the 1940s and 1950s, then, one can (1) account for that curious fact; (2) see how decisively hospital medicine has influenced the American health care system; and (3) understand why Klaus, Kennell, and others sharing Jackson's concerns in the late twentieth century have had, in effect, to "pioneer" all over again.

THE FIRST STEPS TOWARD THE ROOMING-IN RESEARCH PROJECT

Fresh from a six-year training analysis with Sigmund Freud and work in child analysis with Anna Freud, Edith Jackson assumed her part-time junior appointment in psychiatry and mental hygiene at Yale in the fall of 1936 with neither the intent nor a mandate to pioneer. The Yale School of Medicine was then a model of the scientific, somatic, hospital medicine she had learned at Johns Hopkins two decades before.[25] The chair of the Psychiatry and Mental Hygiene Department regarded psychoanalysis as disreputably unscientific;[26] and the Grace–New Haven Community Hospital, where Jackson was psychiatric consultant to the Department of Pediatrics, processed newborns and maternity patients with modern bureaucratic efficiency.[27] Nurses brought infants to their mothers for a twenty-minute feeding every four hours, whether the baby had been sleeping at the appointed moment or crying for hours before; and nursery routines were

---

[24] A survey of rooming-in opportunities, published in the winter of 1956–57, reported that "facilities for rooming-in still are not widely available." Margaret C. Dawson, "Rooming-in: a decade's experience," *Child Study, Quart. J. Parent Education*, 1956–57, *34*: 34.

[25] Charles Rosenberg has written that the Johns Hopkins Hospital in the 1890s "embodied and symbolized a new scientific medicine" in an environment where patients "paid a price in dignity and discomfort for the new clinical skills and efficiency that they hoped would restore them to health." Rosenberg, *Care of Strangers*, pp. 307, 309.

[26] Eugen Kahn, a noted German specialist in "the fundamental sciences which deal with the nervous system," became professor of psychiatry and mental hygiene at the Yale School of Medicine in November 1929. On that occasion, the dean of the Yale medical school, Milton C. Winternitz, announced that the department's work would involve "the fundamental fields of neuro-physiology, neuro-anatomy, and neuro-pathology." *Yale News*, 16 November 1929. Jackson felt "tarred with the brush of psychoanalysis" during her early years at Yale, she subsequently told an associate. E. H. K. [Ethelyn H. Klatskin], "Edith Banfield Jackson, M.D.," *Yale Med.*, 1977, *12*: 13.

[27] In 1936 the New Haven Community Hospital and Grace Hospital in New Haven merged to become the Grace–New Haven Community Hospital.

equally impervious to the possibility that new mothers yearned to cuddle, nurse, or just look at their newborns more often.

Such nursery procedures were standard at American hospitals in the 1930s and reflected not only the bureaucratization of medicine but also the nearly simultaneous repudiation, by child development experts, of Victorian America's sentimental, indulgent attitudes toward children.[28] Since the 1900s, pediatricians such as L. Emmett Holt, Sr.,[29] and psychologists such as John B. Watson[30] had viewed infants as biological units that could be conditioned and unconditioned at will, and their views had "influenced pediatrics momentously."[31] Thus, the received wisdom in the mid-1930s was that infants should have their physical needs for calories, vitamins, immunizations, fresh air, and sunshine satisfied; that they should be fed on a regular schedule; and that they should be left, in between feedings, to "cry it out" lest they become "over-stimulated" and "conditioned" to wail when their wants were not gratified instantly.[32]

Jackson, by means of her Rooming-In Research Project, ultimately challenged both those child-rearing prescriptions and current hospital procedures for the care of new mothers, infants, and children. She began modestly, however. In her first year in New Haven, she observed that a surprisingly large number of children were hospitalized for severe feeding disorders,[33] and she asked the New Haven Department of Health for permission to visit some recently discharged mothers and newborns, in the hope of learning how the feeding problems began. "The home situation," Jackson later recalled, "was bad."[34] Repeatedly, she saw what most practitioners in the late 1930s were failing to see, namely, the negative psychological consequences of hospitalization for childbirth: tense, irritable babies; anxious mothers adhering religiously to the "feed-every-four-hours" regimen of the hospital nursery while caring alone for infants with whom they were barely acquainted; and fathers who had never handled their newborns in the hospital and were thus "scared at home and disrupted by the baby's crying."[35] Those new parents, Jackson observed, regarded the hospital's

[28] Celia B. Stendler, "Sixty years of child training practices: revolution in the nursery," *J. Pediatr.*, 1950, *36:* 129–30.

[29] L. Emmett Holt, *The Care and Feeding of Children: A Catechism for the Use of Mothers and Children's Nurses,* 10th ed., rev. and enl. (New York and London: D. Appleton, 1920).

[30] See, for example, John B. Watson, "Psychology as the behaviorist views it," *Psychol. Rev.,* 1913, *20:* 158–77. That paper, according to Ruth Leys, "launched the behaviorist movement in American psychology." Ruth Leys, "Meyer, Watson, and the dangers of behaviorism," *J. Hist. Behav. Sci.,* 1984, *20:* 133.

[31] [Jackson], "Evolution in psychological care," p. 3.

[32] Holt, *Care and Feeding of Children,* p. 187. Similar logic informed hospital protocols for toddlers and children on the pediatrics ward. So that physicians could concentrate on the somatic treatment of hospitalized children's diseases, parents were permitted only a brief, inevitably emotional, weekly "intrusion" into the supposedly efficacious, scientific treatment of their children. For Edith Jackson's pathbreaking views on the deleterious effect of those standard visiting rules in hospital pediatric wards, see Edith B. Jackson, "Treatment of the young child in the hospital," *Amer. J. Orthopsychiatry,* 1942, *12:* 56–65.

[33] Edith B. Jackson, "Prophylactic considerations for the neonatal period: development of home-visit plan for pediatric interns," *Amer. J. Orthopsychiatry,* 1945, *15:* 90.

[34] Edith B. Jackson, interview by Warren Kennison, Dane G. Prugh, and Albert J. Solnit, February 1975. Tape lent to me by Dane G. Prugh, Denver, Colorado.

[35] *Ibid.*

rigid feeding schedule as "more to be obeyed than their instinctive" inclination to feed the newborn when he or she cried, and "more to be respected than the child's unhappy resistance" to being deprived of nourishment when he or she became hungry. Moreover, she hypothesized that the feeding problems of many hospitalized children originated in that "vicious circle of distress" between parents and infants during the first weeks home from the hospital.[36]

She also came to believe that the changes in medical education over the past several decades were as culpable as the rigid approach to infant feeding.[37] With modern clinical training confined "almost wholly within hospital walls" and largely focused on "the recognition and treatment of disease," medical students "no longer had any direct experience with the family situation" and consequently were, in Jackson's view, "without ... much more fundamental knowledge than the parents themselves in the normal vicissitudes of a little child's development."[38] To enable pediatric house officers to "see what happened to their recommendations of every four hour feeding," she invited them to accompany her on visits to newborns' homes.[39] One intern recalled that they saw not only dissatisfied, crying babies and scared, irritable parents but also "the great unreality of much of our pediatric advice."[40] Repeatedly, mothers told Jackson and her young associates that if they had been able to spend more time with their babies in the hospital, they would not have been so scared to care for them at home.[41] The Rooming-In Research Project, Jackson later wrote, "grew out of the realization" gleaned from those home visits that "the hospital had the key opportunity for helping parents at the very important time around childbirth, but

---

[36] Edith B. Jackson, "Theoretic Considerations and Parental Observations Relating to the Unified Hospital Care of Mother and Infant," in *Transactions of the Third American Congress on Obstetrics and Gynecology* [1947], ed. George W. Kosmak and Robert N. Rutherford (Portland, Oregon: Western Journal of Surgery Publications, 1948), p. 9.

[37] For a review and analysis of the changes in medical education, see Kenneth M. Ludmerer, *Learning to Heal: The Development of American Medical Education* (New York: Basic Books, 1985). Note especially Ludmerer's contentions (1) that clinical science had undergone a remarkable scientific revolution in the early 1900s, such that research in these fields, like research in the basic sciences, had become laboratory-based, and (2) that subsequently "although almost all clinical scientists saw patients, their primary goal was to study disease in the laboratory, and some made no secret of the fact that they regarded patient care as a chore because it took time away from research." *Ibid.*, pp. 208–10.

[38] Quotations, in order of appearance, are from Edith B. Jackson, "The old way is new: rooming-in," *Vassar Alumnae Mag.*, December 1948, p. 2; Richard W. Olmsted, Ruth I. Svibergson, and James A. Kleeman, "The value of rooming-in experience in pediatric practice," *Pediatrics*, 1949, 5: 619; Edith B. Jackson, "Childbirth Patterns in the United States," in *Mental Health and Infant Development*, ed. Kenneth Soddy (New York: Basic Books, 1956), p. 95; Jackson, "Old way is new," p. 2. According to Olmsted, Svibergson, and Kleeman, "What little experience with the newborn or the physically well child [pediatric training] does offer" typically "is fragmented and lacks opportunity for follow-up observation," even though a "remarkably large proportion of pediatric practice is concerned with the broad aspects of child health, which is today defined as the physical, mental and emotional well-being of the individual." Olmsted, Svibergson, and Kleeman, "Value of rooming-in," p. 619.

[39] Jackson, interview by Kennison, Prugh, and Solnit.

[40] Arden Miller, "Thoughts about Edith Jackson," telephone conversation with John C. Cobb, 6 June 1977. Transcription courtesy of John C. Cobb. Miller was professor of maternal and child health and former chancellor of health affairs at the University of North Carolina and a past president of the American Public Health Association.

[41] Jackson, interview by Kennison, Prugh, and Solnit.

was failing ... because of the systematized structure of its service" to do so.[42]

Well aware that hospital care had "significantly reduced for both mothers and infants" the "sickness and mortality associated with child-birth,"[43] Jackson understood that "great advances ... seldom occur without some concomitant disadvantages, which in turn have to be overcome."[44] In her view, the primary disadvantage of "hospitalized" childbirth was that "the hospital's institutional need for regularity and regime [had] blocked a recognition" of both the "infantile needs" of the newborn for "nuzzling," "sucking," and "peaceful, undisturbed rest" between feedings, and the "fundamental urges of normal, mature mothers to love, fondle, nourish and watch their babies."[45] By 1938, then, she had set for herself this substantial question: "Cannot the advantages of safety and home-like comfort be combined in the hospital [both] for the welfare of normal healthy mothers and infants, and for the more realistic education of parents, physicians, and nurses in the interrelationship of maternal and infant needs?"[46]

A specific plan for achieving that end suggested itself to Jackson in May 1938 when, quite by accident, a neighbor, Joan Erikson, and her newborn became the first rooming-in pair at Grace–New Haven Community Hospital. Erikson, the wife of psychoanalyst Erik H. Erikson, and herself trained in child analysis, had borne her first two children in Vienna, where rooming-in was "a matter of course."[47] Grace–New Haven authorities had initially denied her request to room-in with an expected third child, but Erikson contracted mumps just before her due date and consequently got what she wanted: the hospital, to guard other mothers and newborns from the disease, decided that she and her infant daughter should stay together in an isolation ward room.[48]

Regular visits to the contented pair in that unconventional setting persuaded Jackson that hospitals should give other mothers and babies the same opportunity,[49] but few colleagues whom she brought to observe the Eriksons were convinced. Obstetricians claimed that a mother's "rest and recuperation would be hindered by the baby's presence and crying"; pedia-

[42] Edith B. Jackson, "Parenthood," remarks to "soon-to-be-parents" at Grace–New Haven Community Hospital [mid-1950s], Jackson Papers, Schlesinger Library.

[43] Edith B. Jackson, interview on "Yale Interprets the News," Radio Station WTIC, 6 August 1950. A transcript of the program is in Jackson Papers, Schlesinger Library.

[44] Edith B. Jackson, "Should mother and baby room together? Psychological considerations for hospital rooming together of mother and newborn," *Amer. J. Nurs.*, 1946, *46*: 17.

[45] Edith B. Jackson, "General reactions of mothers and nurses to rooming-in," *Amer. J. Public Health*, 1948, *38*: 690; Jackson, "Theoretic Considerations," p. 9.

[46] Jackson, "General reactions," p. 690.

[47] Joan Erikson, interview with author, Cambridge, Massachusetts, 11 November 1985. Note that "practically all European hospitals, as well as those in Japan and China, have always had the rooming-in plan. At the Rotunda in Dublin, and other famous European maternity hospitals, nurseries were unheard of" (McBryde, "Compulsory rooming-in," p. 627).

[48] Edith B. Jackson et al., "A hospital rooming-in unit for four newborn infants and their mothers," *Pediatrics*, 1948, *1*: 29.

[49] Erikson, interview with author, 11 November 1985.

tricians feared "increasing the sources of infection or contagion"; and hospital and nursing administrators were sure "that such an iconoclastic 'experiment' would unduly tax and confuse" nurses accustomed to caring separately for mothers and newborns.[50] Those arguments became moot during the next half dozen years, however, when such wartime exigencies as shortages of hospital staff and accelerated teaching programs at the Yale School of Medicine effectively precluded the initiation of rooming-in, or any other new programs for patients, at Grace–New Haven.[51]

THE ROOMING-IN RESEARCH PROJECT IN THE CONTEXT OF ITS TIME

Jackson's plan eventually came to fruition on 28 October 1946, when a cheerful, homelike rooming-in unit for four mothers and their babies opened at Grace–New Haven Community Hospital. Procedures in that experimental space deviated sharply from standard hospital routines for maternity and newborn patients. First, on the grounds that "a nurse who knows both mother and baby can give more effective help,"[52] the rooming-in pair received care from a single nurse,[53] rather than separate, at times inharmonious, attention from obstetric and nursery nurses.[54] Second, because Jackson believed that "physicians and nurses have a responsibility to learn from mothers and infants as well as to instruct them in procedures of infant care," the rooming-in staff encouraged mothers, as soon as they felt able, to care for their babies "in the way best suited to [their] capabilities,"[55] rather than mechanically to implement the standard hospital routines. Accordingly, in sharp contrast to the clock-bound, assembly line regimen of

[50] Jackson, "Should mother and baby room together?" p. 18. For a comparison between the standard, separate care of hospitalized mothers and newborns and their joint care in a rooming-in arrangement, see Marion S. Lesser and Vera R. Keane, *Nurse-Patient Relationships in a Hospital Maternity Service* (St. Louis: C. V. Mosby, 1956).

[51] Edith B. Jackson, "The development of rooming-in at Yale," *Yale J. Biol. Med.*, 1953, *25:* 486.

[52] George R. Barnes, Jr., et al., "Management of breast feeding," *JAMA*, 1953, *151:* 194.

[53] Nursing duties in the rooming-in unit were performed largely by student nurses who rotated through the unit as part of their training. For an assessment, by a Yale School of Nursing professor, of the valuable learning experience the unit offered nurses-in-training, see Kate Hyder, "Basic preparation in obstetric nursing," *Amer. J. Public Health*, 1951, *41(2):* 90–94. Student nurses in the unit were supervised both by a nursing fellow and by rooming-in fellows. Three of the latter described their work in Olmsted, Svibergson, and Kleeman, "Value of rooming-in experience."

[54] Note, for example, that whereas *maternity* nurses were sometimes sympathetic to a mother's wish that feeding periods be long enough to establish a successful breast-feeding relationship with her infant, *nursery* nurses were primarily concerned with getting babies to their mothers and then back to the nursery according to the prescribed schedule. A maternity floor nurse at a large metropolitan hospital told an interviewer: "I feel very left out when the babies are out with the mothers, and I'm not supposed to go near them. I would like to be able to help the mothers with the babies. If the mothers ask the floor nurses questions about the babies, we have to pretend we don't know anything, because we might tell them something that isn't the hospital policy, and the floor nurses don't know what the babies are receiving—the type of formula, or what they're bathed with, or about their weight." Lesser and Keane, *Nurse-Patient Relationships*, p. 200. A nursery nurse from the same hospital offered her perspective: "A half hour isn't much time to get around to twenty some odd mothers and see that all the babies are awake and eating. ... You get a lot of satisfaction out of seeing a mother learning ... to pick up her baby and bubble it like an old trouper. That's fun, but only if you have the time to spend with her." *Ibid.,* p. 197.

[55] Jackson, "Should mother and baby room together?" p. 19; Olmsted, Svibergson, and Kleeman, "Value of rooming-in experience," p. 619. The staff of the rooming-in unit consisted of a full-time medical director, Edith Jackson; a full-time nursing fellow; one or more full-time pediatric fellows; and student nurses who served a rotation on the unit.

the traditional nursery, mothers in the unit breast-fed whenever their infants seemed hungry;[56] and fathers, who before could only look at their infants through the nursery window, were welcome at any time to visit, hold, change, and enjoy their newborns.

The rooming-in unit, then, represented Jackson's clinical response to the fact that maternity care had become "hospital-centered in the first place and patient-centered in the second."[57] It also embodied her judgment, decades before Klaus and Kennell reportedly "pioneered" in this area, that hospitals could both reinstate "the essential values of old-fashioned mother care ... without losing the protection of modern institutional medicine" and thereby help "parents achieve ... warm parent-child relationships."[58]

The Rooming-In Research Project had other goals as well, for Jackson was troubled not only by "the inappropriate care the hospital offered maternity patients" but also by "the lack of appropriate experience the Newborn Service offered pediatricians in training."[59] Medical students, house officers, and student nurses would get a "more realistic education in the management of ... maternal and infant adjustment"[60] in the rooming-in unit, she believed, because in the process of closely observing the enormous variability of *healthy* mothers and babies, they would necessarily shed some of the intense preoccupation with disease and somatic therapies that their "modern" education had engendered and come to see equal wisdom in the nineteenth-century view that "every clinician had to be something of a psychiatrist and family therapist" and that every "patient was more than a manifestation of the disease from which he or she happened to be suffering."[61] In addition, Jackson regarded the rooming-in unit as an opportunity for testing "a method of child guidance which is now on trial."[62] With data from the rooming-in babies and their families, she and her staff planned a longitudinal study of "mental hygiene as respects parents and neonates"[63] in

[56] Francis P. Simsarian and Roberta White Taylor, "Two mothers revolt," *Child Study*, Winter 1944–45, p. 49. A desire to breast-feed was initially among the criteria for admission to the rooming-in unit. As demand and space for rooming-in increased, women who did not wish to breast-feed were admitted as well.

[57] EBJ [Edith B. Jackson] to Miss [Reva] Rubin, 6 November 1951, Jackson Papers, Schlesinger Library.

[58] Jackson, "Old way is new," p. 2; Jackson, "Development of rooming-in," p. 484.

[59] Edith B. Jackson, "Retrospect and tribute: remarks in acceptance of the C. Anderson Aldrich Award," *Yale J. Biol. Med.*, 1970, *43*: 45.

[60] Jackson, "Old way is new," p. 5.

[61] Charles E. Rosenberg, "Body and mind in nineteenth-century medicine: some clinical origins of the neurosis construct," *Bull. Hist. Med.*, 1989, *63*: 188. Grover Powers, chair of the Yale pediatrics department for more than two decades, told prospective pediatric house officers that "Rooming-In would be the most valuable experience [they] could ever have." Dick [Richard Olmsted] to Dr. [Grover] Powers, 27 May 1959, Jackson Papers, Schlesinger Library.

[62] Jackson, "Old way is new," p. 2.

[63] Jackson, "Development of rooming-in," p. 488. Some of the Rooming-In Research Project's publications that addressed the long-range effects of flexible child-rearing procedures are (1) Edith B. Jackson and Ethelyn H. Klatskin, "Rooming-In Research Project: development of methodology of parent-child relationship study in a clinical setting," *Psychoanal. Study Child*, 1950, *5*: 236–73; (2) Edith B. Jackson, Ethelyn H. Klatskin, and Louise C. Wilkin, "Early child development in relation to degree of flexibility of maternal attitude," *Psychoanal. Study Child*, 1952, *7*: 393–428; (3) Ethelyn H. Klatskin and Edith B. Jackson, "Methodology of the Yale Rooming-In Project on parent-child relationship," *Amer. J. Orthopsychiatry*, 1955, *25*: 373–97; and (4) Edith B. Jackson, Louise C. Wilkin, and Harry Auerbach, "Statistical report on incidence and duration of breast feeding in relation to personal-social and hospital maternity factors," *Pediatrics*, 1956, *17*: 700–715.

an effort to determine whether prompt satisfaction of an infant's needs, rather than the rigid routine of hospital nurseries, provided the better foundation for the development of independence and self-discipline.[64]

An editorial review in the *International Medical Digest* in 1949 suggested that Jackson was on a promising course. Characterizing rooming-in as a "radical departure from the conventional nursery routine of the newborn baby," the editor pronounced it "the most progressive step in mental hygiene in the first half of the twentieth century."[65]

While concurring with the *Digest's* claims, any fair-minded treatment of rooming-in must nonetheless address two additional and curious realities: most medical people of the day did not share the *Digest's* lofty assessment of rooming-in; and rooming-in, although posing a radical challenge both to hospital maternity and infant procedures and to contemporary assumptions about child development, neither rested on nor proposed novel concepts.

No one was more aware of the latter point than Edith Jackson herself. "Rooming-in," she often said, was merely "a new word for the return of an old custom" that had "found itself excluded in the hospital setting" where routines had grown "increasingly impersonal and inflexible."[66] Nor did she claim originality for the rooming-in project's hypothesis that the old, "natural" lying-in procedure was preferable to modern, bureaucratically efficient hospital routines.[67] That idea, she pointed out, was already "in the air" when the rooming-in unit opened.[68] Early in the twentieth century, the father of American pediatrics, Abraham Jacobi (1830–1919) had deplored the effects of "hospitalism" on children and asserted that "feeding cannot be regulated by mathematics so well as by ... the wants of the individual child";[69] and in 1922 another noted pediatrician warned that the infant "suffers most from institutional care." Babies, Henry Dwight Chapin declared, "are brought into the world singly and not in droves, and they crave individual care and mothering."[70]

---

[64] Jackson, "Old way is new," p. 2.

[65] Robert Strong, "Editorial review," *International Med. Digest*, March 1949. Clipping in Jackson Papers, Yale University Library.

[66] Jackson, interview on "Yale Interprets the News." The term *rooming-in* first appeared in print in 1943 when Yale pediatrician Arnold Gesell and his colleague Frances Ilg proposed a "rooming-in arrangement for the baby," claiming it would strengthen "the bonds between mother and child." Arnold Gesell and Frances L. Ilg, *Infant and Child in the Culture of Today: The Guidance of Development in Home and Nursery School* (New York: Harper & Brothers, 1943), p. 85.

[67] Jackson regularly acknowledged that hospitalization for childbirth had "significantly reduced ... sickness and mortality ... for both mothers and infants." See, for example, Jackson, interview on "Yale Interprets the News."

[68] Quoted in Dawson, "Rooming-in," p. 31. A popular magazine article recently referred to the "commonsense point of view" that had prevailed until the late nineteenth century and had first been articulated in A.D. 175 by Galen, the Greek physician, who had written that when babies "cry or scream or are upset, we should understand that it means something is disturbing them, and we must try to discover what they need and give it to them before their minds and bodies become more overly excited." Marie Winn, "New fights over spoiling your baby," *New York Times Mag.*, pt. 2, 16 April 1989, p. 61.

[69] Quoted in Grover F. Powers, "Infant feeding: historical background and modern practice," *JAMA*, 1935, *105:* 760.

[70] Henry Dwight Chapin, *Heredity and Child Culture* (New York: E. P. Dutton, 1922), p. 214.

Moreover, Jackson was not the only pediatrician in the 1930s who attributed the alarming increase in childhood feeding and behavioral disorders to the rigid feeding of newborns that started in hospitals and then continued, on doctor's orders, at home. Yale professor of pediatrics Grover F. Powers wrote in the *Journal of the American Medical Association* that colleagues who had an "itch" for "regulation" and "perfection in dietary regime" should "worship ... the measuring stick, the scales, ... and the clock less" and the needs of the infant and mother more.[71] Four years later, C. Anderson Aldrich was even more explicit. When an infant's need for the "warmth and contact of the mother in the first few weeks" and "permission to eat, sleep, and eliminate according to his own individual rhythms ... are minimized or ignored," he told fellow pediatricians, "growth is hampered and warped."[72]

Child analysts reinforced those claims. Therese Benedek in 1938 addressed "the profound effect of early disappointments during the feeding process on later development" and argued that "satisfaction of the baby's demand" does not "increase the need and demands of the child but rather" that it will "pacify the child and ... cause a feeding regulation to develop which is in many respects more satisfactory."[73] Ruth and Harry Bakwin deplored the emotional deprivation experienced by infants in the hospital.[74] Likewise, Margaret A. Ribble, asserting that "the roots of unhappiness ... and unsocial behavior" are "established in earliest infancy," upbraided "our highly impersonal civilization" for "insidiously" damaging "woman's instinctual nature" and "blind[ing] her to one of her most natural rights— that of teaching the small baby to love, by loving it consistently through the period of helpless infancy." The "modern woman," Ribble wrote in 1943, "needs reassurance that the handling and fondling which she gives are by no means casual expressions of sentiment but are biologically necessary for the healthy mental development of the baby."[75]

By the late 1930s a few mothers had begun to speak out, too. In 1938, anthropologist Margaret Mead persuaded her pediatrician, Benjamin Spock,

[71] Powers, "Infant feeding," pp. 760–61. Powers and others who supported his position in the 1930s were influenced by Clara Davis's pathbreaking experiments that showed that infants allowed to choose the amount and type of food they ate invariably selected a balanced diet. Clara M. Davis, "Self selection of diet by newly weaned infants: an experimental study," *Amer. J. Dis. Child.*, 1928, *36*: 651–79. In 1947, Edith Jackson characterized Davis's study as "a complete break from the teaching that the physician alone could estimate exactly what the child needs in terms of proteins, carbohydrates, fats, vitamins, and that these should be given by the clock without regard for the child's wishes as to quantity, quality or interval between feedings." [Jackson], "Evolution in psychological care," p. 4.

[72] C. Anderson Aldrich, "The role of gratification in early development," *J. Pediatr.*, 1939, *15*: 579. In *Feeding Behavior of Infants: A Pediatric Approach to the Mental Hygiene of Early Life* (Philadelphia: J. B. Lippincott, 1937), editors Arnold Gesell and Frances L. Ilg made points similar to those of Powers, Aldrich, and Jackson.

[73] Therese Benedek, "Adaptation to reality in early infancy," *Psychoanal. Quart.*, 1938, 7: 210, 214 n.

[74] Ruth Morris Bakwin and Harry Bakwin, *Psychologic Care during Infancy and Childhood* (New York: D. Appleton-Century, 1942), p. 295.

[75] Margaret A. Ribble, *The Rights of Infants: Early Psychological Needs and Their Satisfaction* (New York: Columbia University Press, 1943), pp. viii, 14, 15.

to circumvent New York Hospital's rigid feeding schedule for her new-born.[76] Six years later, a woman whose doctor had twice allowed her to room-in with her infants at the George Washington University Hospital called on mothers "to revolt against current hospital practices that deprive them of their newborn babies' company."[77]

By 1945–50, along with those lay and medical people who advocated more flexible, personalized maternity and infant care on psychological grounds, a few clinicians had begun to argue that rooming-in would prevent deadly epidemics in hospital nurseries.[78] Their combined voices clearly had an impact, for between 1946 and 1950 about forty teaching, private, and military hospitals throughout the United States offered rooming-in for their maternity patients.[79]

THE ESTABLISHMENT OF THE ROOMING-IN RESEARCH PROJECT

Despite growing support in the 1930s and 1940s for improved hospital care of newborns and mothers, getting rooming-in established at Grace–New Haven Community Hospital was neither smooth nor easy. Jackson supervised three trial ventures on the hospital's maternity ward in the fall of 1944. Two of the participants, multiparae, "greatly enjoyed the arrangement," feeling "comfortable and competent" with their babies beside them. For the primipara, though, the experiment ended unsatisfactorily. The young woman's nurse, clearly hostile to the novel rooming-in experiment, had effectively told her patient, Jackson later reported, "Well, now, you've got your baby; it's up to you to take care of it!"[80]

[76] Jackson, "Childbirth Patterns," p. 94.

[77] Simsarian and Taylor, "Two mothers revolt," p. 49. Simsarian and her pediatrician, P. A. McLendon, used the occasion of her first hospital confinement to experiment with feeding a newborn on a "self-demand" schedule Frances P. Simsarian and P. A. McLendon, "Feeding behavior of an infant during the first twelve weeks of life on a self-demand schedule: a narrative by the mother with discussion by the pediatrician." *J. Pediatr.*, 1942, *20*: 93–103.

[78] In 1945 two physicians, P. A. McLendon and John Parks, wrote that "it has taken epidemics of impetigo, respiratory infections and, more particularly, 'neonatal diarrhea' to initiate a demand for changes in architecture" that would do away with hospitals' "large nurseries for the collective care of their infant patients." P. A. McLendon and John Parks, "Nurseries designed for modern maternity," *Mod. Hosp.*, 1945, *65*: 46. A rooming-in plan was begun in May 1947 at the Community Health Center of Branch County, in Coldwater, Michigan, "as a prophylactic measure" after "a moderately severe case of impetigo developed in the nursery." Shirley E. Lundgren, "A trial rooming-in plan," *Amer. J. Nurs.*, 1947, *47*: 547, 548. At the Jefferson University Hospital in Philadelphia, rooming-in was instituted in July 1947 by the Department of Obstetrics and Gynecology, "hoping that we could prevent epidemic disease of the newborn in our own institution." Thaddeus L. Montgomery and Pauline Shenk, "Further experiences with the rooming-in project of baby with mother," *Philadelphia Med.*, 25 December 1948, p. 757. Doctors at Duke University Hospital adopted rooming-in in 1947, "not primarily for its psychological advantages but in order to avoid the possibility of nursery epidemics." McBryde, "Compulsory rooming-in," p. 625.

[79] Jackson, "Childbirth Patterns," p. 95. Jackson's Rooming-In Research Project can be distinguished from rooming-in arrangements in other American hospitals in several important particulars. First, it alone had both a full-time medical director and full-time nursing and pediatric fellows to plan, oversee, and document its work. Albert W. Snoke, "A hospital rooming-in unit for newborns and mothers," *Stanford Med. Bull.*, 1948, *6*: 143. Second, whereas other new rooming-in operations had exclusively clinical goals—for instance, to prevent nursery infections, to promote breast-feeding, or to facilitate ad-lib infant feeding—Jackson's project had research and educational components as well. See my description of them in this article, pp. 272–74.

[80] Edith B. Jackson, "Pediatric and psychiatric aspects of the Yale Rooming-In Project," *Connecticut State Med. J.*, 1950, *14*: 5.

A year later, in 1945, as the wives of three pediatric residents prepared to try rooming-in on the Private Pavilion,[81] a telling episode underscored the problem. One of the expectant fathers was about to climb a three-story, free-standing staircase to the pavilion when the head Nursery nurse called to him from the top of the stairwell: "Dr. Walcher! I understand that you and your wife are going to try this newfangled idea that Dr. Jackson has been wanting to use for the newborn babies!" Dwain Walcher "was absolutely stunned," he later recalled, "to have this kind of hostility thrown down the stairwell on my head."[82] Hostility to the "newfangled" arrangement, moreover, was not confined to the head nurse. On the fifth morning of baby Susan Walcher's stay in her mother's room, a floor nurse, thoroughly irritated by the unorthodox assignment that had her caring for both mother and newborn, brought the unsuspecting mother a bottle of sour milk to feed her rooming-in infant![83]

The prospects for getting rooming-in established looked no more promising at the start of 1946. To a request that rooming-in units be included in the Grace–New Haven Community Hospital's building plan, hospital director Albert W. Snoke, himself a pediatrician, expressed the views of many in the American medical establishment when he declared: "That's as crazy an idea as I've ever heard!"[84]

Snoke's colorful rejoinder and the nurse's quiet subversion are graphic evidence that, for hospital administrators, nurses, and doctors as well, Jackson's rooming-in plan portended unwanted, radical changes in the way they understood their work and practiced their crafts. Consequently, it took a fortuitous combination of factors to make rooming-in a reality at Grace–New Haven in the fall of 1946. By briefly recounting them, we can clearly see the threats that rooming-in posed to established procedures and received wisdom in American medicine in the middle of the twentieth century.

No factor was more important than the appointment in March 1946 of Kate Hyder as supervisor of the obstetrical and gynecological service at the hospital and assistant professor of obstetrical and gynecological nursing at the Yale School of Nursing. A lively, forty-one-year-old North Carolinian with a graduate degree in nurse-midwifery, she came to Yale "with tremendous zeal for revitalizing the teaching and practice in obstetrical nursing" and soon concluded that rooming-in could be "a direct means to this end."[85] A less energetic, dedicated, and resourceful new appointee would have given up, because the hospital director was deeply "skeptical," the

---

[81] Edith B. Jackson, "The Initiation of a Rooming-In Project at the Grace–New Haven Community Hospital (University Service)," in *Problems of Early Infancy, Transactions of the First Conference, March 3–4, 1947,* ed. Milton J. E. Senn, 2d ed. (New York: Josiah Macy, Jr., Foundation, 1951), p. 46.

[82] Dwain Walcher, telephone conversation with author, 11 April 1984.

[83] The Walchers, horrified by the nurse's behavior, consulted with Jackson and decided to cut the normal ten-day hospital lying-in period in half and take their baby home. *Ibid.*

[84] Jackson, "Development of rooming-in," p. 487.

[85] *Ibid.,* pp. 488, 491.

nursing supervisor thought rooming-in a "luxury," and nurses on the maternity and nursery services were "not even willing to talk about it."[86] Floor nurses, trained to care for mothers and newborns separately, were "afraid to change," Hyder believed, partly because they "thought it meant more work for them" and also because they failed to realize how gratifying rooming-in would be for both mother and baby.[87]

Hyder overcame those obstacles in a matter of months. She responded to the claim that rooming-in would be a costly luxury by initiating a time-study that demonstrated that fewer nursing hours would be expended if a single nurse cared for four mothers and newborns together than if separate obstetric and nursery nurses attended them in the traditional manner.[88] She was equally resourceful in coping with experienced nurses' hostility to rooming-in. Her proposal to staff an experimental four-bed rooming-in unit with a sympathetic graduate nurse and students from the Yale School of Nursing ensured not only that the unit's nurses would be unencumbered by traditional assumptions about postpartum and neonatal care but also that the Yale nursing school could train a new generation of nurses who were familiar with the problems and, most especially, the rewards of caring for mothers and newborns together.[89]

Along with Hyder's ingenuity, another key factor was timely support from Yale's Department of Obstetrics and Gynecology. Unsympathetic to Jackson's earlier experiments with rooming-in and *ad-lib* breast-feeding, obstetricians and maternity nurses at Grace–New Haven, like their obstetrical colleagues around the country, held that new mothers needed rest, not responsibility for their babies, in the first postpartum weeks. They also widely, if quietly, believed that mothers who breast-fed would be a greater nuisance to them.[90] In the spring of 1946, however, Herbert Thoms, a sixty-one-year-old associate professor of obstetrics and gynecology, had begun to think otherwise. Recently persuaded by natural childbirth theorists that better-informed parturients would be more relaxed during labor and thus more likely to deliver safely and without medication, he then realized, after conversations with Jackson, that natural childbirth and rooming-in had in common not only "a basic philosophy of parental education, with emphasis on parents' ... knowledge about processes which affect them and their

[86] Kate Hyder, interview with author, Hamden, Connecticut, 6 March 1984; *idem*, telephone conversation with author, 22 February 1988. Only the dean of the nursing school, Elizabeth Bixler, was "very interested" in Hyder's wish to try rooming-in. *Ibid.*

[87] *Ibid.*

[88] *Ibid.*; Jackson et al., "Hospital rooming-in unit," p. 32.

[89] Hyder, "Basic preparation."

[90] A woman using prepared formula, it seemed clear to obstetricians, would not be phoning them with questions about cracked nipples, manual expression of milk, and the like. That these views were commonly held by obstetricians in the 1940s was reported to me in interviews with hospital administrators (Albert W. Snoke, New Haven, Connecticut, 9 February 1984; Hilda Kroeger, telephone conversation, 3 May 1984), nurses (Kate Hyder, 6 March 1984; Nilda Shea, telephone conversation, 14 June 1986), and obstetricians themselves (Richard Banfield, New Canaan, Connecticut, 2 May 1984; Frederick W. Goodrich, Jr., Southbury, Connecticut, 17 May 1984).

SARA LEE SILBERMAN

infants,"[91] but also the goal of achieving "a natural, happy, full experience for every mother in pregnancy, childbirth, puerperium and homecoming."[92] With those insights, Thoms persuaded his department chair to permit rooming-in on more than an occasional basis; and in June 1946, Arthur H. Morse authorized the newly constituted Rooming-In Study Group[93] to convert an obstetrics ward solarium into a four-bed experimental rooming-in unit as Kate Hyder had recommended.[94]

Morse, however, was not the final obstacle. "I ran the Hospital," Albert W. Snoke recalled proudly, "and I had to agree to the construction [of the rooming-in unit]."[95] A thirty-nine-year-old pediatrician-turned-administrator, Snoke had been director of the Grace–New Haven Community Hospital for less than a month when Jackson came to his office, early in April 1946, to discuss rooming-in. He had "never heard of it," and furthermore, the "old system" that gave mothers a chance to "loaf" during their postpartum stay in the hospital seemed "perfectly logical" to him. Jackson's "gentle, quiet, sensible presentation" of her case, however, and visits from Hyder, Thoms, Powers, and Dean Elizabeth Bixler of the nursing school persuaded Snoke to give rooming-in a try. His decision evoked the "damnedest opposition" from staff obstetricians, local pediatricians, and New Haven health officer (and physician) Joseph Linde, who personally visited the Hospital to upbraid the fledgling administrator for his "crack-brained idea." If Snoke permitted rooming-in at Grace–New Haven, Linde declared, he would be abrogating "the sacred trust that hospitals were supposed to have to protect the mother and baby from infections" that invariably lurked outside the nursery.[96]

A less "cocky" administrator so early in his tenure might have forborne making a decision that was so "*absolutely* against *all* concepts of infant care" and so likely to divide his medical and nursing personnel. Snoke, however, had come warmly to respect Hyder, Jackson, Powers, and Thoms; and in June he authorized conversion of the solarium to begin. Years later, explaining his decision with obvious pleasure, Snoke observed, "If I make up my mind about something that I think is the right thing to do, God damn

---

[91] Jackson, "Development of rooming-in," p. 492. For evidence of the integrated efforts of pediatricians and obstetricians at Yale after 1947, see Herbert Thoms, *Training for Childbirth: A Program of Natural Childbirth with Rooming-In* (New York: McGraw-Hill, 1950).

[92] Jackson, "Pediatric and psychiatric aspects," p. 3. For concrete evidence of the complementarity of "natural childbirth" and rooming-in, note that most of the first 150 women who delivered their babies via the Grantly Dick-Read method at Grace–New Haven in 1947 and 1948 requested permission to spend their lying-in period in Jackson's rooming-in unit. Frederick W. Goodrich, Jr., and Herbert Thoms, "A clinical study of natural childbirth: a preliminary report from a teaching ward service," *Amer. J. Obstet. Gynecol.*, 1948, 56: 882.

[93] The members of the study group were Grover Powers and Edith Jackson from the Department of Pediatrics; Herbert Thoms from the Department of Obstetrics and Gynecology; Dean Elizabeth Bixler from the Yale School of Nursing; Kate Hyder; and the associate director of the Grace–New Haven Community Hospital, Alan Foord. Edith B. Jackson to Larry [Frank], 14 January 1947, Jackson Papers, Schlesinger Library.

[94] Jackson, "Hospital rooming-in unit," p. 32.

[95] Snoke, interview with author, 9 February 1984.

[96] *Ibid.*

it, I do it!"[97] His support, though, was cautious and measured. While permitting the solarium's conversion into an "experimental" rooming-in unit,[98]
Snoke included neither construction expenses nor the unit's staffing costs in
the hospital's operating budget.[99]

Those financial obstacles were surmounted by Grover Powers and
Edith Jackson, who shared a longstanding concern for the kind of patient-
centered hospital care that rooming-in represented.[100] Powers, chair of
pediatrics at Yale since 1921, had become by the mid-1940s "a legend."[101]
Bald, "somewhat corpulent," and "squeaky"-voiced,[102] he chaired "one of
the two or three most prized pediatric centers in the country"; and by 1950,
"Grover's Boys," as his former residents fondly called themselves, headed
roughly half the pediatrics departments in the United States.[103] Powers had
repeatedly used his influence to support Jackson's work during her decade-
long association with his department.[104] He did so again in the spring of
1946, by personally drafting a request to Mead Johnson & Company for
support of an "investigation in mental hygiene as respects parents and neonates"; and when he received the grant, he authorized Jackson to appoint
nursing and pediatric fellows, without whose services the rooming-in unit
could not have been opened.[105]

Jackson herself was responsible for the final development that made
rooming-in possible at Grace–New Haven in 1946. Just before remodeling
of the solarium was to begin in July, she learned that the Kellogg Foundation would not underwrite the cost. "I had the feeling," she later recalled,
"that we might never again capture the moment when members of four
different departments [obstetrics and gynecology, pediatrics, nursing, and

[97] *Ibid.* Snoke's (spoken) emphasis.

[98] Snoke, "Hospital rooming-in unit," p. 143.

[99] Jackson to Larry [Frank], 14 January 1947, Jackson Papers, Schlesinger Library.

[100] Note, for example, that Powers used the occasion of his presidential address to the American Pediatric
Society in 1948 to urge colleagues to "challenge continually" the procedures that "become routinized in
hospitals, to insure that they are performed, not for their own sake but really to help the patient." Grover F
Powers, "Humanizing hospital experiences," *Amer. J. Dis. Child.,* 1948, 76: 367, 377.

[101] Richard H. Granger, interview with author, New Haven, Connecticut, 28 March 1984.

[102] Seymour Sarason, interview with author, New Haven, Connecticut, 1 March 1984.

[103] Granger, interview with author, 28 March 1984. Albert Snoke, when he assumed the directorship of
Grace–New Haven in 1946, was well aware of the "top flight" Department of Pediatrics at Yale and was
"profoundly impressed" by its chair, Grover Powers. Snoke, interview with author, 9 February 1984.

[104] Powers's moral and financial support for Jackson's work can be documented at length. In 1941, when
Jackson's association with Eugen Kahn, chair of the Department of Psychiatry and Mental Hygiene, became
increasingly problematic, Powers gave her both a professorship and an office in the Department of Pediatrics.
Moreover, when Powers learned of hospital administrator Snoke's initial opposition to rooming-in early in
1946, he wrote to the chair of the Building Fund Committee on 1 March 1946, as follows: "I am absolutely
convinced that if we do not set up some units in the new hospital to meet the need of those mothers who
wish to have their babies with them from birth on, we will be making a mistake in full knowledge ... that
mothers in this community are definitely interested, and this interest is increasing." Quoted in Jackson,
"Development of rooming-in," p. 487. Years after Jackson and Powers had retired, Jackson wrote her former
chair: "The longer I live the greater is my realization of what you did for me in giving me a professional entity
[sic] and backing for my work that suited my capabilities. No one could have happier professional and friendly
associations." Edith B. Jackson to Grover [Powers], 26 July 1967, Jackson Papers, Schlesinger Library.

[105] Jackson, "Development of rooming-in," p. 488. Powers told Mead Johnson that he believed the proposed study would "lead to a further understanding of the origin of certain behavior disorders and therefore
to the possibility of their prevention." *Ibid.*

administration] were so ready to work together on a plan of mutual interest and ... of growing importance." And so, with Powers, Hyder, and Bixler all on vacation, Jackson seized the moment herself and personally guaranteed construction costs.[106]

REACTIONS TO THE ROOMING-IN RESEARCH PROJECT

When rooming-in began in the refurbished solarium that October, Jackson not only directed the unit but was its omnipresent inspiration as well. "This great lady could have been anybody's grandmother sitting in the rooming-in unit with a baby in her arms," one of the rooming-in fellows reminisced. "Her chit-chat way of talking to a mother," often while simultaneously diapering a baby, "was hardly what one would expect from a great psychoanalyst," he continued, but Jackson "spared no action that would make a [nursing or medical] student, a mother or a baby more comfortable and self-assured."[107]

In the short run at least, she succeeded grandly. In less than two years, the demand for rooming-in from both ward and private obstetrical patients was so great that Grace–New Haven opened a second four-bed unit. "The happiness of having my baby with me was indescribable," wrote a representative mother.[108] Another, characterizing her experience as "one of the most delightful ... of my life," said that she "went [home] with the sure inner, knowledge that I knew my baby" and that her husband "was as enthusiastic about rooming-in as I."[109]

By all accounts, the Rooming-In Research Project was similarly rewarding and gratifying to the nurses, doctors, students, and hospital administrators associated with it.[110] Inspired by Jackson's example and the obvious pleasure of their patients, nurses took tremendous pride in their novel work.[111] Students rotating through the unit said over and over again that the experience had constituted "the first time in their nursing education that

---

[106] Jackson to Larry [Frank], 14 January 1947, Jackson Papers, Schlesinger Library. The cost was "approximately $1500 for labor and materials." Edith B. Jackson to Dr. [Ernst] Wolff, 25 April 1949, Jackson Papers, Schlesinger Library. Jackson's income from the Yale School of Medicine was $3,000 in 1946. Her total income for that year, however, was $33,937.15. Edith B. Jackson, Internal Revenue Service return for 1946, William S. Jackson, Jr., Papers, Denver Public Library, Denver, Colorado.

[107] John C. Cobb, handwritten obituary prepared for Edith Jackson's memorial service in Denver, Colorado, June 1977. Courtesy of Dr. Cobb.

[108] Virginia M. Galpin, "Dear skeptics," *League [of Women Voters] Leaflet of New Haven,* May 1949, Jackson Papers, Yale University Library.

[109] Barbara S. Backus, "I roomed in with my new baby," *Child,* 1949, *18:* 67, 77. Reporting on a survey of rooming-in literature over the past decade, Margaret C. Dawson found it "full of glowing reactions from mothers—who often choose to repeat the procedure with second, third and fourth babies." Dawson, "Rooming-in," p. 33.

[110] For a sampling of reactions to rooming-in, see Claire Danes, "Report of a panel discussion on rooming-in," *J. Amer. Med. Women's Assoc.,* 1954, *9:* 80–83; Hyder, "Basic preparation in obstetric nursing"; Albert W. Snoke, "Rooming-in and natural childbirth," *Mod. Hosp.,* 1951, 77: 98–110.

[111] Hyder, interview with author, 6 March 1984; Shea, telephone conversation with author, 14 June 1986.

they [had] been able to give what they consider[ed] ideal care to a patient."[112] And members of the Visiting Nurses Association, on their first postpartum home visits, reported finding rooming-in mothers much more confident than those whose babies had stayed in the nursery.[113]

Doctors who treated rooming-in patients were no less enthusiastic. Three rooming-in fellows noted that their work at Yale had "fostered a more mature and sympathetic insight into the patient," and another remarked recently that a "generation or more of physicians ... all were different because of [their] training" with Jackson in the unit.[114] At Duke University Hospital, where rooming-in became compulsory for all white patients in 1947, obstetricians reported "a decrease of about 90 per cent in the telephone calls from new mothers during their first week at home."[115] Similarly, a doctor-and-nurse team assessing the rooming-in experiences of 1,475 women at Thomas Jefferson University Hospital in Philadelphia declared themselves "firmly convinced that the plan offers a logical solution to the difficulties and problems of institutional care of the newborn." Rooming-in worked not only as "a preventive of epidemic infection," they wrote, but also as "a stimulus to breast feeding, ... an implement to improved baby care, and ... a method of education of the mother in the responsibilities and technics of raising a baby" that would likely lead to "an improvement in mother-baby relationships." Accordingly, they confidently predicted, rooming-in "is here to stay."[116]

Finally, director Snoke reported to fellow administrators in *The Modern Hospital* that, after more than two thousand natural childbirths and rooming-in episodes, Grace–New Haven's "experience to date has been satisfactory." Citing studies indicating that "as high as 70 per cent of mothers might desire rooming-in if it were made available," Snoke added that "patient reaction to rooming-in continues to amaze me and to delight the proponents of this program."[117] On another occasion, he confessed that he found himself making daily visits to the unit. "You didn't hear babies crying," and the mothers "were so pleased with what was happening," Snoke recalled. "I enjoyed it, and was very proud of myself!"[118]

---

[112] Jackson, "Reactions of mothers and nurses," p. 694. One student nurse contrasted her experience on the maternity ward with her service in the rooming-in unit in this way: "It was [in the standard setting] a sort of race with time that left no individuality for anyone. There wasn't time to wait and see if the baby had taken the breast nor was there time to stop and encourage the mother with the poor nurser, but rather some impatience with the mother who wanted to finish combing her hair or fixing her face at 6:00 a.m. rather than taking the baby. Rooming-in was a great change. ... Although we were kept busy, we were not rushed." *Ibid.*

[113] Elaine Baumann, "The Visiting Nurse views rooming-in," *Public Health Nurs.*, 1950, 42: 263.

[114] Olmsted, Svibergson, and Kleeman, "Value of rooming-in experience," p. 621; Morris [Wessel] to author, 24 April 1988.

[115] McBryde, "Compulsory rooming-in," pp. 625, 627.

[116] Montgomery and Shenk, "Further experiences with the rooming-in project," pp. 782, 757.

[117] Snoke, "Rooming-in," p. 108.

[118] Snoke, interview with author, 9 February 1984.

ROOMING-IN SINCE 1952

It is thus striking and puzzling—on the surface—that institutional support for rooming-in waned at Grace–New Haven as soon as Jackson's project officially ended on 30 June 1952. To be sure, hospital authorities responded to vigorous public demand the next year and redesigned the new Memorial Unit so that rooms would be large enough to accommodate rooming-in, but subsequent budgets allocated no funds for the special rooming-in fellows and nurses whose work had made rooming-in, under Jackson's direction, so satisfying for its participants.[119] "Family-centered" maternity and infant care did not become the norm during the 1950s and 1960s in other American hospitals either.[120]

Financial constraints were surely a factor but probably were not decisive, at Grace–New Haven or elsewhere.[121] "I think there always has to be somebody who keeps a thing like that afloat, even when there's money," Sally Provence, professor emeritus at the Yale Child Study Center, recently remarked. Rooming-in, regarded by many Yale medical people as "nice but not essential," was, in Provence's view, "one of those marvelous projects that only survives as long as the people who started it make it survive."[122] At Grace–New Haven in 1953, with outside funding gone, Kate Hyder employed in another city, and Grover Powers retired, Jackson by herself could not persuade hospital authorities to offer mothers and infants in the new Memorial Unit the individualized attention their counterparts had received in the experimental rooming-in units.

At bottom, though, the history of Jackson's Rooming-In Research Project suggests that the fate of rooming-in in the 1950s and 1960s was primarily a function neither of finances nor of personnel, but rather of more global forces. Rooming-in, after all, required only modest additions to a hospital's budget; it posed health hazards to neither mothers nor babies; and it deeply satisfied both lay and medical participants. It failed to become the norm in American hospitals, however, because it challenged assumptions and practices that had profoundly transformed American pediatrics, obstetrics, and

[119] In 1977, when Yale–New Haven Hospital (formerly Grace–New Haven) appointed a nurse whose primary responsibilities were to help mothers breast-feed and to teach student nurses how to facilitate breast-feeding, Morris A. Wessel, a New Haven pediatrician and former rooming-in fellow, regarded the appointment as a gratifying *new* development. "How timely to have this happen on the day of Edie Jackson's death. It was as if to say the health care system, indeed, will carry on with the priorities she held so important!" Morris A. Wessel, "Edith B. Jackson, M.D.," draft of an article sent to *J. Pediatr.*, 1 October 1977, p. 11. Courtesy of the author. (The published version did not contain this comment.)

[120] A survey of rooming-in opportunities, published in the winter of 1956–57, reported that "facilities for rooming-in still are not widely available." Dawson, "Rooming-in," p. 34.

[121] In September 1951, Albert Snoke reported to fellow hospital administrators that to change "existing obstetric units to provide for rooming-in can frequently be done at comparatively little expense." He noted as well that while "the cost for an adequate program of rooming-in is greater than for the conventional method, ... the experience so far" indicates that "the cost is not a great deal more." Snoke, "Rooming-in," pp. 102, 106.

[122] Sally Provence, interview with author, New Haven, Connecticut, 19 June 1984.

hospitals several decades before, and it did so in the following substantial ways:

First, rooming-in tilted against the commonly held view that medicine was preeminently a scientific enterprise that required strict adherence to laboratory-tested procedures to be successful. Thus, while somatic pediatricians held that infants would thrive if their physical needs for proper nutrition, rest, immunization, and cleanliness were met, rooming-in advocates deplored the fact that "*essential* psychological needs of both mother and child [had] been disregarded" in the American hospital setting, and hailed psychiatry for having "picked up this neglected link."[123] Furthermore, although the medical mainstream still regarded psychiatry as little more than "malicious animal magnetism," as one physician put it,[124] exponents of rooming-in countered with the claim that psychiatry, as much as bacteriology or pathology, deserved "its *scientific* place amongst the various specialties."[125]

Second, rooming-in rejected the conviction—held by public health officials, hospital administrators, and many pediatricians—that an infant regularly in contact with his or her father and other visitors was far more likely to contract an infection than his or her counterpart reposing in the nursery.[126] That conviction was well warranted at the turn of the century, when maternal sepsis was rampant; but its persistence in the 1950s, even after infectious diarrhea, impetigo, and other diseases had struck many hospital nurseries,[127] suggests that rooming-in was, among other things, victim of what a noted historian of medicine has called "the traditional conservatism of the medical profession."[128] Having believed since the 1920s that isolation of newborns in glass-enclosed nurseries was a health imperative, numerous public health officials, nurses, and pediatricians could not readily discard that view.

Third, exponents of rooming-in thoroughly repudiated the wisdom of

---

[123] Jackson, "Should mother and baby room together?" p. 17. My italics.

[124] This was a favorite characterization of Daniel C. Darrow, Jackson's colleague in the Yale Department of Pediatrics, whose work on infectious diseases was nationally recognized in the 1940s and 1950s. Walcher, telephone conversation with author, 11 April 1984.

[125] Jackson, "Theoretic Considerations," p. 8. My italics.

[126] Grace–New Haven Hospital administrator Albert Snoke described and explained the long-standing procedures in this way: "Over the period of years, many rules, regulations and procedures have been developed by the departments of obstetrics and pediatrics, and by the state health departments that protect the mother and the baby from infection. As a result, the mothers and babies have been kept in quite strict isolation and every effort is made to separate the maternity and delivery units from the rest of the hospital. Visitors and doctors are kept from the babies to the greatest extent possible." Snoke, "Rooming-in," p. 106.

[127] McBryde, "Compulsory rooming-in," pp. 625, 626. Note that Daniel C. Darrow, a nationally known specialist in infectious diseases, told the Associated Press in June 1951 that hospital nurseries "contain too many babies" and thus permit "the rapid spread of certain types of infection." He then commended Grace–New Haven's "rooming-in" service for having prevented epidemics of infectious and contagious diseases among infants there and predicted that "a few years from now, the typical nursery of today will be regarded as archaic." Newspaper clipping datelined New Haven, Connecticut, and dated 13 June 1951, Jackson Papers, Yale University Library.

[128] Erwin H. Ackerknecht, *A Short History of Medicine*, rev. ed. (Baltimore and London: Johns Hopkins University Press, 1982), p. 178.

contemporary child development experts, most of whom still held, with L. Emmett Holt, Sr., that "babies under six months old should never be played with" or comforted, lest their habits become irregular and their characters "spoiled."[129] Launched on the eve of the Spock revolution,[130] rooming-in programs implemented the diametrically opposite view: that a "child's freedom to learn, and his capacity for self-discipline" were in fact "rooted in his infantile and early childhood *satisfactions*."[131] Rooming-in infants accordingly nursed at will. "Baby care on a flexible schedule," as Jackson put it, would "allow a youngster to slip gradually into 'Orderly Behavior' instead of being pushed abruptly into it."[132]

Fourth, rooming-in necessitated radical revision of the "hospital-centered" routine that had regulated infant feeding, maternal rest, and paternal visitation since the 1920s and had well served the institution's bureaucratic imperatives. Jackson's rooming-in project prescribed that hospital maternity and newborn care be predicated on "individualization in each baby's schedule according to his own needs, *and* the needs of his mother."[133]

Fifth, rooming-in entailed "revolutionary changes in nursing care"[134] at a time when hospital nurses, who had been "seeking professional prerogatives" since the 1920s,[135] were deeply protective of their status as nursery or obstetrical specialists. In that context, having the same nurse care for mother and baby "was just not done!" a former rooming-in fellow recently explained.[136] Jackson managed to do it at Grace–New Haven during the life of the Rooming-In Research Project, but she failed permanently to convert the nursing establishment, there or elsewhere, to that approach.

Sixth, rooming-in frustrated what pediatrician T. Berry Brazelton has called the universal drive of all adults who care about babies to be "the primary caretaker of the attractive helpless infant." Physicians and nurses, Brazelton has written, "basically like to help people depend on *us*."[137] Rooming-in, on the other hand, rejected "the harsh denial of parental privileges which the usual present day maternity ward procedures and hospital

[129] Holt, *Care and Feeding of Children*, pp. 192, 193.
[130] The first edition of Benjamin Spock's *The Common Sense Book of Baby and Child Care* (New York: Duell, Sloan and Pearce) was published in 1946.
[131] Edith B. Jackson, "Clinical sidelights on learning and discipline," *Amer. J. Orthopsychiatry*, 1947, *17*: 588. My italics.
[132] Edith B. Jackson, "Do you really understand 'self demand?' " *Baby Talk Mag.*, January 1950, pp. 2, 1. Jackson noted that many babies, started on a flexible schedule, "can be guided to an easy convenient schedule within three months." *Ibid*, p. 1.
[133] Jackson, "Prophylactic considerations," p. 97.
[134] Morris A. Wessel, "Social Action as Spiritual Component: The Relevance of Nicaragua" (paper delivered at Conference on the Secular and Non-Secular Spiritual Issues of Death and Dying, New Haven, Connecticut, 3 May 1986), p. 15. Courtesy of the author.
[135] Barbara Melosh, *"The Physician's Hand": Work, Culture, and Conflict in American Nursing* (Philadelphia: Temple University Press, 1982), p. 16.
[136] Wessel, "Social Action," p. 16.
[137] T. Berry Brazelton, "Comment," in Klaus and Kennell, *Maternal-Infant Bonding*, p. 97. My italics.

nursery care of newborns entail"[138] and embodied the contrary notion that obstetricians, pediatricians, and nurses should help parents to trust their own nurturing instincts and to assume primary responsibility for their infant's care.

Seventh, rooming-in could not gratify the "desire of hospital trustees and administrators for eminence" of the sort that came when staff clinicians made discoveries concerning infectious diseases or cardiology.[139] Rooming-in's results, by comparison, seemed not nearly as important. Well aware of this problem, Jackson and her associates wrote in 1956, "for some, there is validity enough in the spontaneous statements of hundreds and hundreds of mothers that the presence of the newborn baby and attentive care to both mother and baby by a skilled and considerate nurse is more satisfactory than separate nursery and maternity care," but "others seem to feel that such comments do not have scientific validity."[140] Rosenberg, noting that "well-meaning attempts [such as rooming-in] to shape new social programs within the hospital [have] had comparatively little impact" in the age of scientific medicine, recently explained it this way: "The social mission of the hospital seemed to most physicians not so much indefensible as secondary ... to the realms of bacteriology, biochemistry, and pathology."[141]

Finally, there is evidence for speculating that rooming in threatened traditional assumptions about gender roles in the 1950s. In Detroit, for example, physicians "openly hostile" to a rooming-in proposal called fellow practitioners who advocated it "the big bosom boys."[142] Their vitriol suggests that some practitioners reacted to rooming-in on an emotional level rather than a scientific and/or professional level. Thus, in the strange and schizophrenic 1950s,[143] when the nation's popular culture endorsed the "feminine mystique" while middle-class, married women hurried into the work force in record numbers, it appears that some doctors in Detroit and probably elsewhere experienced rooming-in as an assault on their scientific male domain by purveyors of dubious female folkways, and that they responded accordingly. In that context, perhaps one can also see why, in the 1970s, as women organized to demand control over their bodies[144] and young women entered medicine in increasing numbers, hospitals and physicians responded more favorably to Klaus and Kennell's plea for family-centered maternity and infant care than they had to the campaign for rooming-in two decades before.

---

[138] Jackson et al., "Hospital rooming-in unit," p. 29.

[139] Rosenberg, "Inward vision," p. 388.

[140] Jackson, Wilkin, and Auerbach, "Statistical report on incidence and duration of breast feeding," p. 711.

[141] Rosenberg, *Care of Strangers*, pp. 329, 335.

[142] "Cornelian Corner," *Newsweek*, 21 March 1949, p. 52.

[143] See chapter 5, "The Paradox of Change," in William H. Chafe, *The Unfinished Journey: America since World War II* (New York: Oxford University Press, 1986), pp. 111–45.

[144] See, for example, Boston Women's Health Book Collective, *Our Bodies, Ourselves: A Book by and for Women*, 2d ed., rev. and expanded (New York: Simon & Schuster, 1976).

It would be inaccurate to leave the impression that rooming-in, as conceived and implemented by Jackson and her colleagues in the late 1940s, enjoys widespread acceptance in the United States today. An informal survey of some of the first American hospitals that offered rooming-in reveals that whereas rooming-in at the Thomas Jefferson University Hospital "has continued to the present, and has been so successful and satisfying, in general, that people think it has always been this way,"[145] the rooming-in nurseries "were deleted" at the George Washington University Medical Center in 1971 when the maternity unit was renovated, although "the policies for infants being in mothers' rooms has [sic] been quite liberal since that time."[146] At the Duke University Medical Center, "rooming-in (the twenty-four-hour-a-day variety) was never terribly popular," but "a mother-baby nursing plan in which one nurse will care for both mother and infant" has just been implemented, with "the hope ... that this will foster rooming-in."[147] At Yale–New Haven Hospital (formerly Grace–New Haven), on the other hand, "the one nurse concept for mother and baby has more or less disappeared," but there is "much more flexibility with the babies in and out of the mother's room, fathers in and out."[148] Yale hospital authorities have decided to close the nurseries adjacent to the four-bed units, however, and they are reinstituting a central nursery, "just what Edie [Jackson] tried to abolish, and thought she had."[149] Jackson herself, having surveyed the situation in 1966, was doubtless right when she wrote that "the shortness of the maternity patients' stay seems ... to be working against strong interest in the mother-infant relationship on the part of the pediatric resident staff. The young pediatricians simply do not find it worthwhile to involve themselves with personal contact with the maternity floor patients beyond the duty of admission and discharge examination of the infant."[150]

CONCLUSIONS

The history of Edith B. Jackson's Rooming-In Research Project at Yale, then, adds to our understanding of twentieth-century American medicine in several particulars. It shows, first, that the professionalization and bureaucratization that so profoundly reshaped hospitals, childbirth, infant feeding, and other American institutions early in the century did not progress inexorably or go unchallenged. On the contrary, there were doctors in the 1930s and 1940s who believed that the psychological needs of newborns and their families were not served well by the new developments; and those clini-

---

[145] Maureen C. Edwards to author, 6 June 1989.
[146] James H. Lee, Jr., to author, 11 May 1989.
[147] Peter C. English to author, 7 April 1989.
[148] Morris Wessel to author, 24 April 1988.
[149] Morris Wessel to author, 16 March 1990; idem, 4 July 1989.
[150] Edith B. Jackson to Dr. [Gerd] Biermann, 6 June 1966, Jackson Papers, Schlesinger Library.

cians, decades before Klaus and Kennell reportedly pioneered in "family-centered" lying-in arrangements at American hospitals, and decades before the women's movement, urged that mothers be re-empowered in the birthing and feeding of their young and worked vigorously and intelligently to humanize hospital care.

The mixed and still uncertain fate of rooming-in in the United States in the second half of the twentieth century makes it equally clear, though, how deeply rooted the "transformations" detailed by Leavitt, Apple, and Rosenberg have become. In a recent book, a professor emeritus of psychiatry and pediatrics at the University of Colorado School of Medicine has written pessimistically of "the unhappy fact . . . that many hospitals have become tightly knit, hierarchical, regimented institutions run by administrators (some of them doctors) who often exhibit little concern for people in general, let alone children."[151] Others, however, are more hopeful. "Although things are not where they should be," a former rooming-in fellow observed recently, "they never are." He added, "We are further along because of Edie's insistence on what she believed."[152]

---

[151] Dane G. Prugh, *The Psychosocial Aspects of Pediatrics* (Philadelphia: Lea & Febiger, 1983), p. 502
[152] Morris Wessel to author, 24 April 1988.

The Rise of the Free Standing Birth Center: Principles and Practice

Pamela S. Eakins, PhD

ABSTRACT. The last decade witnessed a movement toward out-of-hospital birth. Licensed free standing birth centers (FSBCs) proliferated and, by 1984, over 100 were operating in the U.S. This paper details the history of The Birth Place in Menlo Park, CA. Over a three year period, 251 women in labor were admitted to the clinic. Of these women, 200 (80%) completed delivery at the center. Of these, four mothers and three babies transferred to the hospital postpartum for treatment. Fifty-one women (20%) transferred to the hospital intrapartum primarily as a result of prolonged or arrested labor. There were 11 forceps deliveries (4%) and six cesarean sections (2%). Of 51 babies born at the hospital, nine had complications requiring treatment. Overall, clients expressed a strong sense of satisfaction regarding their birth experience. The FSBC, with its alternative philosophy, serves as an important experiment testing out-of-hospital birth outcomes in a carefully screened low risk population.

INTRODUCTION

From the early 1970s to the present, out-of-hospital birth centers have mushroomed throughout the U.S. A free standing birth center (FSBC) is "an adaptation of a home environment to a short-stay, ambulatory, health care facility with access to in-hospital obstetrical and newborn services; designed to safely accommodate participating family members and support people of the woman's choice; and, providing professional preventive health care to women and the fetus/newborn during pregnancy, birth and puerperium" (Cooperative Birth Center Network News, 1981). FSBCs are "free stand-

Dr. Eakins is Affiliated Scholar, Center for Research on Women, Stanford University. Address reprint requests to: P.S. Eakins, PhD, Center for Research Women, Stanford University, Stanford, CA 94305.

Women & Health, Vol. 9(4), Winter 1984
© 1984 by The Haworth Press, Inc. All rights reserved.
49

ing" in that they operate independently from hospitals in the official, financial, and physical sense (Note 1).

During the period of the proliferation of these centers, they were strongly applauded by some groups and bitterly opposed by others. Yet, however controversial, the exponential growth of FSBCs in the United States is unquestionable. Begun "as a response to families who were engaging in do-it-yourself home birth rather than submit to in-hospital obstetrical care" (Lubic, 1982), the idea caught on rapidly. In 1972, one FSBC, offering nurse-midwifery care to the rural poor, is known to have been in existence in Texas. By 1975, at least four more were operating in California, New Mexico, New York, and Oregon (Lubic, 1982; Stewart and Stewart, 1979).

At present, there are over 100 FSBCs in the United States. In addition, the National Association of Childbearing Centers (formerly the Cooperative Birth Center Network) is keeping files on more than 300 physicians and midwives, consumer groups, institutions, and health agencies endeavoring to open free standing birth centers in their communities. These groups are at various stages of the planning process (Cooperative Birth Center Network News, 1983).

The FSBC, however rapidly expanding at present, is not a new idea in the U.S. Between 1944 and 1970, for example, nurse-midwives at the Catholic Maternity Institute, an out-of-hospital birth center in Santa Fe, attended more than 6,000 births (Carroll, 1979). What renders recent interest in out-of-hospital birth different is the fact that the current movement addresses issues stemming from both the forty year old natural childbirth movement initiated by the publication of Dick Read's *Childbirth Without Fear* (1959) which advocates unmedicated birth, and the recent consumer health care movement which advocates more humane, less costly, and less centralized methods of health care. The latter movement has resulted in community based clinics and mental health centers, hospices, free standing emergency and surgical centers and, ultimately, the FSBC.

In 1979, the American Public Health Association (APHA) adopted a position endorsing demonstration projects (FSBCs) for "alternatives in maternity care." In 1983, the APHA, reporting that "births to healthy mothers can occur safely outside the setting of an acute care hospital," adopted a set of guidelines for licensing and regulating birth centers. To ensure a reasonable approach to safety, the APHA guidelines emphasize that only clients with a normal, uncomplicated prenatal course should be accepted, and that these women should be attended only by licensed midwives and physicians. The physicians should have hospital obstetrical privileges. The facility must have the capability to initiate emergency procedures in life threatening situations, which, at the very least, consists of cardiopulmonary resuscitation equipment, oxygen, positive pressure mask, suction, intravenous equipment, equipment for maintaining infant temperature and ventilation, blood expanders and emergency medications. Systems for rapid transport to the hospital must be established. The FSBC is not an ambulatory surgical center and "surgical procedures should be limited to those normally accomplished during uncomplicated childbirth, such as episiotomy and repair, and should not include operative obstetrics or cesarean section." General and conduction anesthesia should not be administered. Clients should be fully informed about the benefits and risks of the FSBC and should provide written consent (American Journal of Public Health, 1983).

Whereas the American Public Health Association has adopted guidelines to accommodate the growing movement toward birth center deliveries, the American Academy of Pediatrics (AAP) and the American College of Obstetricians and Gynecologists (ACOG), in their joint publication entitled *Guidelines for Perinatal Care* (1983), offer the simple statement: "Until scientific studies are available to evaluate safety and outcome in free-standing centers, the use of such centers cannot be encouraged" except in particularly isolated geographical situations. This paper addresses the history, safety, and outcome at one urban free standing birth center in an attempt to shed further light on the unresolved birth center issue.

CASE STUDY: THE BIRTH PLACE
IN MENLO PARK, CALIFORNIA

History and Philosphy

It is not sufficient merely to describe the "medical outcome" of births at The Birth Place, Inc. without illuminating its unusual history as a provider of health care services. One of the women who initially masterminded the project was activist, Suzanne Arms. Early in the 1970s, as the recent movement toward out-of-hospital birth was taking shape, she authored *Immaculate Deception* (1975) in which she called for a dramatic restructuring of the circumstances of childbearing in the United States. In that book Arms presented her vision for a free standing birth center in the form of a story about a woman in labor who reflects on the history of the FSBC in which she will give birth:

> The town passed a bond issue at the insistence of a vocal parents' group and raised the money necessary to purchase one of the sturdy older homes near the center of town. . . . They organized a non-profit corporation, then cleaned and painted and equipped the home for births. An obstetrical nurse was hired to supervise the home. . . . The nurse handles all the business of clean and sterile linens and instruments, all on rotating loan from the city hospital twenty minutes away. . . . The home includes a small emergency room with a resuscitator, an incubator, oxygen, and a small supply of hormones and IVs. The nurse-administrator could help in a pinch, or until one of the on-call obstetricians or the ambulance arrived. . . . But what the young woman likes most about the center is that all of the emergency equipment is kept out of sight. And the three large birthing rooms remind her of her parents' home. (pp. 294-295)

Arms, however, did more than compose a story. Beginning in 1977, she worked to realize this dream. She began to organize in her community. Sixty people attended an initial meeting which resulted in the formation of a "Birth Action Group" headed by seven women.

The first target of this "Birth Action Group" was to establish an "alternative birth center (ABC)" in a local hospital. When this group, which quickly grew to 75, approached hospital administrators with their idea, they were informed that the possibility for establishing an ABC in the hospital was at least five years off. The "Birth Action Group" was not prepared to wait. Each member contributed $75 as seed money for establishing an FSBC. They used the funds they generated to advertise their cause and soon obtained donations amounting to several thousand dollars. In 1978, the "Birth Action Group" incorporated as a non-profit organization which allowed them tax exempt status and a Board of Directors was assembled to carry out the mandate.

The first act of this group, now The Birth Place, Inc., was to open a Resource Center to "educate the community." This center opened in a climate of skepticism and, in some cases, outright opposition voiced by local obstetricians. Nonetheless, by 1980, the Resource Center had expanded to 500 paying members. It received over

5,000 visitors and phone calls annually requesting information and referrals in the areas of "alternative" childbirth and early parenting.

In two years, the Resource Center had stabilized financially, and, in 1979, only one and a half years after the initial call to organize, The Birth Place FSBC had opened its doors as a fully-equipped, state licensed facility for unmedicated childbirth. Arms' vision, albeit more modest than the center she described, had come to pass. Today, over a hundred babies are born at The Birth Place each year. In 1983, the number of infants delivered at the center increased 17% over the previous year. Thus, The Birth Place is currently in a state of expanding services and a broadening financial base.

The Birth Place distinguishes its style of practice from that of the "traditional hospital" on "philosophical," "environmental" and "psycho-social" levels (see Table 1). Essentially, The Birth Place views childbirth as a "physical, emotional, social and spiritual rite of passage" for mother and baby. Only secondarily is childbirth seen as a medical event.

Description of the Facility

The clinic itself is a three bedroom house which has been renovated to meet state and county requirements for emergency exits, ambulance and wheelchair access. During the first three years of operation, thirteen medical practitioners including one obstetrician, three family physicians and nine certified nurse-midwives were granted membership on the medical staff where the staffing pattern was similar to that of a hospital. The medical practitioners were supervised by a Medical Director, an MD who was responsible for maintaining the technical capabilities of the facility and staff. These capabilities included continuous assessment of maternal, fetal, and newborn well-being; emergency medication and equipment, maternal and newborn resuscitation and rapid transport to the hospital four miles away. All medical staff personnel were required to demonstrate CPR capability for adults and infants and the ability to intubate neonates.

Obstetrical nurses, on call 24 hours a day, and trained assistants, as well as supplies and equipment, were provided for practitioners by the birth center for a package fee. Clients delivered with the attending physician or midwife of their choice, selecting from among those who had been granted privileges at The Birth Place.

TABLE 1: APPROACHES TO BIRTH*

_____

Traditional Hospital   **The Birth Place**

- -

Philosophical

1. Emphasis on physician.

2. Emphasis on conformity and routine.

3. Protocol predicated on expectation of complications: fetal monitors, routine I.V.s, drugs, forceps, episiotomies.

4. Pain relief through drugs (known to affect infant) and anesthetic blocks which commonly result in forceps delivery or cesarean.

5. Labor often artificially induced or stimulated with drugs.

1. Emphasis on family.

2. Emphasis on individuality and education for informed choice throughout the birth process.

3. Protocol for handling problems and emergencies is detailed but usually not applied: women are healthy. Careful screening and observation with close proximity to hospital if transfer is indicated. I.V.s started and episiotomies performed only as mutually agreed upon and indicated.

4. Pain relief through drugs is made unnecessary by ample preparation and continuous support.

5. Labor never artificially induced or stimulated. Walking, baths and showers, and nourishment are encouraged. Non-intrusive methods are always the first to be used.

- -

Environmental

6. Equipment for convenience of health professionals in expectation of surgery and emergencies: high narrow bed or delivery table, stirrups, bright lights.

7. Environment traditionally austere, sterile, rushed, noisy and intrusive. No windows or access to fresh air.

6. Furnishings to enhance family experience and protect the normal process. Queen size beds, flowered sheets, comfortable chairs, options for low light, daylight and music.

7. Environment quiet, relaxed and private. Doors that open into gardens for walking, sunlight and fresh air.

- -

Psycho-Social

8. Intermittant attendance by nurses and doctor. Routine change of shifts. Shortage of nurses common.

9. Staff unfamiliar to family and their concerns.

8. Constant one-to-one attendance by nurse, more frequent attendance by doctor or nurse-midwife with same nursing staff remaining throughout birth whenever possible.

9. Staff known by family and dedicated to respecting family's choice and individual autonomy in every aspect of their birth.

Traditional Hospital	The Birth Place
10. Lack of primary emotional support for woman or couple.	10. Extra support provided for physical and emotional needs of parents by trained non-medical birth assistant.
11. Separation of baby from mother – immediate cutting of cord with babies taken to nursery for washing, weighing and routine prophylactic medication.	11. No separation of baby from mother/father. Relaxed time for cutting of cord (often done by father), baby put to breast immediately, washing and weighing of baby only after ample time is given for mother-father-infant bonding. No routine prophylactic medication.
12. No provisions for home care or support during post-partum period.	12. Home medical visits and non-medical care, 'post-partum education and support included in services.

*source: Birth Place Brochure

Client Screening and Preparation

Women verified as "low risk" by their physician or certified nurse-midwife could use the center. The Birth Place protocol outlined 49 criteria which would preclude use of the center. These included (1) *prenatal* high risk factors such as chronic hypertension or renal disease, (2) risk factors in *obstetric history* such as previous cesarean section, (3) risk factors in the *present pregnancy* such as preeclampsia or gestational diabetes, and (4) *intrapartum* risk factors such as prolonged ruptured membranes (> 24 hours) or an abnormal fetal heart rate (Note 2).

Clients were required to be well-informed about childbirth and committed to an unmedicated birth as demonstrated by a willingness to attend three general orientation sessions at The Birth Place and a prepared childbirth class, generally teaching the Lamaze or Bradley method of natural childbirth, offered elsewhere in the community. Further, it was required that clients begin prenatal care during the first trimester (and in no case later than 20 weeks of pregnancy) with a certified nurse-midwife/physician team or physician. Clients were required to become familiar with reasons why transfer to a hospital may be necessary and agreed to transfer if these indications arose.

Fees

Between 1979 and 1982, fees for service at The Birth Place were approximately half that of the hospitals in its vicinity, although, by 1983, fees had become more commensurate with local hospitals. The Birth Place employed a sliding fee scale and was covered by Medicaid. Coverage was offered by all major insurance companies. Clients were also provided with the option of bartering (e.g., painting a room; doing clerical work) for birth services.

Socio-Demographic Characteristics of the Population

Nearly all of the women who delivered were caucasian and 90% were married. An analysis of census tract data revealed that the number of single mothers delivering at The Birth Place was only slightly lower than the proportion in the general population in the two county area serviced by the center. The racial consituency was unrepresentative, however, as a significant proportion of the general childbearing community was Black (7%) and Mexican-American (23%).

Two additional areas in which the birth center population was not representative were age and education. Primiparas ranged in age from 18-39 with a mean age of 27 and a median age of 28. This was significantly older than the general population wherein the median age at first birth was between 20 and 24 and over one third of the primiparas fell into this category. Multiparas ranged from 22 to 42 with a mean age of 30 and a median age of 31. Seventy-five percent of the population ranged between 25 and 34.

With regard to education, data were only available for the women completing delivery at the birth center. Of these, 105 (53%) had college educations and 57 (29%) had formal educations which extended beyond the baccalaureate level. The remaining 16% had high school educations, but this figure strongly correlated with age. Fifteen mothers were students at the time of delivery. Several women held PhD, MD or JD degrees.

Of the most prominent occupational categories, 13% identified their occupation as homemaker, 12% of the mothers were teachers,

10% were employed in the health sciences (primarily as RNs and medical assistants), 10% were clerical workers, and 9% were social and behavioral scientists.

Medical Outcome

Over a three year period, 251 women in labor were admitted to the center. Of these women 172 (69%) were primiparas and 79 (31%) were multiparas; 200 (80%) completed delivery at the birth center and 51 (20%) were transferred to the hospital for complications arising during labor.

Obstetricians attended 94 (37%) of the deliveries, 72 (29%) were attended by family physicians and 85 (34%) were attended by certified nurse-midwives. On six occasions, midwives were assisted by physicians.

Fifty-seven percent of the women completing delivery at the birth center had completely unmedicated births. Regional anesthesia was not employed at the center. Where medication was used, the most common form was a local anesthetic (xylocaine) applied to the perineum for suturing after birth which was used in just over one third of the total cases. Pitocin, a drug given to increase the intensity of contractions, was administered to about one fifth of the mothers after the baby was born to facilitate the delivery of the placenta or to control postpartum bleeding, but Pitocin was not used to augment labor (see Table 2).

The majority of the deliveries (182 or 91%) occurred without episiotomy. An intact perineum was preserved in 26% of the cases, while 64% had minor lacerations which were repaired, and 2% had third degree lacerations.

There was no major maternal or neonatal morbidity or mortality at The Birth Place during its first three years of operation. There were some complications including 22 cases of excessive blood loss (> 500 cc.) wherein Pitocin or Methergine was administered, three cases of retained placental tissue and one case each of perineal hematoma and urinary retention. Four women were transferred to the hospital postpartum. All four cases were processed routinely (e.g., manual removal of placenta) and the outcome was good.

Infants born at The Birth Place ranged in weight from 2495-4876 gr. (5.5-10.7 lbs.) with a mean weight of 3580 gr. (7.9 lbs.) On the ten point Apgar rating scale, which assesses heart rate, respiratory effort, muscle tone, reflex irritability and color, 186 babies (93%) had high scores of 7-10 at one minute after birth and at five minutes after birth, 198 (99%) fell into that range (see Table 3).

For 191 (96%) of the newborns, no complications were apparent. In nine cases (4.5%), complications were evident. Four newborns had tight nuchal cords. There were four cases of severe bradycardia (a heart rate of less than 100 beats per minute lasting for 10 minutes) and four cases of respiratory distress.

In 32 cases, meconium staining was noted and five babies were intubated at the center for possible meconium aspiration. Two babies required major resuscitation. Resuscitation procedures were begun at The Birth Place and the babies were transferred to the hospital. Both babies stabilized in transit to the hospital. From the moment of decision to transfer until the baby arrived in the emergency room the time elapsed was 11 and 13 minutes, respectively. A third baby who was also transferred to the hospital appeared abnormal and was later diagnosed as having Downs Syndrome.

Of the 251 women admitted to The Birth Place, 200 completed delivery at the FSBC and 51 (20%) were transferred to the hospital.

TABLE 2: PLACE OF BIRTH, PARITY AND MEDICATION DURING LABOR

MATERNAL MEDICATION

PLACE OF BIRTH		No Medication	Local Only	Other: analgesics, sedatives, etc.	
Birth Place	Primips	47 (19%)	49 (20%)	33 (13%)	129 (52%)
	Multips	39 (16%)	22 (9%)	10 (4%)	71 (29%)
	(Subtotal)	(86 (34%))	(71 (28%))	(43 (17%))	(200 (71%))
Hospital	Primips	1 (3%)	16 (6%)	26 (10%)	43 (16%)
	Multips	2 (1%)	3 (1%)	3 (1%)	8 (3%)
	(Subtotal)	(3 (1%))	(19 (8%))	(29 (12%))	(51 (21%))
	Total	89 (36%)	90 (36%)	72 (28%)	251 (100%)*

*Percentages are rounded off, therefore columns may not total 100%.

TABLE 3:　APGAR SCORES BY PLACE OF BIRTH

		APGAR SCORES			
PLACE OF BIRTH		0-3	4-6	7-10	
Birth Place	1 min.	2 (1%)	12 (6%)	186 (93%)	200
	5 min.	1 (.5%)	1 (.5%)	198 (99%)	200
Hospital	1 min.	6 (12%)	4 (8%)	41 (80%)	51
	5 min.	0	2 (4%)	49 (96%)	51

Over half of these women were transferred as a result of prolonged or arrested first stage of labor. This included maternal fatigue and secondary uterine inertia. In eight cases, the primary indication for transfer was heavy meconium staining. There were five cases of prolonged rupture of membranes. Four women requested analgesia which could not be provided by The Birth Place. Only one woman transferred solely on the basis of a request for analgesia (see Table 4).

Two thirds of the women were given Pitocin at the hospital. Regional anesthesia was administered to half of the transferred women. Six delivered with perineum intact and 28 (55%) had episiotomies. Of the hospital deliveries, 17 were instrumental: 11 by forceps, 6 by cesarean section. The figure for instrumental deliveries represents 31% of the admissions to the hospital and 7% of the total Birth Place admissions. The indications for cesarean included three cases of cephalopelvic disproportion, two cases of fetal distress and one case of failed Pitocin augmentation. In total 2% of the women admitted to The Birth Place ultimately delivered by cesarean section.

There were 51 babies born at the hospital. Newborn complications existed in nine cases (4%). These included three cases of fetal distress, three cases of meconium aspiration, one tracheoesophageal fistula and one cephalohematoma. These babies were admitted to the neonatal intensive care unit (NICU) for observation. Length of stay in the NICU ranged up to several days, but most babies were

TABLE 4: INTRAPARTUM TRANSFERS

PARITY

INDICATIONS FOR TRANSFER	Primiparas	Multiparas	
Prolonged/Arrested Labor	22 (43%)*	4 (8%)*	26 (51%)
Meconium	6 (12%)	2 (4%)	8 (16%)
Prolonged Rupture (Membranes)	2 (4%)	0	2 (4%)
Pain Medication Requested	1 (2%)	0	1 (2%)
Multiple Conditions	12 (24%)**	2 (4%)	14 (27%)
	43 (84%)	8 (16%)	51 (100%)

* Two primiparas and one multipara with prolonged or arrested labor requested pain medication.

** "Multiple Conditions" generally meant meconium coexisting with a prolonged or arrested labor (eight cases). Two "multiple conditions" cases included an abnormal fetal heart rate.

discharged home after a few hours. In sum, a total of 12 babies of mothers who were initially admitted to The Birth Place (5%) required emergency treatment after birth.

Satisfaction with the Birth Experience

A great deal of preparation went into the childbearing experience and a great deal of satisfaction was the result. Clients completing delivery at The Birth Place (n=200) evaluated their experience in five broad areas including (1) people at the birth; (2) birth center facilities; (3) services and fees; (4) general satisfaction; and (5) general dissatisfaction. The first three areas were assessed using Guttman scaling techniques. Respondents selected answers ranging from extremely satisfied to extremely dissatisfied on a five point scale.

Clients gave the FSBC a high rating: 97% were satisfied with physician's nurse-midwive's, nurse's, partner's, and labor supporter's participation in the birth, 91% were satisfied with the services; 77% were satisfied with the fees. A few clients, however, expressed philosophical concern about having to pay for birth services at all, given their view of birth as a "natural part of everyday life."

In response to the essay question "What I liked most about my experience," 43% cited the "supportive environment," 29% "being in control" or "freedom to do things my way," an additional 29% liked the "home-like setting" or "non-threatening environment." Twenty-one percent felt that the FSBC was relaxed or felt a "lack of pressure" and 48% of the respondents used words such as "caring," "calm," "nonintrusive," "quiet," and "sensitive" to describe their experience. While 13% appreciated the "presence of family" and/or "friends," 10% lauded the "skill" or "expertise" of the practitioners. To the question "What I liked least about my experience," 48% answered with a succinct "nothing," and 10% experienced a lack of privacy. Others (6%) felt pressured by a time limit or felt that the environment was "too hot" or "too cold."

DISCUSSION

Several progress reports for FSBCs have appeared in the professional and lay literature (Bean, 1975; Bennetts & Lubic, 1982; Cohen, 1982; Cooperative Birth Center Network News, 1983; De-Jong, Shy, & Clark, 1979; Faison, Lubic, 1975; Norwood, 1978; Pisani, & Douglas et al., 1979; Reinke, 1982; Shy, Frost, & Ullom, 1980). These studies demonstrate that women selecting the birth center alternative tend to be well prepared for childbirth via formal childbirth education. They have more prenatal visits than a home birth population or the population at large, and there is, in general, a favorable medical outcome when medical protocols are strictly adhered to (Bennetts & Lubic, 1982; DeJong, Shy, & Clark, 1979; Shy, Frost, & Ullom, 1980).

Criteria for admission and intrapartum and postparatum transfer to the hospital, as well as reasons for transfer and transfer rates, were comparable in the investigations appearing in the literature between 1975 and 1982 (Bean, 1975; Bennetts & Lubic, 1982; De-Jong, Shy, & Clark, 1979; Faison, Pisani, & Douglas et al., 1979; Norwood, 1978; Reinke, 1982; Shy, Frost, & Ullom, 1980). The rate of intrapartum transfer to the hospital was about 16-20% in each of these reports, with the primary indication for transfer cited as prolonged or arrested labor.

A 1983 study of 62 birth centers reported an average transfer rate of 13%. The authors of this study hypothesize that the low transfer rate may reflect a greater use of Pitocin and forceps at some centers (Cooperative Birth Center Network News, 1983).

The medical outcome for The Birth Place closely parallels that presented in analysis of 1,398 births in 11 FSBCs cross-nationally (Bennets & Lubic, 1982). In this study, as at The Birth Place, about 90% of the births were spontaneous vaginal deliveries. In both cases, 4% of the babies were delivered by forceps. However, 5% of the infants in the 11 birth centers were delivered by cesarean section, whereas cesarean section comprised 2% of the deliveries at The Birth Place. Cross-nationally, and in deliveries completed at The Birth Place, 60% of the births were unmedicated. In both studies, about 95% of the newborns suffered no complications. The neonatal mortality rate for these birth centers was 4-6/1000, compared to 13/1000, the national figure for the U.S. This discrepancy seems to be a result of the selection procedures which screen out high risk cases.

These results are consistent with other assessments of medical outcome which conclude that FSBCs appear to provide a medically safe alternative to the hospital (Faison, Pisani, & Douglas et al., 1979; Reinke, 1982). It is cautioned, however, that risk can only be minimized if a very strict protocol for screening and transfer to the hospital is implemented (DeJong, Shy, & Clark, 1979).

CONCLUSIONS

The precise risks of out-of-hospital delivery remain indefinite and further investigation is imperative (DeJong, Shy, & Clark, 1979; Institute of Medicine and National Research Council, 1982; Shy, Frost, & Ullom, 1980). It is clear, however, that for the specific clientele selecting this option, the vast majority deliver safely and successfully and emerge deeply satisfied with the experience.

The movement toward FSBCs has been criticized from two standpoints. One contingent fears the possibility of undue medical risks to mother or baby incurred outside of a hospital situation. The other enumerates risks, both of a physical and psychological nature, encountered in a hospital environment and claims that the birth center "movement" itself coopts activists as they become extensions of the rules of the medical establishment from which they are trying to escape (Rothman, 1982; Ruzek, 1980).

There may be truth on both sides. At the present time, however, the FSBC experiment will help to clarify what risks, if any, may be encountered for a carefully screened population delivering out of the hospital in an environment which is, in a manner of speaking, medically controlled. The FSBC experiment is, in a sense, a "controlled" experiment. Outcomes at these demonstration projects will, over time, have major repercussions regarding the structure and definition of childbirth in the U.S. What is needed, at this time, is a cumulation of reports.

In the meantime, it is critical to be aware of the fact that women have diverse needs in childbearing (Nelson, 1982) and that the FSBC is not claiming to be the "right way." As we have seen FSBCs tend to address themselves to the needs of a narrowly circumscribed risk classified socio-economic group. This, in itself, may prove to be a shortcoming.

The FSBC demonstrates not *the answer,* but *a possibility.* For some, such as the "Birth Action Group," it is a dream realized in the context of a culture in flux.

REFERENCE NOTES

1. The MacNeil Lehrer Report: "Med Stop," October 9, 1981.
2. The Birth Place Protocol is available from The Birth Place, 1220 University Drive, Menlo Park, CA 94025.

REFERENCES

American Academy of Pediatrics and American College of Obstetricians and Gynecologists (1983). *Guidelines for Perinatal Care.* Evanston, Illinois: American Academy of Pediatrics and American College of Obstetricians and Gynecologists.
American Journal of Public Health (1983). 8209 (PP): Guidelines for licensing and regulating birth centers, *73*, 331-334.
Arms, S. (1975). *Immaculate Deception: A New Look at Women and Childbirth in America.* Boston: Houghton Mifflin Company.
Bean, M. (1975). Birth is a family affair. *American Journal of Nursing, 75,* 1689-1692.
Bennetts, A. B., & Lubic, R. W. (1982). The free-standing birth center. *The Lancet, 1,* 378-380.
Carroll, M.H. (1979). Starting a childbearing center in your community. In: D. Stewart and L. Stewart (Eds.). *Compulsory Hospitalization or Freedom of Choice in Childbirth?* Vol. 2. Marble Hill, Missouri: National Association of Parents and Professionals for Safe Alternatives in Childbirth (NAPSAC).
Cohen, R. (1982). A comparative study of women choosing two different childbirth alternatives. *Birth, 9,* 13-20.
Cooperative Birth Center Network. (1982). *Participants' Manual: How to Start a Freestand-*

ing Birth Center. National Association of Childbearing Centers, Box 1, RD 1, Perkiomenville, PA.

Cooperative Birth Center Network News. (1981). *1,* 1.

Cooperative Birth Center Network News. (1983). *1,* 4.

DeJong, R. N., Shy, K., & Clark, K. C. (1979). An out-of-hospital birth center using university referral. *Obstetrics and Gynecology, 58,* 703-707.

Dick Read, G. (1959). *Childbirth Without Fear.* 2nd Edition. New York: Harper and Row.

Faison, J. B., Pisani, B. J., Douglas, R. G., et al. (1979). The childbearing center: An alternative birth setting. *Obstetrics and Gynecology, 54,* 527-532.

Institute of Medicine and National Research Council. (1982). *Research Issues in the Assessment of Birth Settings.* Washington, D. C.: National Academy Press.

Lubic, R. W. (1975). Developing maternity services women will trust. *American Journal of Nursing, 75,* 1685-1688.

Lubic, R. W. (1982, January). The rise of the birth center alternative. *The Nation's Health,* 7.

Nelson, M. K. (1982). The effect of childbirth preparation on women of different social classes. *Journal of Health and Social Behavior, 23,* 339-353.

Norwood, C. (1978, May). A humanizing way to have a baby. *Ms,* 89-92.

Reinke, C. (1982). Outcomes of the first 527 births at the Birthplace in Seattle. *Birth, 9,* 231-241.

Rothman, B. K. (1982, September). Anatomy of a compromise: Nurse midwifery and the rise of the birth center. Paper presented at the American Sociological Association, San Francisco, CA.

Ruzek, S. B. (1980). Medical response to women's health activities: Conflict, accommodation, and cooptation. Research in the Sociology of Health Care, *1,* 335-354.

Shy, K. K., Frost, F., & Ullom, J. (1980). Out-of-hospital delivery in Washington state, 1975-1977. *American Journal of Obstetrics and Gynecology, 137,* 547-552.

Stewart, D. & Stewart, L. (Eds.). (1979). *Compulsory Hospitalization or Freedom of Choice in Childbirth?* Vol. 3. Marble Hill, Missouri: NAPSAC.

MARY STEWART

PAT ERICKSON
University of Missouri–Kansas City

The Sociology of Birth: A Critical Assessment of Theory and Research

Although sociologists have applied their theoretical and analytical abilities to many stages of the life process — childhood, adolescence, transition to marriage and family, widowhood, aging, and death — the life entry stage has been virtually ignored by sociologists. Demographers have traced rates of fertility and fecundity, and anthropologists have given fairly extensive attention to the process of pregnancy and birth in different cultures.[1] The greatest interest in pregnancy and birth has been evidenced by physiologists, embryologists, and pharmacologists, and the bulk of the research appears in such journals as the *American Journal of Nursing, Journal of Psychosomatic Research,* and *Journal of Obstetrics and Gynecology*. Psychologists have not altogether neglected the area of birth, although their concentration on the individual and internal states may be somewhat limited.[2] Even the popular press has been more attentive to pregnancy, labor, and birth than has sociology.[3] A review of the literature, however, indicates that within sociology the attention which has been given this area comes from the deviance theorists' research on illegitimacy or abortion and from the superficial coverage offered by marriage and family literature, which is more likely to discuss the impact of the infant on the extant family. The inevitable conclusion is that there remains a curious lack of interest in birth within the discipline of sociology.

There are various reasons why such an obvious and important area has been neglected within sociology long after the acceptance of a sociological analysis of death, an equally natural and ordinary, albeit more inevitable, process.[4] Perhaps because these events and processes have been taken for granted and have been so intricately woven into the social fabric, they have not been sifted out as something which merits our attention and have thus evaded analysis by researchers. Yet their very pervasiveness, their unquestioned existence, indicates their imposing weight, their importance in the formation of the infrastructure of the social system. Yet why has a phenomenon that is so pervasive become a taken-for-granted reality?

One of the most obvious reasons for the neglect is that pregnancy and birth are experiences specific to women. Furthermore, they are viewed as the natural expression of and integral to being a woman in our society. Those women who do not have these experiences are met with either suspicion or sympathy.

Just as with other experiences or exigencies that are specific to women, pregnancy and birth have not been viewed as significant topics of investigation, relegating them to the role of "women's issues," women's problems, occupying much the same interest as "women's stories" in literature.[5] Feminists have decried the treatment of women by health care experts. Authors such as Seaman[6] and Frankfort[7] not only point out the neglect of women's health issues, but also illustrate the misconceptions about women and their bodies perpetuated by training programs for physicians, especially obstetrics-gynecology practitioners. The neglect of women's health issues has led some feminists to demand that males be denied further entrance to obstetrics-gynecology residencies.[8]

The evidence that suggests that women's health was not a significant factor in the production and proliferation of potentially death-dealing and crippling birth control devices, or that treatment of breast cancer has not been more adapted to women's needs than to the surgeon's skill, or that such female-specific diseases such as endrometriosis have not been investigated for either cause or successful treatment all merely illustrate the politically disenfranchised position of women. The neglect of issues within the sociology of birth provides further evidence of the powerlessness and social insignificance of women.

If we define pregnancy and birth as processes which are inseparable from being a woman, as an extension of the female role, and if these processes are so much a part of the definition of woman as to be her presumed nature, then we cannot even perceptually differentiate them as processes significant for study. The mere fact that pregnancy and birth are processes experienced (at least most intimately and, until recently, almost inevitably) by women has been partially responsible for the neglect of these areas by social scientists. An indication of this is the realization that male-specific or male-related diseases or risks, from prostate problems to impotency and heart failure, have been far more likely to attract the attention and interest of researchers and policymakers. One simply does not gain status by working with processes or problems related to low-status people.

Sociologists, along with economists, historians and psychologists, have paid scant attention to women. There are several reasons for this in addition to the general devaluation of and disinterest in women. First, most sociologists are male and most theorists and methodologists within sociology are male. Consequently, their work, the areas they choose to investigate or analyze, have reflected male interests. In addition, as sociology has become a more specialized field, the areas of specialty not only reflect the selection by male sociologists of what is a significant area of study, but as a consequence provide interest and research in areas in which males have been the primary and most powerful participants.

A glance at the many areas of specialization illustrate this point: Complex Organizations, Occupations and Professions, Industrial Sociology, Sociology of Sports, Criminology, Sociology of Work and Stratification. Women seem to have interested them only if they are deviant in some fashion (lesbian or prostitute) or as they fill their role or prepare for their potential role of a man's wife or someone's mother. Women's lives have not been seen as significant enough to warrant study, with some important exceptions.[9]

Another related consideration within sociology is that on the prestige scale, study of women ranks fairly low. Such areas as marriage and family are most likely to deal with the lives and experiences of women. Yet even in this relatively low status sub-field, males dominate in both research and authorship, while women may be asked to teach the courses because it is consistent with their "nature," interests, or "natural abilities," much as women have been encouraged to enter the compatible professions of nursing, teaching, and, within medicine, pediatrics. Only recently have women abandoned the notion that marriage and family courses must be avoided if one is to be a serious sociologist and have come full circle to the understanding that this area and the topics included therein require the elucidation which can be provided by conscientious women sociologists. Thus, the attempt by sociology to gain acceptance as a significant science and the attempt by sociologists to gain prestige and status within their field contributed to the neglect of issues of pregnancy and birth (women's issues) within the field.

During the past several years, however, significant social changes have provided an atmosphere in which the emergence of a sociology of birth seems more possible. Certainly the Women's Movement has generated an enormous amount of research on women, sex roles, etc., and the specific issues raised by the Women's Movement, such as inadequate health care, oppression by institutions in which women operate, and denial of rights over self, body, and life, have provided a wealth of research topics and have led to the allocation of monies to fund studies. A related movement, which could be termed "back to the earth," ritualistic, reactionary, and mostly antithetical to the Women's Movement, has also focused upon the damage perpetrated upon women by hospitals and their personnel. The interests of the very traditional earth-mother women in this movement, the work of professionals and others in the development of prepared childbirth and encouragement of home births, the inclusion of the father in the pregnancy and the birth process, and the legalization of nurse-midwifery have dovetailed with the criticism being voiced by various segments of the Women's Movement that the medical establishment consistently oppresses, degrades, and damages them through its organizational structure and emergent definitions.

These broad social factors have, it seems, provided a climate in which the sociology of birth can emerge as a legitimate area of study, and indeed a growing number of sociologists in this and other countries are doing research on the life entry process. The sociology of birth can be broadly defined as the application of sociological theory and methodology to that significant life process which chronologically incorporates the period from decision-making through the first year of an infant's life. The possible topics for investigation are numerous, as the field is largely untrammeled and is one which can incorporate such diverse research as the study of "products of the womb" to the changing self-image of the woman throughout the pregnancy stage.[10] The area can be delineated into six stages or phases: (1) the decision to or not to become pregnant, (2) the pregnancy phase, (3) labor and delivery, (4) the post-delivery stage, (5) the first six weeks, and (6) the first year.

The task now is to more clearly delineate this field of study and to provide analysis and areas for analysis. This process may be enhanced by outlining at least one possible form that the sociology of birth might take. In the following discussion, attention will be focused on two of these phases: (1) pregnancy and (2) labor and delivery.

PREGNANCY

In light of the prevalence of the phenomenon of pregnancy, it is surprising to note the paucity of attention and information on the subject within the discipline of sociology. This neglect of the topic of pregnancy is evidenced by the minimal attention given to this phase in marriage and family textbooks as well as by the lack of attention devoted to pregnancy in related journals.

A survey of some of the most widely used texts in the area of marriage and the family discloses either no discussion of the phenomenon of pregnancy[11] or a cursory examination of the subject.[12] Though the subject of children is usually given extensive coverage in such texts, it is often assumed that the transition from pre- to post-parenthood is a relatively smooth one, although there is some recognition of the temporary disruptiveness caused by the infant. Some attention may be given to difficulties or changes experienced during the pregnancy period, such as anxiety about the prospective parent role, but no systematic treatment is offered whereby the social reality of pregnancy is understood.[13]

The sociological research that has been done in the area of pregnancy reveals a narrowness of scope in the analysis of this phenomenon. Miller has classified research in the area of pregnancy as centering about five major themes.[14] First, a social problems orientation exists, where the major focus has been the analysis of deviant pregnancies (e.g., the unwed pregnant teenager). Second, there is a socio-medical orientation, where the major focus is on the "health issues" of pregnancy (e.g., prenatal care, diet, poverty). Third, a personal adjustment theme is stated, where psychoanalytic concepts are applied to pregnancy. Fourth, a social planning focus is defined, which emphasizes a demographic analysis of fecundity and fertility rates and is often concerned with the consequences of "excessive" numbers of births. Fifth, there is an ethnographic approach, which describes pregnancy in various cultures. Miller's bibliography on pregnancy substantiates the classifications presented above.[15]

From these classifications, it is apparent that *sociological* research in the area has been extremely limited in terms of the types of pregnancy "issues" that have been analyzed. For the most part, sociological analysis of pregnancy stems from a deviance or demographic orientation. Outside the discipline of sociology, medical, psychoanalytic, and anthropological orientations predominate. The reasons for this "narrow" treatment of pregnancy within the discipline of sociology have already been discussed. It is the intent in this section to demonstrate the potential benefits of a broader sociological approach through a description of the applicability of role theory to pregnancy. This analysis will primarily focus on some of the "unique" features of the pregnant role and examples of sociological research in the area of pregnancy.

Role Entrance

Traditionally, there have been tremendous cultural pressures for married women to enter the pregnant role. There has also been little that women could do to prevent the physiological reality of pregnancy. With the availability of contraception and the emergence of the Women's Movement, the inevitability and desirability of entrance into the pregnancy role is being seriously questioned by many women. For women who do enter the pregnant role, the mechanisms for entry can vary in terms of whether entrance into the role was planned, accidental, or coerced (e.g., rape). The reactions to and interpretations of the pregnant role may therefore be expected to vary, depending on the mode of entry.

The conditions under which women enter this role can also vary in terms of the legitimacy of role entrance. Normatively, pregnancy has been "reserved" for married women, and there have also been implicit age prescriptions in terms of the appropriate time for the assumption of this role. In contemporary American society, the pregnant teenager or the pregnant woman over forty may be viewed as occupying a deviant role for her age. These traditional definitions of deviant pregnancies are being questioned by an increasing number of women who opt for the adoption of the pregnant role outside the traditional marital structure. The reasons for and consequences of their choice of a deviant role would be an interesting subject for sociological research.

Entrance into the pregnancy role may also be expected to vary by socioeconomic position, race/ethnicity, and religious affiliation. For example, the number of times entrance into this role is considered appropriate and the type of decision-making involved in role entrance may be predicted to vary with each of these three variables.

These considerations indicate that entrance into the pregnant role is an extremely complex process. The analysis of the process is further complicated by the interplay between a physiological reality and a social reality. Entrance into the pregnant role is preceded by a physiological diagnosis of pregnancy, either by self or by an expert. This physiological condition must then be interpreted and translated into a social reality.

Miller questions the assumption of an equivalence between the physiological reality and social reality of pregnancy.[16] She treats the issue of acquiring a pregnancy identity as problematic and focuses on the process through which pregnant women acquire the pregnancy identity and became socially defined as pregnant. Utilizing panel interviews as a basis for analysis, Miller makes a distinction between "true-planners," "sort-of-planners," and "non-planners" in terms of the extent to which their pregnancy was a planned event. The con-

clusion is that these groups differed in important ways in terms of their acquisition of a pregnancy identity. For example, the non-planners saw physical
signs of pregnancy cues only retrospectively—after they had been medically
diagnosed as pregnant, while the true and sort-of-planners made their own
initial diagnoses. The non-planners entered into use of medical facilities for
sickness, not for pregnancy, while the sort-of/true-planners sought obstetrical
care. The non-planners had no new identity to reveal to friends, relatives,
husbands before diagnoses, while the true and sort-of-planners discussed their
probable new identity with others. Finally, the non-planners had a much
weaker attachment to their new pregnant status.

In sum, the process of entrance into the pregnant role is one which could
benefit from many kinds of sociological analyses, ranging from an examination of the decision-making process and of the structural conditions surrounding entrance into the pregnant role to the acquisition of a pregnancy identity.

Role Expectations

The pregnant role has some unique features associated with it in comparison with other types of roles (e.g., marital, occupational). The pregnant role
is one which lasts for a relatively short period of time. Progression in the role is
accompanied by a tremendous number of physiological changes, and the
most visible of these changes end when the role is terminated. The "successful" completion of the pregnant role results in the immediate acquisition of
another role—motherhood. These features of the pregnant role lead one to
ask about the set of expectations of that role. How do the temporariness, the
physiological manifestations, and the acquisition of a new role when the pregnant role is "successfully" completed affect the set of expectations of the pregnant role?

Rather than assuming that the pregnant role is characterized by role
clarity and harmony, the features of the pregnant role described above would
lead one to argue that the role is characterized by role ambiguity and inconsistency. The temporariness of the role may mean that there is not sufficient
time to feel comfortable in the role. Indeed the temporariness and the knowledge of when the role will terminate may mean that a clear set of expectations
for the role have not been completely developed, i.e., it is characterized by
role ambiguity.

The physiological changes occurring may be interpreted in a variety of
ways. On the one hand, pregnancy may be defined as an illness. Since, in contemporary American society, the appropriate "handling" of a pregnant role
requires regular visits to a physician and the termination of the role occurs
within a hospital setting, there does exist an "illness" expectation attached to
that role. This expectation is intensified by physiological changes which may
result in morning sickness, toxemia, etc. The interpretation of this "illness"
definition may result in the expectation that other roles of the pregnant
woman (e.g., sexual, occupational) should be curtailed or terminated.

On the other hand, pregnancy has been conceptualized as a time during which women reach the "peak" of their femaleness. Such an inconsistent set of expectations not only implies difficulty for the pregnant woman in assessing what behavior is appropriate for the role (sickness or radiant health) but also implies that physiological changes occurring will have consequences for the pregnant woman's self-image.

Finally, Alice Rossi has suggested that although pregnancy is viewed as a time of anticipatory socialization for the role of mother, in comparison with occupational and marital roles, there is a lack of any realistic training for the role of mother. Rossi argues that the preparation time that exists is "confined to reading, consultation with friends and parents, discussions between husband and wife and a minor nesting phase in which a place and the equipment for a baby are prepared in the household."[17]

It is not suggested that all pregnant women will experience role inconsistency and role ambiguity. But rather the degree of role ambiguity and inconsistency will vary in terms of the interpretations that the pregnant women attach to their experience. For example, women who have "successfully" completed several pregnancies may experience less role ambiguity. Women with "problem" pregnancies may accept the illness conceptualization of the role more readily. In addition, the expectations attached to the pregnant role may vary by marital status, socioeconomic position, and race/ethnicity.

For example, women engaged in deviant pregnancies whose financial resources are limited may view the anticipatory socialization expectation of the pregnant role as a source of anxiety. Likewise women who are employed full-time in a career may also view the pregnant role as a cause of anxiety. Therefore, the expectations of the pregnant woman cannot be assumed to be well-defined. Rather the characteristics of the pregnant role outlined above suggest that the pregnant role is characterized by ambiguity and inconsistency and further variations may be anticipated due to differences in marital status, socioeconomic position, and race/ethnicity.

Role Relationships

One of the interesting features of the pregnant role is the degree of isolation the pregnant woman experiences from others who are experiencing the same process. Even if friends happen to be or have been pregnant, it is not likely that these friends will be at the same stage of the pregnancy process. Unlike other preparatory roles (e.g., graduate school), where there emerges a "fellowship of suffering" among those experiencing or enduring the same process, the pregnant woman can share little of her concerns, anxieties, etc., with others who are also in the pregnant role.[18] There is no pregnancy subculture for most women.

Most role relationships of the pregnant woman are therefore with others who are not in the role. These others are likely to be her spouse, friends, relatives, employer, and physician, all of whom have a set of expectations about the pregnant role. Since, as indicated in the last section, the expectations for the pregnant role are ambiguous and inconsistent, it is likely that others' expectations conflict with one another and with the pregnant woman's own set of expectations. Even more significantly, because of the physiological manifestations of pregnancy, the major status variable that others are likely to be typically reacting to is the pregnant one. Hence, the focal identity for others is likely to be the pregnant identity, and other identities of the pregnant woman may not be viewed as relevant and important.

Furthermore, interpretation of her behavior may be linked to her pregnant role. Her emotions may be taken "lightly" by others because they are seen as stemming from her pregnant status.[19] If a woman defines the pregnant role as her most salient role, then no difficulty may arise. However, if other identities are equally or more salient, then the pregnant woman may encounter role strain. For example, La Rossa examined the relationship between first pregnancy, role salience, and marital strain.[20] Using a systems approach, he argued that the degree to which marital partners have occupational versus familial orientations is of critical import in assessing the impact of the first pregnancy on the marital relationship. Where the occupational identity is primary for one or both partners, it is highly likely that the first pregnancy will create a great deal of marital strain, while a familial orientation of both partners lessens the strain of the first pregnancy.

Obviously, the role relationships of the pregnant woman are in need of further analysis and elaboration. For example, how does the socioeconomic position of the pregnant woman affect the relationship she has with her physician? What are the role relationships of women engaged in "deviant" pregnancies? The preceding discussion has illustrated some of the major issues that are open for investigation.

Role Exit

The typical mechanism for exit from the pregnancy role is through the "successful" completion of that role and entry into the role of motherhood. The pregnant woman, however, has little control over the timing for exit from this role, outside of knowing that it will usually end in nine months. Exit from the role in this manner therefore means little control over the termination of one role and entrance into another role.

Exit from the role may also occur before the "successful" completion of the role where the exit is involuntary—miscarriage. Exit in this manner not only means that the pregnant role has been terminated early, but entry into the mother role is no longer a possibility at that time. This "unsuccessful" completion of the role and the lack of control over its termination would be expected to have important implications for definition of self.

Finally, exit from the role may be accomplished through voluntary termination before the "successful" completion of the role through abortion. Abortion as a mode of exit indicates a rejection of the pregnancy and/or motherhood identity. An important question for research is ascertaining under what conditions is abortion as a mode of exit chosen by the pregnant woman. For example, Rosen and Martindale analyzed the relationship between contraception, abortion, and self concept, using data collected on 1,746 women with "problem pregnancies."[21] They concluded that significantly more aborters reported the use of contraception than was true of the group who have the child, and women who had contracepted and/or who had chosen abortion were significantly higher in perceived competence and lower in traditional female role orientations than those who had not contracepted or had not chosen abortion. They interpret these findings as indicating that both a decision to contracept and a decision to abort indicate activism rather than passivity and that among the forces resulting in activism are a sense of competence and a manifest concern for one's own rights.

Rosen and Martindale's analysis provides an assessment of the interplay between mode of entrance, role expectations, and mode of exit. That is, the use of contraception and the rejection of traditional female role is associated with abortion as a mode of exit. Several other research questions concerning the interplay among the various aspects of the pregnant role emerge. For example, if the mode of entrance is coercive, as in rape, what is the probability that the mode of exit will be abortion? Even more significant, what is the socially constructed reality which intervenes between this mode of entry and exit? Or if the mode of entry is planned and the exit is miscarriage, what are the implications for the woman's self-image? These questions suggest that not only is each aspect of the pregnant role, the entrance, expectations, relationships and exit, filled with research possibilities, but also that the relationships among them is an exciting area for inquiry.

LABOR AND DELIVERY

Descriptions of birth experiences vary enormously. Some women recall it as the most gruesome, bloody, and horrible experience of their lives. Others indicate that they had the most satisfying, deepest orgasm during delivery. Surely the manner in which women describe their labor and delivery varies by many factors, including such things as the setting, the difficulty of the labor, their definition of themselves as sick or healthy, their expectations, and how well these were met.

A complete sociological analysis of labor and delivery would take into account such factors as the impact of different organizational settings, role relationships within those settings, support structures, and the impact of such characteristics as socioeconomic status, marital status, definition of the pregnancy as problematic or not, race, and age. All of these would affect both the experience and the interpretation of that experience by self and others. Although there are many research questions to be posed about labor and delivery, one way of delineating the area for investigation is to look at the process of entering the birth setting and then at labor and delivery, recognizing that these would vary by institutional requirements as well as by many other characteristics of self, relationships, and social structure.

Entry

Whether the mother chooses home or hospital birth, she is very likely ill-prepared for the role of mother. Regardless of the number of previous children, there is almost a total lack of knowledge and control over the process of "giving birth," which is one of the most powerful processes many women will ever experience. This failure leaves a woman unprepared for the reality into which she is so quickly and irreversibly thrust, especially if she, like the vast majority of women, enters an institutional setting for labor and delivery.

Beginning with their redefinition in terms of social and biological history upon admission, through the increasing loss of control which they experience as labor becomes heavier, women are transformed from adults with identities to faceless children. The transformation can be rapid because the woman is encouraged to perceive the situation as one of crisis which demands her co-operation. Family members, from whom she will soon be almost entirely isolated, encourage her to submit and cooperate. High status persons on whom she is dependent for information and help also encourage cooperation. This process is similar to the process of becoming a mental patient described so well by Goffman as a process in which the pre-patient cooperates in his/her own capture and is then angry and humiliated for having done so.[22] During this entry phase, the woman is often unaware of procedure, and her lack of knowledge makes her more vulnerable and more dependent on the very people who will prep and drug and otherwise manipulate her for their convenience and for the smooth operation of the institution. It is interesting to note the patient's lack of information, considering that she may have had nine months of contact with an obstetrician, a person quite familiar with hospital procedure. It is plausible that the obstetrician had nothing to gain by informing the patient, since he maintains a separation between the other activities that take place in the labor setting and his more important work of delivering.

Scully and Bart report that our official experts on women, gynecologists, are unbelievably condescending to women, often casting them in roles of frigidity and usually seeing them as narcissistic, masochistic, and passive.[23] These characteristics do not enhance communication with women on an adult level and make meaningful communication with women, who are viewed as driven by their hormones and likely to be emotionally unstable, even less likely.

During contact with the obstetrician and the transition from woman to child, when the change from autonomous decision-maker to dependent begins, role relationships of differential power, authority and knowledge are clearly established, and these ease the transition which is expected in the hospital. Women who walk into hospitals are soon wheeled through the halls in wheelchairs and are assigned a bed in a labor room which may be occupied by several women in various stages of labor and responding quite differently. Whether they are prepped or not, what sort of prep they receive is controlled by the staff according to such factors as hospital policy or financial status. The decision to have drugs, either pain killers or drugs that affect labor, is a decision in which women have only minimal, if any, say. The staff may encourage submission to drugs during their most vulnerable labor times and may cajole and convince when the woman is least resistant and most reliant upon the judgment of others. These others are likely to make decisions based upon organizational requirements, routine practices, or preference rather than the desires or plans of the woman.

A growing awareness of this has led to the questioning of the hospital as an appropriate place for giving birth. In tracing the development of the dependence upon hospitals, researchers have indicated that the process was heavily influenced by political power struggles rather than by concern with improving health care for women during labor and delivery.[24] Women, such as those interviewed by Caterine Milinaire, are rejecting the notion that birth is unnatural and a form of sickness, and they are questioning the institutional treatment of this process as a sickness.[25] Because women in our culture receive extensive obedience training and because their socialization leads to dependence, easy acceptance of guilt, and feelings of inadequacy or incompetence, they are especially vulnerable to degradation by the labor and delivery situation. During a period of pain and powerlessness, they are more susceptible to institutional intervention than they might otherwise be.

Labor and Delivery

It is difficult to separate labor from entry since most women do not enter the hospital until they are well into labor. This is why women who enter hospitals are so vulnerable to institutional requirements. They are involved in a process over which they have less control than they usually have. They anticipate some pain, but they cannot form any clear picture of what lies ahead or how long, or how hard the labor and delivery might be and what the outcome will be. It is reasonable to assume, as did Bernstein, Kinch, and Stern in a study of anxiety and length of labor,[26] and Fox in his study of the relationship between degrees of neuroticism and length of labor, that the length and difficulty of labor may be associated with individual characteristics such as desire to have a child, general tolerance of pain, fear, and definition of pregnancy as a sickness or a healthy state.[27] However, it is more important to look at the interactional and structural factors which may effect both labor and delivery.

The work of such authors as Kovit,[28] Rosengren and Devault[29] and Paige and Paige[30] encourages further analysis of the organizational characteristics and definitions that affect labor and delivery. Just as importantly, the disappointments and experiences of women who have labored and given birth in these institutions encourages further careful research. The description of the almost total objectification of 'the woman during labor and delivery as "primips," "multips," or as patients who will "precip," "dump" or provide an "interesting or routine or textbook" case, and the determination of such things as length of labor, type of prep, or whether or not to perform Caesarean section by the availability of personnel, changing shifts, work load, need for training, and other obligations is one of the major contributions of Kovit's work.

265

This coincides directly with women's damning evaluation of their treatment by doctors and nurses, their lack of decision-making ability, and their feelings of powerlessness. Because the woman is experiencing a total institution with all of its control and coercion mechanisms during a period of pain and transition, she is especially susceptible to organizational demands. Furthermore, the very techniques that are viewed as necessary, such as the administration of drugs or strapping down, increase her powerlessness and impair her abilities to control her situation. This process of systematic degradation, the transition from responsible adult to incompetent child, and the ever greater imposition of institutional demands resulting in her increasing powerlessness is worthy of study, both in terms of status degradation and radical resocialization. The oppressive treatment of women in hospitals needs to be examined not only in organizational terms, but also with emphasis on the relationship between the woman's sex-role socialization and the demands placed on her during labor and delivery. The impact of this process; how it relates to her definition of self as capable and competent; and how it affects subsequent feelings about self, the child's father, and the child all need investigation. What is the long-term impact of the experience, whether severe humiliation or exhilaration, on her relationship with others and subsequent treatment of the child or other children?

Despite the fact that most labors and deliveries are not problematic, the establishment of a crisis orientation in hospitals simultaneously leads to and serves as justification for the dehumanization of the patient. The responses to an actual crisis or complication and the factors which effect that response would be an interesting research area. Characteristics of the woman, such as marital status, response to pain, and social status, may be expected to influence the responses to her. In addition, how interesting or informative the case is, how instructive it might be, and other such considerations apparently influence behavior of others toward the woman and thereby interact with the problem.

It would be of some interest to study the degree of pain experienced by women in labor and delivery and their response to it, as these are related to various characteristics of the physical/social setting. The situation, whether it be private and comfortable or crowded and unpleasant, can be expected to affect not only the amount of pain, but also the expression of pain and the woman's feeling about herself because of her response (i.e., shame, guilt, relief, or gratification). Social characteristics of the woman will also affect the situation she is placed in and thereby the other variables and will influence others' responses to her expression of pain. Exploratory interviews suggest that black women, especially young, unmarried black women, may be seen as "deserving" their pain by paying for their sexual misconduct. An interpretation may apply on a more subtle plane to all women: "Women shall give birth in sadness" in payment for original transgression.

The isolation experienced by the woman throughout these processes must be especially severe during delivery. Separation from significant and familiar others during a period of such social consequence is unique to the birth experience. During grave illness, even during death, others are allowed to participate, to oversee, or to merely be present. This physical and social isolation must have significant consequences on the mother's response. The subsequent separation of her from her baby probably increases her feeling of being in a transitional status of having given birth but not yet being a mother socially. A question presents itself: When does a woman define herself as a mother, and what are the structural and interactional factors that affect that definition? This also calls for extensive research, for the questions to be explored are numerous.

IMPLICATIONS FOR FUTURE RESEARCH

In the foregoing sections, discussion has centered on the neglect of the sociology of birth within the discipline of sociology and the reasons why it is an important area for sociological research. Focusing on the areas of pregnancy and labor and delivery, it has been demonstrated that the utilization of sociological perspectives can enhance understanding of each of these areas and point to numerous research possibilities.

It has also been argued that the sociology of birth is not an area limited to pregnancy and the labor and delivery process. The decision to or not to become pregnant, the immediate post-delivery phase, the first six weeks after birth, and the first year are also areas that should be included. Numerous sociological research questions can be asked about these latter four areas. For example, in the area of decision-making, little is known about the pressures to become parents. Pressures are both explicit and implicit from parents, peers, or the media, and these pressures may vary by class, age, sex, religion, and career pattern. In terms of the post-delivery stage, it is important to investigate the factors that affect the parents' initial reaction to the child (e.g., sex of child, immediate contact, behavior of hospital staff, difficulty of labor, or multiple births). For the first six weeks, the focus of investigation could be on the changes in interaction, attitudes which may be the result of the infant's behavior or characteristics (e.g., colicky or irritable) and/or the mother's health (soreness, fatigue) and social situation (physical and social isolation). Finally, the areas to investigate during the first year would include an examination of the parent role in terms of parents' expectations and evaluations of the child, strains caused by the presence of the child, and coping behavior.

In short, it is argued here that the neglect of sociological research in the area of sociology of birth is due not to an absence of research potential, but rather to an explicit and/or subtle unconcern with women's issues. It is hoped that with an awareness of the importance and potential of research in this area, sociologists will begin to apply theoretical perspectives and methodologies to it.

NOTES

1. See Lucille F. Newman, "The Anthropology of Birth," *Sociological Symposium*, vol. 8 (Spring 1972), pp. 51-63, for an elaboration of anthropological contributions.

2. See, for example, Fox's study of the relationship between degree of neuroticism and

length of labor, Warren Fox, "Psychological
Factors in Childbirth" (Ph.D. dissertation,
New York University, 1964).

3. Niles Newton, "Childbirth and Culture,"
Psychology Today, vol. 4 (Nov. 1970);
Richard L. Krebs, "Mother and Child: Inter-
rupters," *Psychology Today*, vol. 3 (Jan.
1970); Melissa Stones, "Giving Birth," *Ram-
parts*, vol. 13 (Sept. 1974); Boston Women's
Health Book Collective, "Woman's
Body/Woman's Mind; Post Partum Blue—As
Natural As Natural Childbirth," *Ms.*, vol. 4
(Mar. 1976).

4. The earliest and best known study is
David Sudnow's *Passing On; The Social Or-
ganization of Dying* (Englewood Cliffs, N. J.:
Prentice-Hall, 1967).

5. See Elizabeth Hardwick, *Seduction and
Betrayal; Women in Literature* (New York:
Vintage Books, 1975).

6. Barbara Seaman, "Pelvic Autonomy:
Four Proposals," *Social Policy*, vol. 5
(Sept./Oct. 1975), pp. 43-47.

7. Ellen Frankfort, *Vaginal Politics* (New
York: Quadrangle, 1972).

8. Seaman, pp. 43-47.

9. For these exceptions, see Jessie Bernard,
Academic Women (New York: Meridian, New
American Library, 1964); Helena Lopata,
Occupation: Housewife (New York: Oxford
University Press, 1971); and Anne Oakley,
*Women's Work: The Housewife Past and
Present* (New York: Pantheon, 1974).

10. Leonard Kovit, "Babies As Social Products" (paper delivered to the Seventy-first Annual Meeting of the American Sociological Association, New York, Aug. 1976).

11. Rose L. Coser, *The Family; Its Structure
and Functions* (New York: St. Martin's Press,
1964); Robert F. Winch, *The Modern Family*
(New York: Holt, Rinehart and Winston,
1963).

12. Bert N. Adams, *The American Family*
(Chicago: Markham Publishing Co., 1971);
Robert R. Bell, *Marriage and Family Interac-
tion* (Homewood, Ill.: Dorsey Press, 1971);
Carolyn C. Perrucci and Dena B. Targ, *Marri-
age and the Family; A Critical Analysis and
Proposals for Change* (New York: David
McKay, 1974); Ira L. Reis, *The Family System
in America* (New York: Holt, Rinehart and
Winston, 1971); Arlene S. Skolnick and
Jerome H. Skolnick, *Family in Transition*
(Boston: Little, Brown, 1971).

13. Bell, pp. 423-26.

14. Rita Seiden Miller, "The Social Con-

struction and Reconstruction of Physiological
Events: Acquiring the Pregnancy Identity"
(paper delivered to the Annual Meeting of the
Midwest Sociological Society, Chicago, Apr.
1975).

15. Rita S. Miller, "The Social Aspects of
Pregnancy: A Preliminary Bibliography"
(paper delivered to the Annual Meeting of the
American Sociological Association, Montreal,
Can., Aug. 1974).

16. *Ibid.*, pp. 41-43.

17. Alice S. Rossi, "Transition to Parenthood," *Journal of Marriage and Family*, vol.
30, no. 1 (Feb. 1968), p. 30.

18. See, for example, the discussion of graduate training by Wilbert E. Moore, *The Professions; Rules and Roles* (New York: Russell
Sage Foundation, 1970).

19. See Everett C. Hughes, "Dilemmas and
Contradictions of Status," *American Journal
of Sociology*, vol. 50, no. 5 (Mar. 1945), pp.
353-59.

20. Ralph La Rossa, "The First Pregnancy
As a Marital Crisis: What We Know and Don't
Know About the Effect of the First Pregnancy
on the Husband-Wife Relationship" (paper
delivered to the Seventy-first Annual Meeting
of the American Sociological Association, New
York, Aug. 1976).

21. R. A. Rosen and Lois O. Martindale,
"Contraception, Abortion and Self-Concept"
(paper delivered to the Seventy-first Annual
Meeting of the American Sociological Association, New York, Aug. 1976).

22. Erving Goffman, "The Moral Career of
the Mental Patient," *Asylums* (Garden City,
N. Y.: Doubleday, 1961), pp. 125-69.

23. Diana Scully and Pauline Bart, "A
Funny Thing Happened on the Way to the
Orifice: Woman in Gynecology Textbooks,"
American Journal of Sociology, vol. 78, no. 4
(Jan. 1973), pp. 1045-49.

24. Karen Paige and Jeffrey Paige, "The
Politics of Birth Practices: A Strategic Analy-
sis," *American Sociological Review*, vol. 38
(Dec. 1973), pp. 663-76.

25. Caterine Milinaire, *Birth* (New York:
Harmony, 1974).

26. Irving Burstein, R. Kinch, and L. Stern,
"Anxiety, Pregnancy, Labor and the Neo-
nate," *American Journal of Obstetrics and
Gynecology*, vol. 118 (1974), pp. 195-99.

27. See Fox.

28. Leonard Kovit, "Labor Is Hard Work:
Notes on the Social Organization of Childbirth," *Sociological Symposium*, vol. 8 (Spring
1972), pp. 11-21.

29. W. Rosengren and S. Devault, "The Sociology of Time and Space in an Obstetrical Hospital," in E. Freidson, *et al.*, *The Hospital in Modern Society* (New York: The Free Press, 1963), pp. 266-92.

30. Paige and Paige, pp. 663-76.

Modeling the Quality of Women's Birth Experience

SUSAN G. DOERING
Environmental Programs, Inc., Baltimore

DORIS R. ENTWISLE
Johns Hopkins University

DANIEL QUINLAN
Bucknell University

Journal of Health and Social Behavior 1980, Vol. 21 (March):12–21

A longitudinal study of 120 couples over the period when they became first-time parents reveals that formal preparation for the birth event (learning in classrooms and from books) improves women's birth enjoyment. Such preparation often involves husbands and encourages them to participate at the birth. A recursive model was estimated supporting the notions that being able to remain in control is a major benefit conferred upon a woman by preparation and that the social support afforded by the husband's presence at the birth contributes both directly and indirectly to the enhancement of the woman's birth experience. The findings are interpreted in line with Janis' stress theory.

Until lately the sociology of birth, like the sociology of death, received little notice. Social scientists have frequently pointed to birth as a "life cycle event," of course, but there is little research that begins to study families at a time before the birth of their first child and then continues through the birth crisis and on into the child's early life. (Exceptions are found in the psychiatric and psychological literature: Meyerowitz and Feldman, 1966; Shereshefsky and Yarrow, 1973. See also Eichler et al., 1977, Feldman and Rogoff, 1977, and Grossman, 1978, for brief reports of ongoing studies). A few cross-sectional studies on this topic in the early sociological literature led to somewhat equivocal outcomes (e.g., Dyer, 1963; LeMasters, 1957). To fill part of this gap, we have undertaken a longitudinal study of family formation emphasizing variables of interest to sociologists. This paper, first in a series of reports from this research, focuses on how preparation of the wife during pregnancy and the

This research was supported by National Institute of Mental Health grants MH 25172 and MH 12525 and by a Guggenheim Fellowship to Doris Entwisle. The authors are grateful to an anonymous reviewer for helpful comments on an earlier version of this paper.

Address communications to: Dr. Doris R. Entwisle, 304 Barton Hall, Johns Hopkins University, Baltimore, MD 21218.

husband's participation in the birth of their child affect the wife's reaction to the birth event. As will be made clear in what follows, the quality of a woman's birth experience not only is important for her own well-being but is increasingly recognized to be of importance for the marital relationship and parenting as well.

The Birth Event

The crisis character and critical nature of a first pregnancy and childbirth in a female's life have long been recognized (Benedek, 1970; Bibring et al., 1961; Haas, 1952; Larsen, 1966; Menninger, 1943). Shainess (1963), in fact, referred to this period as a "crucible tempering the self" and recognized the possibility that the tempering process might go awry, resulting in damage to the self and, by implication, to the self's relationships with others. Chertok (1969) speaks of pregnancy as a progressively developing crisis that has the labor and delivery as its peak—both because of the final results of the confinement (separation of the mother and child) and because of its isolation in time as an event.

Other considerations as well have sparked interest in the birth event. The feminist movement, with its emphasis on female achievement, strongly recommends an active role for women in childbirth—many women now wish to "give birth" rather than to be passively delivered, and there is an undercurrent of feeling among feminists that the treatment of obstetric patients at the hands of (mostly male) obstetricians can denigrate the woman's role in the birth process (Corea, 1977). Broadened sex roles for men have focused male attention on the birth event also. Many young men now wish to share in tasks formerly designated as the exclusive domain of the female, including pregnancy and childbirth.[1] Still another reason for current interest in birth is that close and immediate contact between mother and child, starting at the moment of birth, is considered to be crucial for the optimal growth of attachment (Klaus and Kennell, 1976a, 1976b; Sosa et al., 1976), and the birth event can be managed in ways that foster or inhibit such contact. The birth event, then, intersects a number of important theoretical and practical concerns.

There is an extensive literature suggesting that women who are prepared for childbirth weather the crisis better than women who are unprepared. Whether "preparation" denotes Lamaze[2] training (psychoprophylaxis) or some less intensive form of preparation, evidence points to physical benefits such as shorter labors, less medication, fewer forceps deliveries, and the like (Laird and Hogan, 1956; Miller et al., 1952; Pearse et al., 1955; Thoms and Wyatt, 1951; Zax et al., 1975). A handful of more recent studies point to psychological benefits as well (see, e.g., Chertok, 1969; Huttel et al., 1972; Tanzer, 1968). Yet, though one careful evaluation of the literature judges preparation for childbirth to exert positive effects net of background factors (Charles et al., 1978), it is not clear exactly how preparation confers its benefits. Also, despite recent changes in hospital procedure that permit husbands to be present during the birth of their child, there is not much information concerning how social variables, including the extent to which husbands participate in labor and delivery, affect women's coping with birth.

A previous cross-sectional study (Doering and Entwisle, 1975) used Janis' (1958) stress theory as a source of suggestions to account for the effectiveness of childbirth-training classes. Drawing again upon that perspective and extending it, this paper proposes and tests a structural model designed to explicate the mechanisms by which women's preparation during pregnancy and the joint participation in birth of husband and wife affect the psychological and physical quality of the woman's experience during birth.

Rationale for the Model

As previously mentioned, a positive association between preparation for childbirth and the pleasurableness of women's birth experience is frequently reported, although the exact mechanisms by which preparation achieves its salutary effects are not clear. Janis (1958), in research on surgical patients who had knowledge about their operations in advance, concluded that psychological preparation was a major defense against stress. Individuals forewarned by their physicians of likely unpleasant aspects of surgery were much less disturbed than other individuals whose physicians minimized unpleasant aspects or told them nothing. Janis (1958:353) postulated that the "unpleasant task of mental rehearsal" is apt to be shirked unless patients are given "approximate preparatory communications before being exposed to potentially traumatizing stimuli."

From a psychoanalytic perspective, the "work of worrying" is a healthy phenomenon. It mobilizes the individual's psychological resources in a way to allow effective coping with stress. Janis (1958:384) also noted the importance of the physician informing the patient of "overt actions he can execute" to minimize aches and pains. Although Janis emphasized the "active control" notion less than the "work of worrying" notion and did not attempt in his analysis of surgical-patient data to disentangle the two as precursors of more positive responses to surgery, in his discussion he explicitly distinguished between control and worrying.

The application of Janis' theory to childbirth is relatively straightforward. Preparation classes teach women what to expect during labor and delivery and forewarn them of unpleasant events that may occur. Classes encourage women to air their concerns ahead of time, and teach pregnant women and their partners many techniques that will help during childbirth. Furthermore, the possibilities of "active control" and the benefits to be derived from self-help are far greater for childbirth than they are within a surgical context. A surgical patient can help him- or herself to a limited extent in the postoperative period, but a parturient woman can take direct action during labor and delivery itself as well as in the recovery period.

In addition, the more intensive kinds of preparation classes strongly encourage active husband participation in labor and delivery. Such social support, of course, is rarely feasible for patients undergoing surgery, and consequently Janis does not consider it.

Women in childbirth thus have potentially greater opportunities and means for coping with stress than surgical patients—a greater freedom to act themselves and wider sources of social support. Recent reports are consistent with these arguments.

Henneborn and Cogan (1975) found that in a group of 40 women who had attended preparation classes before birth with their husband, those whose husband elected to remain through delivery reported less pain and required less medication than those whose husband chose to remain only through labor. And recently Norr et al. (1977) offered evidence that both preparation in pregnancy and husband's presence were positively associated with the quality of a woman's birth experience, although the husband's presence seemingly had no direct effect on pain perception. The conclusion from these two studies is that, with preparation level held constant, the husband's presence is an additional bulwark against stress.

Our earlier cross-sectional study revealed not only that the quality of a woman's birth experience was associated with the extent of her preparation for childbirth but also that the effect of preparation on birth experience was not altogether direct (Doering and Entwisle, 1975). A considerable portion of preparation's positive effect seemed to be mediated indirectly through the woman's "awareness" level or level of consciousness during delivery (reflecting the amount and type of medication received). The conclusion drawn from this study was that preparation operates through two control mechanisms to enhance the birth experience: The first mechanism acts to provide the requisite psychological support (which has a direct effect); the other entails an increase in physical and mental awareness, allowing the woman to be more actively in control.

Drawing upon Janis' stress theory and the previously discussed empirical studies of birth experience, we formulated the model portrayed in Figure 1 to explain the quality of a woman's birth experience. In the model both woman's preparation level and husband's participation are taken as exogenous variables. A plausible argument can be made for assuming correlation between the two, since, as mentioned earlier, the more intensive kinds of preparation classes strongly encourage prospective fathers to attend classes with their wife and to be present during labor and delivery. During these classes men as well as women are taught skills that aid in coping with labor and delivery. It seems doubtful, however, that woman's preparation is the only cause of husband participation, since a wife's preparation by no means guarantees her husband's participation. Some men who wish to take an active role in the birth event, furthermore, may be the ones providing encouragement for the couple to enroll in preparation classes rather than the reverse.

Direct paths link both woman's preparation level and husband's participation to pain. Earlier work, already alluded to, documents the possible influence of women's preparation on pain. In addition, one would suspect that the husband, by encouraging and comforting his wife, would reduce her anxiety (closely related to pain), and that pain would be more bearable in any case with the husband present to work with the parturient woman in controlling contractions.

Both pain and the two variables prior to it are expected to act directly upon level of awareness—with less pain, less medication is required. Also, a husband might persuade his wife to, or support her decision to, use less medication either because of danger to the fetus or because of prior commitments to avoid medication as much as possible, thereby yielding a direct path from husband participation to level of awareness. Finally, our earlier work points to a direct effect of woman's preparation level upon level of awareness, probably attributable to techniques women learn in preparation classes to reduce or control pain so that they are less likely to request medication.

FIGURE 1. Model explaining the quality of women's birth experience (BESCL) in terms of level of awareness (AWARE), severity of pain in the first stage of labor (PAIN1), husband's participation (HPART). and woman's preparation level (WPREP)

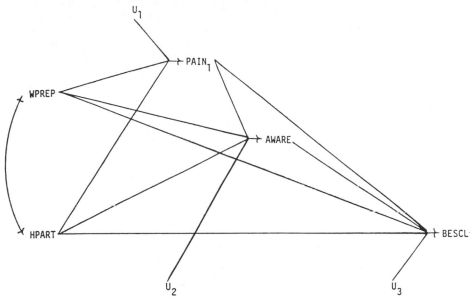

Woman's birth enjoyment, the ultimate endogenous variable, is assumed to be directly affected by all of the prior variables for the following reasons. First, preparation covers many topics in addition to methods of coping with pain and avoiding medication, and these and other effects of preparation are represented by the direct link between preparation and quality of birth experience.[3] Second, husband participation has the potential of enhancing birth experience directly, apart from any influence it has on pain or level of awareness, in that the simple sharing of the experience could make the birth experience more gratifying to the woman, everything else being held equal. Next, the level of pain would obviously be expected to have a direct effect on the quality of the woman's birth experience. Last, there is direct evidence from our prior study linking level of awareness directly to the quality of the woman's birth experience. Moreover, a woman assuming an active role via maintaining a high level of awareness would be expected, on the basis of Janis' thinking, to derive more pleasure from the birth experience, and in line with feminist thinking, women who actively work in the birth process may find childbirth more gratifying than women who are passively delivered.

This rationale yields the model depicted in Figure 1, fully recursive, woman's preparation level and husband's participation jointly exogenous, and with pain, level of awareness, and quality of woman's birth experience as successive endogenous variables.

DATA SOURCE AND MEASUREMENT

In the longitudinal study referred to at the beginning of this paper, 120 Maryland women delivering a first child were interviewed twice before birth and also again in the early postpartum period. In addition, 60 of the women's husbands were interviewed before birth and 57 afterward. Half of the women can be classified as blue-collar and half as middle-class. One-third of the women belonged to each major religious group. The average age of the women in the sample was 24.7; ages ranged from 18 to 31. (Couples in the sample, although not a random sample, seem reasonably representative of white persons in the United States having a first child when compared in terms of demographic and psychosocial characteristics with several nationwide surveys [U.S. Bureau of the Census, 1975, 1976; U.S. Department of Labor, 1975; see also Yankelovich, 1974].) All the women and their husbands were white volunteers. The women were attended by 65 different physicians, 3 midwives, and 12 residents; one baby was delivered by its father. In addition to five planned home births, deliveries occurred at 15 different hospitals in the Baltimore-Washington-Annapolis area. Because the women in the sample were cared for in many different facilities, their birth experience may represent what "average" women experience, rather than what happens in large teaching hospitals, the source of most data on childbirth experience. At any rate, data from this panel of women were used to estimate the model in Figure 1.

One further fact deserves notice. Because women undergoing caesarean sections have birth experiences markedly different from those of women delivered vaginally, the 20 women in the panel who were delivered by surgery were excluded from the analyses reported here.

A brief description of how each variable in the model was measured follows.[4]

Woman's preparation level (WPREP) combines all sources of a woman's knowledge about what to expect in labor and delivery and how to implement this knowledge. It includes information obtained from books, movies, medical training (if a woman is a nurse or medical technician), and preparation classes. It was measured initially in the first interview when the woman was six months pregnant, and then measured, and re-scored if necessary, in a second interview three to four weeks before her due date. The preparation level·of women in this sample varied from zero, literally, or reading a book or two, to full Lamaze preparation. The scoring was derived from several long-answer questions.

Husband's participation (HPART) is based on a 6-item scale measuring husband's participation in labor and delivery in both behavioral and emotional terms.[5] Because only about one-half of the husbands in this sample were interviewed, this variable was constructed using information gathered from wives. Ordinarily, one would prefer to use information

about husband participation gathered from *both* husbands and wives.[6] However, a careful investigation of the overlap between a husband's and a wife's replies to questions about the husband's participation, as well as a comparison of parameter estimates using information obtained directly from husbands versus those using information about husbands supplied by wives, suggests that the differences in this sample are inconsequential.[7] Accordingly, the variable HPART was constructed from data supplied by wives, leading to a case base of 96, the set for which complete information was available on all other variables.

The measure of pain (PAIN1) is extracted from questions soliciting a description of the worst pain that a woman experienced during the first stage of labor at any one point. Women were asked to rate the most severe pain they experienced and to indicate whether it lasted for a contraction or two, or went on for a considerable period.

Level of awareness (AWARE) is a subjective measure, derived from careful evaluations of women's replies to several long-answer questions about medication received and level of consciousness during the actual delivery. It should be emphasized that "awareness" refers to both mental and physical consciousness. Thus a woman who had been given a saddle block was scored in the middle of the scale because, although her mind was clear, she had lost consciousness of physical sensations in the "saddle area."

The quality of women's birth experience (BESCL) is represented by a score on a 5-item scale.[8] It covers how the woman felt both physically and emotionally immediately after the birth, how she felt 30–45 minutes later in recovery, and what she thought, right after birth, about having another baby.

RESULTS

Table 1 provides both the standardized and metric regression coefficients estimated from the panel data for the recursive model in Figure 1. Although the respondents do not form a probability sample, coefficients exceeding twice their standard errors are tagged in Table 1 for the reader's convenience. The coefficients estimated for this model suggest a

TABLE 1. Predicting the Quality of Women's Birth Experience (BESCL) (C-sections not included)

	Dependent Variables					
	PAIN1		AWARE		BESCL	
Independent Variables	Metric Coefficients	Standardized Coefficients	Metric Coefficients	Standardized Coefficients	Metric Coefficients	Standardized Coefficients
Women's preparation level (WPREP)	−.090	−.197	.429*	.451*	−.144	−.055
Degree of husband participation (HPART)	−.005	−.041	.062*	.226*	.193*	.254*
Worst pain in first stage of labor (PAIN1)			−.309	−.148	−1.035*	−.178*
Women's level of awareness at delivery (AWARE)					1.446*	.522*
Variance accounted for:	5.0%		43.7%		52.0%	
Constant term:	4.026		1.969		13.196	

* Coefficient at least twice its standard error.

number of interesting linkages among these variables.

As found earlier, preparation acts to increase the likelihood of a woman manifesting a higher level of awareness at the time of delivery, as the .451 standardized regression coefficient indicates. However, the direct effects of preparation on birth enjoyment are small relative to other variables, as indicated by the size of the standardized coefficient (−.055) and its sign.

Husband participation contributes both directly and indirectly to the woman's birth enjoyment. The size of the standardized coefficient linking husband's participation to level of awareness (.226) suggests that the husband's participation enables a woman to manage with less medication. A sizable standardized coefficient linking husband participation directly to birth enjoyment (.254) also exists. In this case, however, the direct effects of husband's participation on the quality of the woman's birth experience seem to surpass its indirect effects through level of awareness (.254 vs. .118), although the indirect effects are substantial enough to consider seriously.

As would be expected, the effects of pain on birth enjoyment are negative. Pain directly reduces the quality of the woman's birth experience (the standardized coefficient computed is −.178); also, more pain seemingly reduces the level of awareness (more medication is required), although the coefficient here fails to

exceed twice its standard error. Neither preparation nor husband's participation is observed to have much effect on the worst pain a woman reports, and only about 5% of the variance in pain is explained by these two factors.

The importance of level of awareness in predicting the quality of the woman's birth experience is clearly revealed in this analysis. The standardized coefficient of .522 connecting BESCL to AWARE is more than twice the absolute size of all other estimated coefficients. The maintenance of a high level of awareness thus seems to increase the likelihood of a woman's experiencing an enjoyable birth. Furthermore, it appears that remaining in control (receiving less medication) is much more important to the pleasurableness of a woman's birth experience than simply experiencing less pain.

Some comment is needed about the overall effects of preparation. Its direct effects on the quality of women's birth experience are small and negative, despite a zero-order correlation of .457 (see Table 2). Its indirect effects, however, through awareness and through husband's participation, are relatively large. The zero-order correlation can be decomposed, of course, into a direct effect, here negligible, plus the product of the two indirect effects (.254 × .590 = .150 and .522 × .617 = .322). This sum obviously exceeds .457. It therefore appears that preparation improves the quality

TABLE 2. Zero-Order Correlation Coefficients (listwise present) (N=96)

	WPREP	HPART	PAIN1	AWARE	Mean	S.D.
WPREP					4.76	2.07
HPART[1]	.590				22.38	7.20
PAIN1	−.222	−.157			3.48	0.94
AWARE	.617	.516	−.283		4.32	1.97
BESCL[2]	.457	.519	−.354	.670	19.47	5.46

[1] α reliability = .842; correlation with scale based only on husband's response = .832.
[2] α reliability = .734.

of women's birth experience in this sample entirely by acting to improve social support and women's "active measures," i.e., control. To the extent that the "work of worrying" is represented by a direct effect of preparation on birth enjoyment, it appears inconsequential here, although the "work of worrying" may have operated earlier to persuade women to learn how to retain control and also to persuade husbands to participate.

All in all, then, it appears that the major impact of preparation on a woman's birth enjoyment is by way of increasing level of awareness, which is observed in this analysis to be the most critical determinant of the quality of women's birth experience. Husband's participation seems to exert both a direct effect and, through AWARE, an indirect effect on birth enjoyment, the former effect probably one of social support at the time of delivery. Neither preparation nor husband's participation, however, seems to exert any substantial effects on pain. The worst pain felt during the first stage of labor nevertheless seems to be only weakly and negatively related to the quality of a woman's birth experience. And, finally, it is noteworthy that this model accounts for over half of the variance in women's birth enjoyment.[9] This is no modest achievement, considering that physiological and other medically related variables are not included in the model.

DISCUSSION OF THE MODEL

In both the present study and our earlier study, Janis' (1958) theory provides a powerful means for explaining the benefits of preparation. Janis found that surgical patients who weathered the crisis well were those who were given information in advance about what would happen during surgery and who had prepared themselves by doing the work of worrying. By contrast, he found that surgical patients who dealt poorly with the crisis either denied the importance of the coming surgery or were so overwhelmed with anxiety that they were unable to prepare themselves for it. Other researchers have also noted that counseling before surgery confers significant benefits (see Andrew, 1970; Egbert et al., 1964).

"Preparation" as defined for the group of women in this study included reading books, attending movies, and other forms of self-preparation as well as enrolling in formal classes. Such preparation is presumed to stimulate the "work of worrying," since it causes women to air their concerns and to ask questions about what is likely to happen. The converse may also be true: Those who are doing the "work of worrying" will choose to acquire information by reading, attending classes, and so forth. But such preparation also teaches women how to help themselves in labor and delivery. For meeting the birth crisis, this present model suggests that preparation is effective mainly because it leads women to retain active control in labor and delivery. It is the patient's efficacy in that regard which seems to lead to favorable outcomes. In Janis' data, "control" and "worrying" were confounded. Here they can be separated to some extent by examining the direct and indirect effects of preparation on a woman's birth enjoyment. In our study, it appears that "control" is by far the more important factor in accounting for the quality of the woman's birth experience.

The model also elucidates how social supports, mainly in the form of the husband's presence, may help. The husband's participation probably is beneficial in three regards: (1) His very presence is comforting, and the couple together appreciate the birth experience more fully than would be possible alone (a direct effect); (2) most husbands who participate have attended some preparation classes, where they learned how to assist in implementing techniques designed to help their wife remain in better control, especially late in labor when fatigue and confusion can complicate matters (an indirect effect); and (3) the husband's presence may lead to better relationships between the woman and the hospital staff, because he can lessen his wife's demands on them and also because his presence enables his wife to retain control (both direct and indirect).

Norr et al.'s (1977) careful and comprehensive study, based on a single postpartum interview with women delivered at the Michael Reese hospital in Chicago, also offers evidence that the husband's presence in delivery positively affects the quality of a woman's birth experience. Their findings agree with ours in that the husband's presence has no significant effect on pain but does have a significant impact on the woman's enjoyment in giving birth. However, contrary to our observation that preparation has no significant effect on pain, they found a significant partial regression coefficient between preparation and pain. Their analysis, though, does not conceptualize level of awareness separately. The specification of paths from preparation to pain, from pain to level of awareness, and from preparation to level of awareness is a more complete structural analysis of how these three variables are related to the quality of a woman's birth experience. Our analysis indicates that there is an indirect path from preparation through level of awareness to birth enjoyment, implying that preparation aids in coping with pain and remaining in control and that coping and remaining in control substantially enhance the birth experience. This path is much larger than the two indirect paths of preparation through pain to birth enjoyment. Hence our results suggest that pain is a relatively independent factor and that the benefits which accrue to those women who are prepared are those of coping more successfully with pain and of remaining in active control in delivery. Despite these divergent findings, both Norr et al.'s analysis and our model are able to account for over half the variance in women's birth enjoyment, and both agree in finding social support factors (husband's presence) to be of critical importance.

The relative sizes of effects for the present set of cases are somewhat different from those based on a simpler model estimated earlier (Doering and Entwisle, 1975). In particular, relatively greater effects of preparation on "attitude toward childbirth" (roughly similar to the quality of women's birth experience in the present study) were uncovered. However, since the earlier model was incompletely specified and different measurement strategies were followed, no fruitful comparison of coefficients can be pursued. At any rate, the structural connections revealed by the two studies are broadly similar.

Conclusion

The structural model advanced to explain the quality of women's birth experience suggests, for this panel of women, that a primary mechanism explaining the relation between preparation and the quality of the woman's birth experience is awareness at delivery, rather than the reduction of pain per se. The model also suggests that stress can be diminished by patients' direct action and that overt action may overshadow "work of worrying" as a protection against stress. "Overt action" was a factor mentioned by Janis but was of less applicability in the surgical patients he studied than it appears to be for women giving birth. In addition, the model offers further confirmation of the widely held notion that the husband's participation contributes considerably to the woman's birth enjoyment, and points to social support as an additional defense against stress.

NOTES

1. This kind of sharing is apparently very gratifying to women as well as men. For example, in the sample of couples who are the subject of this report, 94% of the women expressed a strong desire to have their husband present in labor, and after delivery only one woman had changed her mind about the desirability of having her husband present.
2. One of many good descriptions of Lamaze training can be found in Chabon (1966).
3. In particular, by informing women of what to expect and encouraging them to ask questions, it is likely that much apprehension is avoided. Women take tours of hospitals, see movies about pregnancy and childbirth, and are put in contact with other women who have successfully weathered the crisis.
4. Due to space limitations, we are unable to offer a more detailed description of the questions asked

to obtain these measures, their coding formats, and the like. The authors will be happy to furnish this information upon request.

5. The alpha reliability computed for this scale is .83.

6. It could be argued, however, that women's perceptions of their husband's performance emotionally and behaviorally are more important than the husbands' own perceptions of their performance in affecting their wife's birth experience. For example, the husband could disguise his anxiety during labor and delivery and thereby create a favorable impression of his performance in the mind of his wife, whereas, given his anxiety, his own evaluation of his performance might be considerably lower.

7. The correlation obtained from the common sample of husband and wife respondents between a husband participation scale derived from husband responses and a husband participation scale derived from wife responses is .83, equivalent to the alpha reliability of HPART.

8. The alpha reliability coefficient of BESCL is .734.

9. When the model in Figure 1 was reestimated by FIML techniques (Jöreskog and Sörbom, 1978) so as to incorporate measurement error, the coefficient of determination for BESCL was .78. This suggests that the model is well specified and, especially, that the influence of any variables omitted from the model is not very consequential.

REFERENCES

Andrew, J. M.
1970 "Recovery from surgery with and without preparatory instruction for three coping styles." Journal of Personality and Social Psychology 15:223–26.

Benedek, T.
1970 "The psychobiology of pregnancy." Pp. 137–52 in E. James Anthony and Therese Benedek (eds.), Parenthood: Its Psychology and Psychopathology. Boston: Little, Brown.

Bibring, G. L., T. F. Dwyer, D. S. Huntington, and A. F. Valenstein
1961 "A study of the psychological processes in pregnancy and of the earliest mother-child relationship." Pp. 9–72 in Psychoanalytic Study of the Child, XVI. New York: International Universities Press.

Chabon, Irwin
1966 Awake and Aware. New York: Dell.

Charles, A. G., K. L. Norr, C. R. Block, S. Meyering, and E. Meyers
1978 "Obstetric and psychological effects of psychoprophylactic preparation for childbirth." American Journal of Obstetrics and Gynecology 131:44–52.

Chertok, Leon
1969 Motherhood and Personality. London: Tavistock.

Corea, Gena
1977 The Hidden Malpractice. New York: Morrow.

Doering, S. G., and D. R. Entwisle
1975 "Preparation during pregnancy and ability to cope with labor and delivery." American Journal of Orthopsychiatry 45(5):825–37.

Dyer, E. D.
1963 "Parenthood as crisis: A re-study." Marriage and Family Living 25:196–201.

Egbert, L. D., G. E. Battit, C. E. Welch, and M. K. Bartlett
1964 "Reduction of postoperative pain by encouragement and instruction of patients." New England Journal of Medicine 270:825–29.

Eichler, L. S., S. A. Winickoff, F. K. Grossman, M. K. Anzalone, and M. H. Gofseyeff
1977 "Adaptation to pregnancy, birth, and early parenting: A preliminary view." Unpublished paper presented at APA meetings, San Francisco.

Feldman, H., and M. Rogoff
1977 "Correlates of changes in marital satisfaction with the birth of a first child." Mimeographed. Department of Child Development and Family Relationships, Cornell University.

Grossman, F. K.
1978 "Fathers are parents too." Mimeographed. Department of Psychology, Boston University.

Haas, S.
1952 "Psychiatric implications in gynecology and obstetrics." Pp. 90–118 in Leopold Bellak (ed.), Psychology of Physical Illness. New York: Grune & Stratton.

Henneborn, W. J., and R. Cogan
1975 "The effect of husband participation on reported pain and probability of medication during labor and birth." Journal of Psychosomatic Research 19:215–22.

Huttel, F., I. Mitchell, W. M. Fischer, and A. E. Meyer
1972 "A quantitative evaluation of psychoprophylaxis in childbirth." Journal of Psychosomatic Research 16:81–92.

Janis, Irving L.
1958 Psychological Stress. New York: Wiley.

Jöreskog, K. G., and Dag Sörbom
1978 LISREL: Version IV. Chicago: International Educational Resources.

Klaus, Marshall H., and John H. Kennell
1976a "Parent-to-infant attachment." No. 5 in D. Hull (ed.), Recent Advances in Pediatrics. Edinburgh: Churchill Livingstone.
1976b Maternal Infant Bonding. St. Louis: Mosby.

Laird, M. D., and M. Hogan
1956 "An elective program on preparation for childbirth at the Sloane Hospital for Women: May, 1951 to June, 1953." American Journal of Obstetrics and Gynecology 72:641–47.

Larsen, V. L.
  1966 "Stresses of the childbearing year." American Journal of Public Health 56(1):32–36.
LeMasters, E. E.
  1957 "Parenthood as crisis." Marriage and Family Living 19:352–55.
Menninger, W. C.
  1943 "The emotional factors in pregnancy." Bulletin of Menninger Clinic 7:15–24.
Meyerowitz, J., and H. Feldman
  1966 "Transition to parenthood." Psychiatric Research Reports 20:78–84.
Miller, H. L., F. E. Flannery, and D. Bell
  1952 "Education for childbirth in private practice." American Journal of Obstetrics and Gynecology 63:792–99.
Norr, K. L., C. R. Block, A. Charles, S. Meyering, and E. Meyers
  1977 "Explaining pain and enjoyment in childbirth." Journal of Health and Social Behavior 18:260–75.
Pearse, R. L., E. B. Easley, and K. A. Podger
  1955 "Obstetric analgesia and anesthesia." North Carolina Medical Journal 16:18–24.
Shainess, J.
  1963 "The structure of the mothering encounter." Journal of Nervous and Mental Disease 136:146–61.
Shereshefsky, Pauline M., and Leon J. Yarrow
  1973 Psychological Aspects of a First Pregnancy. New York: Raven.

Sosa, Roberto, J. H. Kennell, M. Klaus, and Juan J. Urrutia
  1976 Breast-feeding and the Mother. New York: Elsevier-North-Holland.
Tanzer, D.
  1968 "Natural childbirth: Pain or peak experience." Psychology Today 2:17 ff.
Thoms, H., and R. H. Wyatt
  1951 "One thousand consecutive deliveries under a training for childbirth program." American Journal of Obstetrics and Gynecology 61:205–9.
U.S. Bureau of the Census
  1975 Current Population Reports, Series P-25, No. 613, November. Washington, D.C.: U.S. Government Printing Office.
  1976 A Statistical Portrait of Women. Current Population Reports, Series P-23, No. 58, April. Washington, D.C.: U.S. Government Printing Office.
U.S. Department of Labor
  1975 1975 Handbook on Women Workers. Women's Bureau, Bulletin 297, p. 19.
Yankelovich, Daniel
  1974 The New Morality: A Profile of American Youth. New York: McGraw-Hill.
Zax, M., A. J. Sameroff, and J. E. Farnum
  1975 "Childbirth education, maternal attitudes, and delivery." American Journal of Obstetrics and Gynecology 123:185–90.

BONNIE B. O'CONNOR

THE HOME BIRTH MOVEMENT
IN THE UNITED STATES

ABSTRACT. The home birth movement in the United States is an alternative
health belief system that promotes a model of pregnancy and childbirth contradictory to the conventional biomedical model. The alternative model stresses
normalcy and non-intervention and is informed by an ideology that promotes
individual authority and responsibility for health and health care. It is founded
in an epistemological system that assigns primacy and goodness to the Natural,
fuses moral and practical injunctions in the arena of health behavior, and
valorizes subjective as well as objective sources of knowledge. (*Natural* = as
found in nature without technical intervention). Differences of opinion with the
conventional medical model of childbirth do not spring from misunderstanding
of this model, but from disagreement with it. Members of this movement are
typically educated, middle class, and white.

Key Words: alternative childbirth, home birth, midwifery, out-of-hospital birth

INTRODUCTION

The home birth movement in the United States is somewhat over
twenty years old. Though it serves a small proportion of the total
childbearing population in this country, it remains a vigorous and
vocal movement promoting an alternative to the conventional
medical model of birth in the hospital with its routine preventive
and facilitative interventions. The home birth philosophy does not
require or encourage wholesale rejection of conventional
medicine. Indeed the need to work *with* medicine is stressed,
though with specific caveats that particularly emphasize a redefinition of the client-practitioner relationship (Weitz and Sullivan,
1986). Members of the home birth movement mediate their
encounters with conventional medicine by minimizing their
number and frequency (at least with respect to perinatal visits), by
retaining personal authority for decision making, and by controll-

*Bonnie B. O'Connor, Ph.D., Assistant Professor, Department of Community and
Preventive Medicine, Medical College of Pennsylvania, 3300 Henry Avenue, Philadelphia, PA 19129, U.S.A.*

ing disclosure of beliefs and intentions likely to meet with medical disapproval. Central to the movement's philosophy is a rejection of the medical model of childbirth and all of the practices which that model entails. This rejection is grounded in a coherent system of deeply held convictions that fundamentally contradict the medical model and that regard standard medical management of low risk labors as unnecessary and dangerous (Table 1).

Basic features of the alternative childbirth model are: (1) that pregnancy and birth are non-pathological, normal body functions, (2) that they are inherently safe in the majority of cases, (3) that each labor is unique and must be responded to as such (4) that interference in the natural course of labor is undesirable and likely to provoke problems and (5) that family bonding is an integral part of perinatal experience, serves a natural and essential function, and must be facilitated as a part of the total birth process. These premises are supported by reference to various authoritative and evidentiary sources: scientific studies (including medical studies), academic and advocacy literature, popular wisdom, personal experience and observation, and overriding higher authorities. Higher authorities invoked are God (in religious belief contexts) or Nature (in secular contexts); the claim of inherent rightness of creation or natural design is made for both.

Evidence cited in substantiation of claims includes individual and cumulative observation (empirical evidence) and testimonial accounts (i.e., personal experience narratives) of others; direct personal experience carries the greatest evidentiary authority (see also Sagov *et al.*, 1984; Weitz and Sullivan 1986; Oakley and Houd 1990). Decisions are made and conclusions reached by the use of ordinary inference, introspection, reflection, comparative and probabilistic reasoning, and occasionally as a result of a direct apprehension of knowledge (which I have labeled "just knowing," following the conversational usage of members of the movement). Personal experience provides the most frequently cited clinching evidence in support of claims to knowledge about the true nature of childbirth. A central feature of the home birth movement at organizational, practitioner, and client levels is its valorization of subjective knowledge, which is accepted as having equal or greater authority than objectively derived knowledge in certain circumstances.

Table 1. Summary of the Home Birth Movement Philosophy

Fundamental assumptions	Corollary
What is natural is good; natural is equivalent to normal, and is inherently effective for its purposes.	Natural processes seldom need alteration, and should be altered as little as possible.

Basic beliefs about birth	Conclusions re hospital birth
Pregnancy and birth are normal body functions; as such they are inherently natural (therefore good) and effective.	Normal birth does not belong in hospitals, and medical management is not necessary.
Under ordinary circumstances, birth is inherently safe; the majority of births fall into this category.	The medical model of childbirth as inherently dangerous or pathological is incorrect, and exaggerates the rate of occurrence of serious problems.
Accompanying health problems may cause difficulties which are rightly defined as medical problems.	Medical care is proper for medically complicated labors (but not for others).
Labor can be defined in advance only in its broadest generalities; each labor is unique in its particulars.	Standardization of expectations and responses to labor is undesirable and unrealistic.
The natural course of labor should be shaped or interfered with as little as possible.	Unneeded [medical] intervention itself complicates labor and introduces danger; this sets up a chain reaction of subsequent interventions.
Family bonding after birth is a natural and important human (animal) need.	Hospital procedures interfere with bonding and are therefore damaging to the well-being of all family members.
Subjective sources of knowledge are valid (even critical) sources, and may be used as a basis for decision-making in labor. *Only* the laboring woman is truly in a position to know certain things during labor.	The judgments and interpretations of medical personnel do not necessarily constitute the most authoritative or appropriate sources of information upon which to base decisions during labor. Objective sources are at times inferior to subjective sources for information which is most germane.

Table 1 (continued)

Accompanying moral principle	Conclusions re birth settings
Individuals should exercise responsibility for and authority over their own health and health care.	Parents are primary actors and authorities in their home births; midwives serve as informed assistants. [Desirable.] In hospital births, physieians assume (usurp) authority and relegate parents to roles of incompetence and spectatorship. [Undesirable].

A. HISTORICAL BACKGROUND

In the early 1970's the social movement promoting childbirth at home began to gather momentum in the United States. This movement built upon the earlier prepared childbirth and natural childbirth movements, which had stressed the importance of prenatal education and labor training for parents in setting the stage for a delivery with minimal medication. Avoidance of analgesics, anesthesias, and other drugs that dull sensation or awareness was positively valued. In their place came pain control through regulated breathing, relaxation, and other personally executed techniques. These philosophies viewed birth as a momentous event to be approached in a natural (as opposed to drug-altered) frame of mind and body and to be accomplished by means of natural strengths and capabilities, honed through preparation and training (Dick-Read, 1944, 1957; Lamaze, 1958; Karmel, 1959). Still, the hospital was its setting.

The home birth movement, however, has carried the concept of "natural childbirth" to a new and much broader level of meaning, taking as its central tenet the proposition that childbirth is *inherently* natural, and that "natural" equates with "normal". Under ordinary circumstances, neither pregnancy nor birth is seen as a medical event but as normal – if demanding – female body processes. As such, they can be handled properly and safely at home. Medical intervention is defined as necessary (or even appropriate) only when specifically *medical* conditions or complications are involved. To varying degrees, the movement has drawn upon and interacted with the women's health and holistic health movements, feminist politics, back-to-nature ideology, and health consumerism. All of these movements stress the possibilities and importance of "personal awareness, self-care and informed choice" (Sagov *et al.*, 1984, p. 3).

The social structure of the home birth or alternative childbirth movement consists of formally constituted organizations of local, national, and international scope; health care professionals sympathetic to the movement's position and aims; midwives serving as principal birth-attendants;[1] and parents and families with home births in their histories and futures. Maintenance and dissemination of the beliefs and values central to the movement's philosophy are accomplished through both "official" and "unofficial" channels. The larger scale organizations sponsor speakers, meetings and conferences; organize political lobbying efforts; publish advocacy, reference, and training literature; and endorse the work of authors and scholars the results of whose studies support movement aims and positions. Less formal affiliations of midwives and other sympathetic birth attendants provide for training, consensual standard setting and validation (Peterson, 1983), as well as exchanges of ideas and narratives comprising a shared body of knowledge about the variations and possibilities in childbirth. Personal experience narratives told and retold by clients of the system give immediacy to the message of the movement, play a part in the self-recruitment of new participants, support the word-of-mouth referral network of midwives, and help to sustain the home birth epistemology at the individual, group, and movement levels.

Midwives have been the traditional birth attendants through history and across cultures, becoming supplanted over time by physician specialists in many developed nations.[2] Childbirths of urban upper and middle class American women, though still remaining in the home, began increasingly to be attended by physicians from the early to mid-nineteenth century (Sullivan and Weitz, 1988). At the turn of the twentieth century, birth began to move into the hospital, beginning in the poor and working classes. Hospital births had become the norm among white women across all social classes in the United States by the 1950's (Wertz and Wertz, 1977). Concurrently, the public image of midwifery came to be associated primarily with rural populations, poorer social classes, immigrant and ethnic minority groups, and certain religious communities (Wertz and Wertz, 1977; Sullivan and

Weitz, 1988). By contrast, the home birth (or alternative childbirth) movement and the reinvigoration of midwifery are recognized as largely white, middle class phenomena (Cobb, 1981; Nelson, 1983; Simmons and Bernstein, 1983; Sullivan and Weitz, 1984, 1988; Weitz and Sullivan, 1986; McClain, 1987). Since 1970, rates of home birth in the United States have increased slightly for white women at the same time as rates for ethnic minority women have declined (McClain, 1987). The total rate for home birth remains small, having stabilized (to the best of our statistical ability to track it)[3] at approximately 1% of all births recorded nationally (McClain, 1987). This rate also holds for a number of individual states reporting statistics (Simmons and Bernstein, 1983; Sullivan and Weitz, 1984; Schneider, 1986; Weitz and Sullivan, 1986; Schramm *et al.*, 1987; Meyers *et al.*, 1990). This small minority is nevertheless very firm in its convictions, and participates in an alternative childbirth services network whose beliefs and practices are in many respects directly contradictory of the orthodox model of perinatal events, their meaning, and their proper management.

B. SAMPLE HOME BIRTH POPULATION

Between January and April of 1981 I interviewed twelve Philadelphia area couples who had had at least one child born at home. All of these couples had been attended by a lay midwife, i.e., in Pennsylvania, a non-licensed birth attendant. Potential interviewees had been suggested to me by a locally practicing lay midwife whom I had located through word-of-mouth referral. With their prior permission, the midwife gave me names and telephone numbers of several client couples. Her selection was intended to encompass a range of birth experiences, so as not to bias my sample toward accounts of short or easy labors with flawless deliveries. I interviewed all referred couples who remained willing to participate after my initial contact with them. Interviews were tape-recorded and later logged thematically or transcribed verbatim. Description and analysis of the home birth movement presented here are drawn from this field sample and from the extensive literature on the home birth movement.

All of the informants were between the age of 20 and 35, white, with a minimum of high school education, and in "middle-income" range. Educational and occupational data are incomplete for the sample, but at least four of the mothers had attended or completed college; one of those had completed all but her dissertation for a doctorate in psychology and one other mother had attended (but not completed) nursing school. Fathers' occupations included skilled craftsmen and tradesmen, salesmen, businessmen, a small business owner, and a dentist. The majority of the mothers worked in the home full time, and the fathers were the principal breadwinners for the family. None of the women identified themselves with feminist politics, and only two of the couples had a consciously "counter-cultural" lifestyle. The couples were rarely acquainted with one another except through their common experience of home birth, did not see each other socially (with the exception of two women who were sisters), and were not part of an alternative childbirth "community". These patterns appear typical of the membership of the home birth movement (Hazell, 1974; Cobb, 1981; Weitz and Sullivan, 1986).

C. THE BIOMEDICAL MODEL OF CHILDBIRTH

Biomedicine conceives of childbirth as a stressful process that is potentially hazardous for both mother and child (Peterson, 1983; Rothman, 1983; Weitz and Sullivan, 1985; Oakley and Houd, 1990). Professional surveillance and management are promoted in the interests of maternal and infant safety – in terms of both preventive actions and rapid responses to developing or potential problems. Responsibility and authority for ongoing evaluation and decision making rest with the physician in attendance. The medical model organizes labor and delivery into three stages or phases which are defined by specific physiological events: the first stage is characterized by the process of dilation and effacement of the cervix which makes possible the baby's passage out of the uterus; the second, by the passage of the baby through the vagina and its birth; and the third, by delivery of the placenta. Each stage is conceptualized as an ideal sequence of events. The events and stages are believed properly to take place within an idealized time frame based upon statistical norms derived from observations of labors and computation of average durations for each medically defined phase (Friedman, 1959; Rothman, 1983; Sagov *et al.*, 1984).

The process, if "normal", is seen as continuous. Arrests in labor, departures from the normative timetable (and especially time frame "overruns"), and non-normative events and developments are "complications". Complications are by definition abnormal and may prompt interventions (such as labor augmentation by medication, use of forceps, and so forth) aimed at keeping the labor on course (Rothman, 1983). These in turn may require other interventions (episiotomy, partial anesthesia) to facilitate medical management. Attention is focused on present or potential risk to both mother and baby throughout the process, and medical interventions of a preventive and management nature (e.g., fetal monitoring) are undertaken with sufficient frequency as to be considered routine in current hospital practice (Cobb, 1981; Rothman, 1983; Weitz and Sullivan, 1986).

D. THE ALTERNATIVE MODEL OF CHILDBIRTH

The home birth movement constructs a radically different model of childbirth, one whose broad features are shared across the domains of "official" movement organizations, midwives (individually and in their informal peer groups), and individual clients. The alternative model conceptualizes birth as a normal, non-pathological process, which is not inherently dangerous. Underlying the model is a fundamental (and often tacit) belief that "natural" (at least in this specific context) is proper and good, is preferable to "not natural", and should be interfered with as little as possible. The role of the specialist practitioner, in this case the midwife, is not to "manage" the labor but to provide supportive assistance and expert monitoring and advice. With the midwife's assistance the parents, with whom final responsibility and authority for all decisions rest, may make informed choices in response to presenting sensations and events as the birth process unfolds. Parents and birth attendant work together in a "therapeutic alliance" (Sagov *et al.*, 1984, p. 72).

The medical model's division of the birth process into phases is accommodated in the home birth movement's model, though largely as a descriptive convenience with identifiable physiological referents. Labor as a general physical event is conceptualized within these broadly defined parameters, while each individual labor is seen as unique in its specific timing, details of progress, and character. A particular labor may be difficult or smooth, lengthy or brief overall; it may stop (perceived as the body's taking a needed "rest" – see also Rothman, 1983) and start again; it may change over its course in character and intensity, and so on. Standardization of response to actual labors is therefore undesirable (even logically impossible), for it is felt to be based upon false premises. Intervention in the natural course of any labor is discouraged unless absolutely necessary and is believed to promote or exacerbate complications when inappropriately applied.

Pregnancy and childbirth, though they entail important considerations of health, are emphatically defined as being neither illness conditions nor health problems in themselves (although they do entail health in ways to be discussed below). In the home birth movement's lexicon, both pregnancy and birth are defined as normal, though specialized and demanding, female body processes. As such, they are not believed to require medical intervention or management *unless* there are attendant health problems. "Complications" in labor, defined as developments emergent in a particular birth which cause some difficulty to the mother or baby, are believed to be largely self-limiting, self-resolving, or readily manageable. This view is principally legitimated by reference to cumulative empirical evidence: the experiences and observations of hundreds of parents and scores of midwives participating in successful births at home. At the organizational level, academic studies comparing outcomes in maternal and infant morbidity and mortality for home and hospital births are also cited as supporting evidence; additionally midwives and parents observe that midwife-attended home birth has global and historical success on its side.

Home birth proponents positively value watching, waiting, and continuous, conservative evaluation as responses to the presentation of complications. The range of events and possibilities qualifying as "normal" is much broader than that set forth in the conventional obstetric model. It is acknowledged that complications to labor which call for medical intervention do sometimes arise, but their rate of occurrence is perceived, on the whole, to be quite small. It is an important feature of the belief structure that such problems are defined as *possibilities* ancillary to normal labor and delivery, and not as *probabilities* inherent in the process. Parents electing home birth use probabilistic reasoning in their decision making process, basing their assessment of danger on this view of the natural course of normal labor (see also Sagov *et al.*, 1984; Thompson, 1987). Movement rhetoric criticizes medicine for taking an alarmist, risk-based view of all childbirth, which permits the process to be defined as safe or "normal" only in retrospect

(Rothman, 1983; Weitz and Sullivan, 1984). The alternative view is that childbirth in low risk pregnancies is inherently safe and may be said to have been dangerous only in retrospect.

The concept of risk is part of both the alternative and conventional medical models of childbirth, but it is differently applied in the two systems (Sagov *et al.*, 1984; Oakley and Houd, 1990). Midwives accept clients for home birth at least partly on the basis of low risk or low probability of serious complication in the pregnancy or delivery. Their risk assessment follows some of the same criteria that obstetrics uses. Indeed, all of the midwives in my contact group insisted on an initial screening and bloodwork by a physician[4] as a condition for accepting a client. Physicians' findings were central, but they were not necessarily ultimately decisive in the midwives' own client screening and selection processes. Midwives also weighed such factors as prospective clients' dietary, smoking, and lifestyle patterns. They were hesitant to accept those with unhealthy practices who seemed unwilling or unlikely to change, because client responsibility and accountability for health is an important ideological feature of the movement. In addition, personal qualities such as extreme anxiety or nervousness (in general or in relation specifically to the pregnancy and birth), emotional immaturity, or general disorganization were considered indicative of a client's likely inability to "take charge" of the birth with confidence when the time came, and were therefore contraindications for home birth. These qualities were subjectively assessed on the basis of conversational interaction and, frequently, a home visit during the pregnancy. Trustworthiness (also subjectively assessed or intuited) was an important consideration as well, since the legal safety of the midwives depended on it.

Typical medical factors for exclusion from home delivery are breech or other anomalous presentations, multiple births, development of toxemia, anemia, pre-eclampsia, Rh sensitivity, hypertension, diabetes, heart disease, third trimester bleeding, abnormalities of the amniotic fluid, and active venereal infection within two weeks of onset of labor (Brooks and Bennett, 1976). These conditions if present are considered to be health problems which are concurrent with the pregnancy and birth and which introduce the element of risk. As health problems, they call for medical oversight during the pregnancy and, if persistent, at the birth. Maternal age over 35 at the time of a first birth, and premature and post-mature births (2 weeks before and 2 weeks after due date by medical definition) may not be accepted for delivery at home (Brooks and Bennett, 1976), as these circumstances are recognized as having the potential to produce or result in health problems for either mother or child.

Individual midwives vary widely in their willingness to consider attending a home birth in the presence of any of these factors. Some in the group of midwives serving my interview sample were willing to attend a woman whose potentially complicating health or gestational developments were monitored by a physician throughout the pregnancy and appeared stable or under control at onset of labor; others felt capable of such monitoring themselves. One birth in my sample was attended precisely *because* there were likely complications, and the couple refused for religious reasons to consider a hospital delivery. Under the circumstances the midwife did not feel that she could ethically refuse to assist them.

For some in this group of midwives, "postmaturity" was considered to be more a medically created categorization imposed upon pregnancy than a firmly reliable guideline derived from the natural history of gestation itself (see also Rothman, 1988). Individual women's "natural" due dates were considered to be as variable (within a range of weeks) as their individually varying menstrual cycles, frames of mind, or states of general "readiness" (a concept encompassing physical, mental, emotional, and sometimes spiritual aspects, and subjectively or intuitively evaluable by both client and midwife). Maternal age at primiparity was likewise a negotiable criterion, the most important corollary considerations being general state of maternal health and subjective evaluation of the woman's personality and frame of mind. Personal qualities such as a calm, easygoing, flexible demeanor, or strength of character, tended to be evaluated as being indicative of the attitude the woman would take when in labor. On the principle of mind and body unity, such attributes were though to have or to promote their physical counterparts; thus strength of character and flexibility were considered favorable to the birth process.

E. AFTER THE BIRTH

The alternative childbirth movement perceives both parental-infant bonding and breastfeeding to be integral perinatal events.

Citing animal models, advocates point out that mother's milk is the natural source of sustenance for infants, and that infant-maternal imprinting is critical to survival and development of newborns of warm-blooded species (Sullivan and Weitz, 1988). Midwives encourage mothers to nurse their infants immediately upon delivery, sometimes before the umbilical cord is cut. Postpartum examination of the infant is conducted without removing the baby from the mother's arms, or with the infant lying on the mother's stomach. Following the birth, the midwives and other non-family guests withdraw from the birth-room, leaving the parents and any siblings present alone for an extended period of familial bonding time (up to 1 hour may be common). The five couples in my interview sample who had had both home and hospital births all reported feeling a "special" connection to their home-born children, and felt they were calmer and more self-assured than their hospital-born siblings. Mrs. F theorized that not having been separated from his mother or subjected to frightening hospital procedures or impersonal handling meant for her home-born son that "all he's ever known is love". Most parents in this group refused to have silver nitrate drops instilled in their newborns' eyes, at least partly out of concern that the resulting inflammation would interfere with bonding. Siblings who were included in the home birth (some had roles as towel-carriers, or cold drink providers to their mothers) were universally felt to have experienced little or no resentment of the newborn. In these respects, home birth is seen as contributing to the well-being of the whole family; its benefits are not restricted to mother and infant.

F. COOPERATING WITH NATURE

The views of pregnancy and childbirth taken by members of the home birth movement emphasize the innate correctness of natural processes. Proper conduct of labor involves cooperating with and responding to those processes and avoids attempts to reshape or redirect them unless other factors – including anxious or fearful responses, or underlying health problems –, cause them to go awry. Ignorance and poor health can interfere with the natural order of labor and birth. Personal knowledge and good health are promoted as critical contributions to successful childbirth, setting the stage for nature to take its smoothest course. Regular prenatal care is considered an essential preventive and health maintenance regimen. Participating in a regular program of care is typically a requirement for securing the services of a midwife at one's birth. The choice of prenatal care provider is a matter of client preference, and it is the responsibility of the client to arrange and pursue a prenatal regimen. The importance of good diet and nutrition are especially emphasized by midwives, with a preference expressed for a healthful nutritional program based on high protein intake, whole (unprocessed) foods, and foods as free as possible from synthetic additives.[5]

Self-education and participation in childbirth preparation classes are also strongly promoted as contributing to facilitation of the natural process of birth. Fear and anxiety are felt to inhibit the "opening up" which is intrinsic to giving birth; they are believed in turn to result from ignorance of natural body processes, as well as from years of misguided social conditioning regarding pregnancy and birth. These beliefs contribute to the critique of hospital delivery: the unfamiliar atmosphere, regulatory pressures, and interventions of the hospital make it, in the words of Mrs. B, "so tense – such a wrong place to have a baby". Being well informed helps to reduce anxiety, and is seen as crucial to acting on one's own authority, a central value in the home birth movement. Clients are encouraged to read and ask questions, as well as to enroll in a six-week series of preparation classes. Several of the midwives in my contact group taught such classes, and were certified as childbirth educators by the Association for Childbirth at Home, International (ACHI), a movement training and advocacy organization. Childbirth classes of this type unite clients, midwives, and movement organizations in a "community of ideas", and provide a venue for the dissemination of movement ideology.

G. PERSONAL VARIATIONS ON THE THEME

In the membership of any system of beliefs and values, there are personal variations in acceptance and interpretation of particular points, and other belief contexts into which the system is integrated. At the time I interviewed them, all of the members of my sample held personal beliefs congruent with the home birth movement's model of childbirth. Not all had conceptualized childbirth this way from the beginning of their childbearing careers, however. Six of the eleven couples had had their first

birth at home,[6] half of them having had more than one home
birth. The remaining five had "switched" after one or more
hospital deliveries. No one had opted for a hospital birth following a home birth. Individuals had arrived at their positions as
result of several factors. Common to most respondents were
reading (most often cited was Suzanne Arms' *Immaculate Deception*, 1985), hearing one or more first-hand accounts of home
births, discussing the option with the women who eventually
became their midwives, and attending ACHI childbirth education
classes (ten of the couples attended). For three women, a strong
dissatisfaction with hospital obstetrics, based on personal experience, had prompted them to seek alternatives. Two others
simply found their hospital births unsatisfying and began to
explore other possibilities for subsequent births.

Among the interviewees, there was a variety of reasons given
for seeking a home birth in the first place, and the alternative
childbirth philosophy was integrated into a number of different
personal belief frameworks. Mr. and Mrs. I were very young
when their first child was born, had a meager income and no
health insurance. These factors, coupled with an existing confidence about childbirth, led them to choose a physician who
would attend them at home inexpensively. (Their subsequent
home birth was attended by lay midwives.) Mrs. H was raised as
a Christian Scientist. She did not feel she had "decided" to have a
home birth but rather the thought of having a hospital birth had
simply never entered her mind. She had been looking for a
Christian Science nurse to attend her birth when she was introduced to her midwife. Couples J and K were followers of Eastern
spiritual philosophies, which committed them to a low technology
lifestyle lived as closely as possible in accordance with nature, and
to family-centered values. Non-technological childbirth, accomplished naturally and in the home, fitted an existing value
system which guided all aspects of their lives. Like Mrs. H, both of
these couples felt that home birth followed naturally from their
larger personal philosophy, and did not constitute a separate,
conscious choice. Mrs. A participated in her sister's home birth
and the experience, coupled with a personal distaste for medical
interaction style and invasive procedures, was convincing for her.
Mrs. E was sympathetic to the women's health movement, had
parents who had in recent years become enthusiasts of a holistic
approach to health care, and valued personal independence and

accomplishment. She chose home birth birth even though "[her] upbringing said 'hospital'." Each of these couples had their first births at home.

Religious considerations entered into the choice of home birth for eight women or couples. For five of these (including the three mentioned above), religion played a central role in their selection of home birth whereas for three others it was a collateral consideration. Couple G identified themselves as "Christians", and believed in "doing things as close [as possible] to how the Lord created them". It was implicit in their faith that God would not have created an inherently incorrect or dangerous way for people to fulfill the commandment to multiply and be fruitful. Mrs. G concluded that acceptance of the medical model of childbirth in the absence of identifiable complicating factors would entail doubting the perfection of creation. The couple did not take their decision lightly, but read scripture, prayed, and consulted with members of their congregation for guidance. Among their concerns were moral qualms owing to the legal status of lay midwifery. Through prayer and scriptural consultation they reached the conclusion that the laws of humanity were imperfect and in this case, in error. The Bible and principles of faith provided a higher authority for the G's choice. Mrs. G's two previous pregnancies (both also planned for home birth) had ended in premature labor, one resulting in the loss of twins. On both of these occasions, the couple went willingly to the hospital. They viewed medical care as having its place among the healing resources provided by divine providence, but regarded it as an option to be used judiciously and conservatively in the case of childbirth. Within this belief framework, Mrs. G's history of prematurity was not a deterrent to their plans for another try at home birth.

Couple F were Jehovah's Witnesses. Mrs. F's birth history was significant for post-partum hemorrhage of increasing severity with each of three successive births. The couple determined to have their fourth baby at home *because* they felt that another severe hemorrhage was likely. They reasoned that the probability of an enforced transfusion in a hospital setting was high, believing that physicians would be overwhelmed by the possibility that this young mother of four might die – "needlessly", in medical judgment. Mrs. F accepted the possibility of her own death, and considered the outcome to be a matter of God's will. She explained, "I knew I wasn't somebody that couldn't be replaced".

For several months Mrs. F searched unsuccessfully for a physician willing to attend her home birth. In the meantime, she began a regular course of prenatal care at a nearby naturopathic clinic. By her seventh month of pregnancy the couple had determined to handle the birth on their own, and enrolled in childbirth education classes to prepare themselves to meet their challenges knowledgeably. Their classes, selected on the basis of convenience of location and schedule, were ACHI classes, taught by a midwife. When the F's intentions and situation became known to the midwife, she and two colleagues offered to attend the couple's birth.

For three other women, religious convictions contributed, but were not critical, to their decisions to give birth at home. Mrs. D. dearly wanted a home birth but, while Mrs. D. was very attracted to the idea in principle, she remained nervous about the possibility that something might "go wrong". (Mrs. D opined that this nervousness was the result of the time she spent in nursing school, which she felt had inculcated a disproportionate focus of attention on potential problems.) As the couple's discussions progressed, Mrs. D became more confident about home birth, reminding herself that "the Lord built in a procedure". Mrs. B and Mrs. C, sisters and near neighbors, were both Jehovah's Witnesses. Mrs. C had an Rh negative blood type, and refused to accept RhoGAM because of the Witnesses' proscription of blood and blood products. She felt that home birth provided the only setting in which she could be certain to be free of pressure to take RhoGAM. Her sister, Mrs. B, felt that home was the best venue as a general precaution against violation of religious beliefs in the event of unforeseen circumstances.

Legal considerations were insignificant to all but the one couple previously mentioned, who resolved their concerns by appeal to religious authority. As Mrs. H summed the matter up, "I don't remember what they said [about legalities]. We didn't think it was that important". All clients were aware that the midwife's practice was illegal in their state. A majority believed that this legal status reflected political issues related to medical hegemony and was unconnected to the actual safety of home birth or to the qualification, knowledgeability, and skill of their midwives. Education, professional training, licensure, and certification were not considered essential or even relevant measures of a midwife's qualifications. Alternative legitimation criteria included: the midwife's breadth of experience in assisting at births;[7] her personal qualities of openness, warmth, and empathy; her capacity for calm and patience (Mrs. A.: "The best midwife is one who can sit on her hands and watch and wait."); an egalitarian attitude leading to the frank sharing of information and of limitations of their knowledge; the capacity to listen, take seriously, and respond to the observations and preferences of the mother during labor; and a personal acquaintance, as a woman and a mother, with what women in labor were experiencing (all of the midwives in my contact group had children). On the basis of these criteria, Mrs. B considered the midwives "qualified – in my opinion more qualified than the obstetrician".

Several women reasoned that the midwives' legal status contributed positively to the safety of employing them as birth attendants. Awareness of their own liability, they felt, prompted the midwives to be very conservative in taking risks with a client's health or well being. With every birth, observed Mrs. B pragmatically, "They're putting their butts on the line". In the same vein, privileged legal status was cited as a factor in making physicians cavalier toward their patients and in shielding their errors from scrutiny. Mrs. F likened physicians to craftspeople who do not make themselves accountable to their customers for the caliber of their work. Respondents felt that their respective legal standings contributed to making the accountability – and thus the ultimate concern for safety – of the midwife greater than that of the physician. All parents interviewed said that they would without hesitation repeat their past experiences with their midwives and the events of their home birth(s); this group included five couples who had experienced at least one significant complication (one delayed placental delivery; one severe post-partum bleed; one baby slow to respond; and two very protracted labors with some uterine inertia, including one requiring transport to a hospital to complete the delivery). All of those who planned to have more children planned to have them at home as well.

H. SUBJECTIVE SOURCES OF KNOWLEDGE

In addition to print and formally organized instruction, midwives and clients place a high value on subjective sources of knowledge (Cobb, 1981; Sagov *et al.*, 1984; Susie, 1988; Sullivan and Weitz, 1988; Oakley and Houd, 1990). Three classes of subjective knowledge were identified in my sample. Certain rapid, strong, interpersonal impressions of character or personality were considered to be reliable as knowledge. These moments of insight played a part in the selection of clients by midwives (or in their rejection as good candidates for home birth), as well as in clients' choice of midwife. Two women felt that their midwife's personality was a clinching factor in finalizing their decision to have a home birth. Their sense of trust did not result from making a reasoned evaluation of the midwife's competence, values, and so forth, but was an instantaneous reaction. Said Mrs. A, "Once I met her, there was no doubt". The instantaneous quality and non-inferential nature of this sense of confidence were valued above deliberate assessment as an indicator of the midwives' "rightness" as birth attendant. In a number of other instances, when respondents' confidences and doubts had balanced each other closely in weighing significant choices, similar kinds of "gut" feelings also proved to be decisive.

A second type of non-objective knowledge stemmed from a shared, unspoken, and gender-based understanding whose sources were taken to be partly instinctual (Mrs. G: "Midwives are women, and [women] know life".) and partly experiential. This intersubjective body of knowledge obviated the need for verbal explanation at many moments in the women's labors. Midwives relied on it along with their other types of knowledge (e.g., training by textbook and apprenticeship, cumulative observational knowledge, and consensual peer-group knowledge) as a basis for decision-making during deliveries. Women giving birth placed a very positive value on this connection through unspoken knowledge, and cited it as an unbridgeable divide between attendance at birth by midwives and physicians.[8]

Most striking is the third category of subjective sources of knowledge. In their birth narratives (both hospital and home accounts), seven women mentioned a special kind of knowing which they had experienced during their labors and some had experienced during pregnancies as well. This was distinguished from feeling, impulse, instinct, and other types of "automatic" response to physiological or psychological stimuli of labor. It was emphatically identified as an intellectual experience: a direct apprehension of knowledge, suddenly and with trustworthy certainty. It is signalled in their narratives by voice emphasis ("you *know* what you have to do") or by some form of the phrase

"I just knew". "Just knowing" might best be described as a secular or non-transcendent version of mystical, unitive knowledge. That is, it has no objective measures, is not attained through ordinary sense-experience, and is not publicly verifiable (Feigl, 1958). The experience is not amenable to legitimation by testing, analysis, intentional replicability, or observation. In some instances, observation may even appear to contradict the content of the claim. For example, when a woman, never having given birth before, suddenly "just knows" that she must take a certain action, physical signs perceptible to the trained observer may not objectively support her contention. For the experiencer, "just knowing" has complete authority; it tells her what to do and it impels action. It overrides objective information. The midwives who assisted these clients recognized "just knowing" as a source of genuine knowledge and considered the knowledge so acquired a reliable basis for decision and action. Indeed, they operated on the assumption that the woman in labor is the *only* one in a position to truly know certain kinds of things. In these cases, they accepted the primacy of direct experience over objective observation as a source of valid information.

Responses to "just knowing" were named as critical differences between home and hospital birth by women who had been through both. Doctors, they said, do not recognize women's claim to this knowledge as factual, while midwives do. In their experience, physicians classified claims of "just knowing" as reactions to the stresses of labor, i.e., precisely *as being* what the women who have the experience insist they *are not*. "Just knowing" is not recognized in the medical epistemology as a valid way of knowing, and so does not qualify as valid grounds for action. Mrs. B recounted with frustration that her hospital physician responded to her claim of "just knowing" by encouraging her to ignore the sensation and reassuring her that it was not a pathological sign: "Don't worry", he told her, "[it] happens all the time". To the doctor, the phenomenon was a commonplace without "real" significance, i.e., it was not taken to give actual information (interpreted as information about potential pathology) about the labor. As such, it was dismissable from attention along with other routine but non-significant concomitants of childbirth such as groaning, sweating, etc. For Mrs. B this constituted an almost unbearable irony. It was an event which she knew by personal experience to be real and authoritative, but

which was dismissed as essentially delusional on grounds of its acknowledged frequency of occurrence. Evidence which in her
belief system supported her epistemic claim was used in the
medical belief system to refute it, by reference to prior definition
of what could "count" as information.

Women who have had the experience of "just knowing" can
obtain intersubjective validation of its epistemological status from
each other, that is, from midwives at the time of its occurrence and
from other mothers when birth narratives are recounted. Midwives who might not have had the experience themselves are
likely nevertheless to provide ideological validation; that is, they
will accept its significance on principle, and act accordingly.
Clients expressed tremendous gratitude for having been "listened
to" by their midwives in this way. All of the women who had had
this experience (regardless of whether they had had any hospital
births at all) listed doctors' attitudes toward this and other subjective ways of knowing as a shortcoming of physicians and counted
it among the reasons for their rejection of hospital obstetrics.

I. RELATIONSHIP TO CONVENTIONAL MEDICINE

The relationship of the home birth movement to conventional
medicine is complex. The two belief systems hold mutually
contradictory models of childbirth and of proper perinatal
routines, and each is a stern (and often heated) critic of the other.
Some key personnel are members of both systems, for example
physicians who are sympathetic to and sometimes participate in
home birth, midwives who have training in nursing or by apprenticeship to supportive physicians and nurse-midwives, clients
who use the services of both physicians (including obstetricians)
and midwives. The home birth movement does not reject conventional medicine in its entirety, although individual members may
go farther in this direction. However interactions with the orthodox system are quite consciously managed to minimize
medical control, reduce friction in dealings with physicians, and
maximize personal autonomy.

Both obstetrics and the home birth movement base their models
of childbirth in part on cumulative empirical evidence, i.e., observations over time of large numbers of births. However, the two
groups' observational claims are mutually disconfirming in that
they strongly disagree on the fundamental definition of the event

which is their focal point. Home birth proponents believe that obstetrics is observing an artificial set of events, artifacts of its own setting and interventions (Oakley and Houd, 1990), while the home birth model is rooted in childbirth as it *is*. They charge that physicians meddle and change the course of events and then take what they have seen as normative; home birth attendants, on the other hand, hold back and take note of how birth behaves on its own. Obstetrics counters that the home birth movement is taking a selective look, leaving out of account many real perils which threaten both infants and mothers. Obstetrics views itself (to use the terminology of the current decade) as proactive, while chastising the home birth approach as merely reactive. Reaction, they assert, is not an adequate *modus operandi* to deal with the range and rapidity of potential problem development during labor. The alternative childbirth movement counters that the home birth model is affirming and responsive, while the approach of obstetrics is crisis-oriented and pre-emptive, changing the natural course of events without taking the time to determine what that course might have been.

Each group uses statistics to support certain of its claims, while criticizing its opposite number for selective application of statistical information. In addition, home birth proponents criticize the medical model for equating statistically normative labor events and phases with individual, physiological normality (Rothman 1988). Each finds the supporting arguments of the other to be guided more by self-interest than by reliable observation and information, and debates between them are often marked by acrimonious rhetoric (see Sagov *et al.*, 1984: xx). A past president of the American College of Obstetrics and Gynecology referred to the movement in its early years as "the home birth crisis" (Pearse, 1967) and a decade later denounced home birth as a form of "maternal trauma" and "child abuse" (Obstetrics and Gynecology News, 1977). Members of my interview sample, on the other hand, found routine hospital obstetric practices "barbaric" (Mrs. I), "bizarre" (Mrs. H), "absurd" and "primitive" (Mrs. J).

Each system defines certain limitations on the basis of a concept of risk, but the notion is differently applied and the probabilities oppositely calculated. Each is alarmed by dangers it believes to be intrinsic to the other's approach to birth. Mrs. J believed the risk of infection was greater in hospital setting where "there is sickness, and so many people moving in and out. I feel like my home is cleaner than a hospital". Mrs. A referred to iatrogenic problems associated with hospital deliveries (including overuse of cesarian section), and said of the home birth alternative, "You never know what you prevent". Mrs. B summed up the opinion of herself and her sister (Mrs. C) on the comparative safety of each method of child birth: "*We* feel that you're taking more of a risk in having the baby in a hospital than you are at home".

Nevertheless the systems interact with regularity, in a number of ways. Physicians who are sympathetic to home birth participate in the movement at various of its social organizational levels, and with varying degrees of openness. In my contact group, two physicians' names came up repeatedly. Dr. S, an obstetrician, had for a number of years attended home births himself and had delivered the first child of Mrs. I at home. He helped to train at least one of the midwives in the group and remained in active contact with her as a consultant. He had referred two of the client group to her and provided all or part of their course of prenatal care to three. Among his own professional colleagues, Dr. S kept a very low profile and no longer assisted at home births himself as a result of previous collegial censure which had included a threat of revocation of hospital privileges. Dr. W, a pediatrician, had made house calls to provide postnatal checkups for four of the infants, and Dr. S for one.[9] At least one of the midwives in the group was a certified nurse-midwife, and another was beginning nursing school at the time of the interviews.

Lay midwives do not reject conventional medical care for their clients, but incorporate it into their total regimen. Their preventive health concerns are the same as those of physicians (smoking cessation, reduced alcohol consumption, obesity, exercise, and so forth) (Sullivan and Weitz, 1988), with somewhat less emphasis on tightly-controlled weight gain during pregnancy and considerably more emphasis on nutritional concerns. The midwives in my contact group required that clients have an initial health screening and bloodwork done by a physician. Copies of the results were used to help evaluate prospective clients' suitability for home birth (in terms of overall health and likelihood of health-compromising developments). In this respect, physicians were used, with or without their knowledge and consent, as consultants. They were recognized as specialists with acknowledged expertise, but also with a "party line". Their suggestions and interpretations were taken under advisement, with personal judgment of both midwife and client always included in formulating a response and plan of action.

Regular prenatal care is required by the midwives, and M.D.'s are among its providers. Three couples in my sample used the services of obstetricians, three of osteopathic family physicians, and one a naturopath; three received all of their prenatal care from their midwife, and four transferred to the midwife's care at some point during their pregnancies. An additional requirement of the midwives is that each client couple make backup arrangements including transport and nearby receiving hospital to be used in the event of emergency medical complications. In all of these interactions, the alternative system is regarded by participants as their primary care system, and medicine as their fallback or adjuvant system.

It is the responsibility of the clients to manage the interaction between the two systems of care in which they participate when planning a home birth. Individual clients take differing approaches to this task, but all aim to reduce friction between the two systems and retain maximum personal autonomy. Many reported meeting with forceful resistance from physicians when (if) disclosing their plans for a home birth; the response of some, anticipating opposition, was simply to avoid disclosure. Four women reported that one or more physicians with whom they had existing relationships (obstetricians, family physicians) refused to provide prenatal care for them if they insisted on going through with their plans for home births. Two voluntarily left their physicians' practices as a result of this refusal, and two more were dropped from their physicians' patient rosters. Mrs. H. called physicians until she found someone supportive, being unwilling to work with a doctor who opposed her or accepted her grudgingly. Mrs. I pretended to capitulate, stayed with her obstetrician through her seventh month (while also working with her midwife), and then withdrew from his care and pursued the rest of her prenatal regimen with her midwife. She considered her withdrawal from the obstetrician's practice to be permanent, owing to its circumstances. Had he been more accommodating of her wishes, she believed that she would not have withdrawn from his practice, and would have consulted him in future pregnancies.

In the arrangement of backup services, similar mediation was involved. Some clients looked for a hospital willing to receive them in full knowledge of the circumstances. This often necessitated making several inquiries. Others selected their backup hospital and mapped out their route, but planned in the event of transport simply to present themselves at the emergency room without prior arrangement. The midwives advised against use of teaching institutions as backup services, whenever possible, believing that in teaching hospitals staff attitudes were more rigidly focused on "correct" procedure, and that these institutions posed a greater risk of numerous interventions undertaken for educational purposes. Most women were very cautious in their disclosures to hospital personnel, fearing hostility and retaliatory treatment in the event of eventual transport (see also Rothman, 1983; Sullivan and Weitz, 1988). Mrs. C believed that apparent *intention* with respect to the birth was a critical factor in the reception one would receive if transported to a hospital. She recounted that, when her second child had been born in the car en route to a birthing center, she was initially received with suspicion and resentment when she presented at the nearby emergency service for postpartum examination. But once the staff had determined that her out-of-hospital birth had not been intentional, the response switched to one of entertainment at the novelty and congratulatory appreciation of her "heroic" performance.

Several of my interviewees were skeptical of conventional medicine in general, and very seldom went to M.D.'s. For four of the respondents, this sentiment predated and contributed to their choice of home birth. For three others, physicians' responses to their home birth plans had contributed or given rise to their negative opinion. A number of the women found it ironic, and even unconscionable, that physicians who criticized home birth as unsafe also refused to provide the prenatal care which all would agree would increase the safety of pregnancy and birth under any circumstances. Some concluded on these grounds that these physicians' motivation must have more to do with self-interest (in terms of power, authority, and money) than with interest in the health and safety of their patients and their babies; by extension, physicians in general were tarred with the same brush. In a similar vein, women who had received prenatal care from both physicians and midwives felt that the midwives had the women's interests much more at heart and found the midwives' care more thorough. Physicians' prenatal care regimens were especially criticized as superficial with respect to nutrition, highlighting the fact that different standards of what constitutes a healthful and adequate diet operate in the two belief systems.

J. SUMMARY

Membership in this non-biomedical health belief system is middle class, well educated, medically well-informed, and predominantly white. Members have chosen their alternative form of care not through faulty understanding of medical principles and practices, but as a result of active and reasoned disagreement with them. The home birth movement is one of a number of lay health belief systems currently flourishing among middle class populations. Collectively, these systems give the lie to the still-lingering stereotypes which locate users of folk or popular healing modalities primarily among the poor, the relatively uneducated, and the medically unsophisticated, or which portray their use as concentrated in ethnic and minority populations with strong indigenous cultural grounds for their beliefs. Ironically, in light of these misleading notions, it is the more mainstream groups which are most assertive of their disagreements with medical orthodoxy and most ready directly to question physicians' explanations, established practices, and authoritative claims to knowledge. Dissatisfaction with specific physicians' responses to their values and needs prompts many home birth proponents to withdraw from the care of those physicians. Those who have once experienced birth at home attended by midwives typically withdraw permanently from conventional obstetrical delivery.

Readily available ethnographic evidence makes it impossible to sustain any longer the fiction that education and acculturation will inevitably lead to the supplanting of lay health beliefs and practices by an obviously superior and preferable modern and scientific medicine. Indeed the opposite proposition – that educated and sophisticated middle class people often have *in common* with poor ethnic minorities and recent immigrants an interest in and commitment to other forms of healing and care – is suggested.[10] This new idea must now be thoroughly explored with an eye to its implications for understanding the meanings of health and illness to all types of people on the receiving end of care.

NOTES

[1] Unless otherwise specified, the term "midwives" as used here refers to independently practicing midwives attending births at home. These practitioners may be lay midwives (licensed or unlicensed, but without formal, accredited educational certification) or certified nurse-midwives. The legal status of independent midwifery is a matter of state regulation (Butter and Kay, 1988).

[2] See Oakley and Houd 1988, for discussion of developed countries in which physician-attended hospital birth and midwife-attended home birth are equally available options, supported by health insurance plans and payors.

[3] In Pennsylvania, parents having home births file birth certificates themselves. Out of concern for their own or their midwives' legal safety, these parents typically list "self" or "relative" as birth attendant. Since statistics are derived from birth certificates on file, these common tactics make the incidence of home births attended by lay midwives impossible to track with accuracy.

[4] Osteopaths were used by two members of the surveyed client group, and a naturopath by one. These practitioners were regarded as equivalent to MD's in qualification to provide thorough and reliable prenatal screening.

[5] Physicians are generally regarded by movement members as lacking in knowledge or understanding of truly health-promoting nutrition. Conventional medicine's view of nutrition is considered inadequate and in many ways incorrect.

[6] I include in this number Mrs. K., who was transported to a hospital for the birth itself, experiencing uterine inertia following close to 48 hours of labor at home. She considers her experience "mostly" a home birth.

[7] Mrs. H, however, was unperturbed to be her midwife's first "solo".

[8] None of the women in my sample had been attended by a female physician. Many stated that physicians cultivate distance, while midwives teach themselves to foster empathy and connection; one believed that a female physician would be more likely to act as "doctor" to "patient" than as woman supporting woman.

[9] Parents of boys who wished to have them circumcised (irrespective of parental religious preference) used the services of a *mohel* recommended by the midwives. The circumcisions were preformed in the home, as is customary in Jewish tradition.

[10] For a discussion of the general prevalence of non orthodox healing beliefs and practices, and the problems of ethnic stereotyping in the folk medicine literature see Hufford, 1988.

REFERENCES

Arms, S.: 1975, *Immaculate Deception*, Houghton-Mifflin Company, Boston, Massachusetts.

Brooks, Bennett, L.: 1976, *Giving Birth at Home*: Association for Childbirth at Home International, Parent Information Handbook, ACHI, Cerritos, California.

Butter, I.H., and Kay, B.J.: 1988, 'State laws and the practice of midwifery', *American Journal of Public Health* 78, 1161–1169.

Cobb, A.: 1981, 'Incorporation and change: The case of the midwife in the United States', *Medical Anthropology* 5(1), 73–88.

Dick-Read, G.: 1944, *Childbirth Without Fear: The Principles and Practice of Natural Childbirth*, Harper & Brothers, New York.

Dick-Read, G.: 1957, 'Childbirth without fear and without pain', *Ladies Home Journal* 74, 72–73.

Feigl, H.: 1958, 'The "mental" and the "physical", In *Minnesota Studies in the Philosophy of Science*, Vol. II, University of Minnesota Press, Minneapolis, Minnesota.

Friedman, E.: 1959, 'Graphic analysis of labor', *Bulletin of the American College of Nurse-Midwifery* 4(3), 94–105.

Hazell, L.D.: 1974, *Birth Goes Home: An Ethnographic and Attudinal Study of 300 Couples Electing Home Birth in the San Francisco Bay Area*, Catalyst Publishing Company, Seattle, Washington.

Hufford, D.J.: 1988, 'Contemporary folk medicine', In Norman Gervitz, ed. *Other Healers: Unorthodox Medicine in America*, Johns Hopkins University Press, Baltimore.

Karmel, M.: 1959, *Thank You, Dr. Lamaze: A Mother's Experience in Painless Childbirth*, Doubleday, New York.

Lamaze, F.: 1958, *Painless Childbirth*, Burke, London.

McClain, C.: 1987, 'Some social network differences between women choosing home and hospital birth', *Human Organization* 42(2), 146–152.

Meyers, S.J. *et al.*: 1990, 'Unlicensed midwifery practice in Washington state', *American Journal of Public Health* 80(6), 726–728.

Nelson, M.K: 1983, 'Working class women, middle class women, and models of childbirth', *Social Problems* 30(3), 284–297.

Oakley, A., and Houd, S.: 1990, *Helpers in Childbirth: Midwifery Today*, Hemisphere Publishing Corporation, New York.

ACOG official: 1977, ' Home delivery, maternal trauma, child abuse', *Obstetrics and Gynecology News* 1:1.

Pearse, W.H.: 1967, 'Home birth crisis', *American College of Obstetricians and Gynecologists (ACOG) Newsletter* July.

Peterson, K.J.: 1983, 'Technology as a last resort: The work of lay midwives', *Social Problems* 30, 272–283.

Rothman, B.K.: 1983, 'Midwives in transition: The structure of a clinical revolution', *Social Problems* 30, 262–271.

Sagov, S. *et al.*: 1984, *Home Birth: A Practitioner's Guide to Birth Outside the Hospital*, Aspen Publications, Rockville, Maryland.

Schneider, D.: 1986, 'Planned out-of-hospital births, New Jersey, 1978–1980', *Social Science and Medicine* 23(10), 1011–1015.

Schramm, W.F. *et al.*: 1987, 'Neonatal mortality in Missouri home births, 1978–1984', *American Journal of Public Health* 77(8), 930–935.

Simmons, R. and Bernstein S.: 1983, 'Out-of-hospital births in Michigan, 1972–1979: Trends and implications for the safety of planned home deliveries', *Public Health Reports* 98(2), 161–170.

Sullivan, D., and Weitz,R.: 1984, 'Obstacles to the practice of licensed lay midwiferey', *Social Science and Medicine* 19(11), 1189–1196.

Sullivan, D.: 1988, *Labor Pains, Modern Midwives and Home Birth*, Yale University Press, New Haven, Connecticut.

Susie, D.A.: 1988, *In the Way of Our Grandmothers. A Cultural View of Twentieth-Century Midwifery in Florida*, The University of Georgia Press, Athens, Georgia.

Thompson, P.: 1987, 'Home birth: Consumer choice and restriction of physician autonomy', *Journal of Business Ethics* 6, 481–487.

Weitz, R., and Sullivan D.A.: 1986, 'The politics of childbirth: The re-emergence of midwiferey in Arizona', *Social Problems* 33(3), 163–175.

Wertz, R.W., and Wertz, D.C.: 1977, *Lying-In: A History of Childbirth in America*, The Free Press (MacMillan), New York.

Oral Traditions and Folklore of Pregnancy and Childbirth

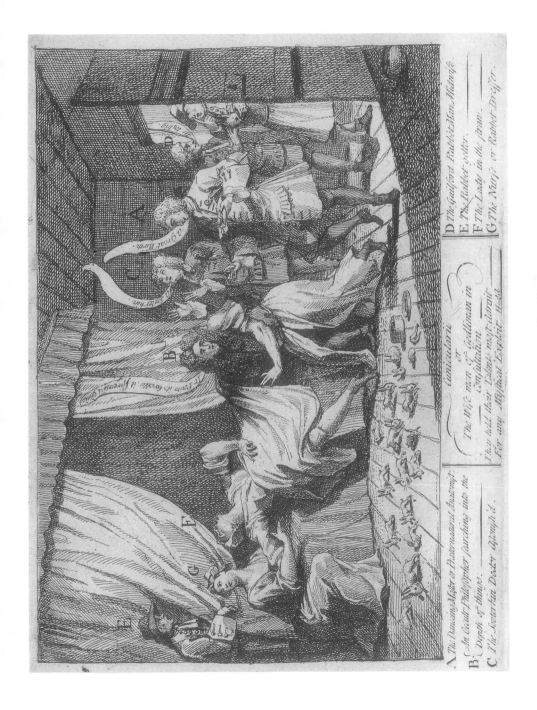

PREGNANCY, PARTURITION, AND CHILDBED AMONG PRIMITIVE PEOPLE.

BY

GEORGE J. ENGELMANN, M.D.,

St. Louis.

As I have already called the attention of the profession to some of the peculiar features in the obstetric practice of savage races, I will now, for the better understanding of these details, completely describe that most interesting period in the life of woman, so important, socially as well as professionally, —the time of pregnancy, labor and childbed.

We will find among the natural habits of primitive people many points of resemblance to the customs of our more advanced civilization. In their views, in their methods of treatment of the parturient, we see rudely depicted the lying-in chamber of to-day; indeed, many a labor in the cellar or the attic of a crowded city, or in the log cabin of a secluded country district, differs but little from that which we will find in the *tepee* of the Indian or the hut of the Negro; in fact, it is here that we often see customs which are rudely indicative of some of the very best of our modern improvements upon which obstetricians greatly pride themselves; observation has taught these children of nature many a lesson of which, in their natural shrewdness, they have profited.

PREGNANCY.

We can trace a certain resemblance throughout; thus a great deal of interest, and I may say of importance, attaches among many tribes to the pregnant state, be it in the jungles of India, in the wilds of Africa, or upon our own prairies. It is to the woman an eventful period of her life, and is appreciated as such by her tribe as important, not only for herself but for all her people. The Andamanese, for instance, are extremely proud of their condition, which in their native state is of course very evident to any beholder, and if a stranger shows himself in their villages, they point with a grunt of satisfaction to the distended abdomen. Among the Hebrews and other people of ancient times, sterility was a disgrace (Gen. xi. 30; Exod. xxiii. 26; Kotelman), and the mother of many children was a greatly envied woman. Conception was favored, although no laws existed upon the subject, by coitus soon after the cessation of the menses, the act being forbidden only during religious service and upon the days of the high feasts.

Abortions as a rule are not numerous; the African tribes in the main are fond of children, and hence rarely destroy them. Among some of our Indians, especially those in closer contact with civilization, laxer morals prevail, and we find abortion quite frequent; some tribes have a reason for it, on account of the difficult labor which endangers the life of the woman bearing a half-breed child, which is usually so large as to make its passage through the pelvis of the Indian mother almost an impossibility.

In old Calabar, medicines are regularly given at the third month to prove the value of the conception. Three kinds of conception are deemed disastrous: first, if resulting in twins; second, in an embryo which dies *in utero;* third, in a child which dies soon after birth; and it is to avoid the further development of such products that the medicines are given; the idea being that, if the pregnancy stands the test of these medicines, it is strong and healthy. In case the ovum is expelled, it must have been one of these undesirable cases of which no good could have come. The medicines are first given by the mouth and the rectum, then *per vaginam,* and applied directly to the *os uteri,* provided that a bloody discharge follows the first doses. For this purpose they use one of three herbs: a Leguminosa, an Euphorbia, or an Amomum. The stalk of the Euphorbia with its exuding juice is pushed up into the vagina; on the same part of the leguminous plant is placed some Guinea pepper, chewed into a mass with saliva: in a few days the abortion takes place. The measures employed are frequently too severe, as constitutional disturbance, and sometimes death follows. Among Indians and Negroes abortion is now and then practised if a suckling mother conceives, as they reason that the living child is the more important and would be harmed by the drain which the new pregnancy necessarily exerts on the strength of the mother.

The seventh month is not unfrequently regarded as dangerous, as many abortions then occur. For this reason, in Old Calabar, the patient is generally sent away, as pregnancy advances, to a country place where she can live quietly and free from the excitement and bustle of the town ; and above all where she can be out of the way of witch-craft. A great many superstitions exist among all peoples in reference to this important epoch, more especially among some tribes of the Finns, for instance the Esthonians ; one of the most amusing of these ideas is the weekly changing of shoes customary among pregnant women, which is done in order to lead the devil off the track, who is supposed to follow them constantly that he may pounce upon the new-born at the earliest moment.

The same great wish prevails for a boy among savage races as among our own people, even to a much greater extent, and naturally so, as in the male child the warrior of the future is looked for ; our own Indians, as well as the Negroes of Africa, have numerous ceremonies by the faithful observance of which they hope to produce the desired sex ; but, however interesting they may be, we cannot now enter upon their further consideration.

Here and there signs of pregnancy are carefully observed : in Old Calabar, as well as in the interior of Africa, pregnancy is counted from the suspension of the menses, and the time is reckoned by lunar months ; among Sclavonians the appearance of freckles is looked upon as a safe sign of pregnancy.

The care which is taken of pregnant women depends, of course, greatly upon their surroundings and increases with the civilization of the people. We see this best illustrated among the North American Indians : very little or no distinction is made among the nomadic tribes, but as soon as we come to a more sedentary population, such as the Pueblos, or the natives of Mexico, we see that they become more considerate. No over-exercise is permitted, warm baths are frequently taken, and the abdomen is regularly kneaded in order to correct the position of the child. This is also the case in Japan, and whether the diagnosis of a malposition is made in the early stages of pregnancy or not, it is a fact that the abdomen is subjected to this treatment, and, unquestionably, in many instances, the position is thus rectified. This is done by massage and manipulation among these somewhat more advanced people, whilst the nomadic Indians of the prairie accomplish the same end by hard work and horse-back riding. The great danger in labor, and to the savage woman *the one* great danger, is a transverse position of the child. This they must use every means to avoid, as with them death is certain if labor is inaugurated with the child in such a position.

I have already described in full the method of rectifying malpositions as practised in Japan, in my paper on " Posture," and will only say that the process, mainly massage, is repeated every morning after the fifth month, the practitioner making the patient stand up and put her arms around his neck. The Andamanese and the Wakamba of Africa, many of the nomadic Indians, and undoubtedly almost all of the women of savage tribes work up to the very hour of labor. Rigby states that he finds the easiest labors, and the best results, when the women work or continue their wonted employments until labor pains are upon them; it always goes worse with those who idle beforehand, with the view of saving themselves and making labor easier. This statement we find constantly verified in our ordinary practice; we know that the working women—and we have many such—who continue their wonted employments until the very moment of delivery, have the easiest labor. It is the lady who is so conservative of her strength and anxious to do everything in her power to promote her health and the welfare of her offspring, who suffers most. At all events we shall not fear evil, and the pregnant woman will fare best in the coming labor, if she will continue as long as possible in the exercise of her usual duties, whatever they may be.

In Mexico, as the old histories tell us, the pregnant woman was forbidden to yield too freely to the desires of the husband, although coitus was indeed ordered to a certain extent, so that the offspring might not prove weakly. In Loango coitus is not forbidden. Some regulations with regard to the act exist among other tribes, and the too free exercise of matrimonial rights is often cautioned against.

40

The well regulated government of old Mexico was careful of pregnant woman in many ways; the Burmese women wear a tight bandage about the abdomen after the seventh month of pregnancy, to prevent the ascent of the uterus, under the idea that the higher the child ascends in the abdomen the farther it will have to travel in labor when it descends, and hence the more painful the delivery will be. In Japan, the midwife is consulted at about the fifth month, and she then binds the abdomen with a cloth which is not removed until labor begins, it being kept there so that the child should not grow too large. It is the same procedure which is followed in India, although the underlying idea is different, and three times a month the abdomen is rubbed. The Nayer women bathe a great deal during pregnancy, taking good care of body and soul. In fact, the frequent bathing of pregnant women is common also to all the higher castes of India. The Nayer perform a ceremony during the first month of pregnancy, but as it so frequently happens that a woman erroneously considered herself in that condition, this ceremony for the preservation of the pregnant woman against the wiles of the devil is usually delayed until the fifth or even the seventh month; and upon the following morning she very properly drinks the juice of tamarind leaves mixed with water.

Here and there some preparation is made to ease the intensity of the coming labor pains. Upon the isle of Jap, in West Mikronesia, they begin to dilate the *os uteri* at least one month before delivery is expected; the leaves of a certain plant, tightly rolled, are inserted into the *os*, moistened by the uterine secretion they distend, and when fully dilated a thicker roll is introduced. They are to act upon the principle of laminaria or sponge tent, slowly dilating the mouth of the womb and making labor more speedy and less painful.

A very pretty idea exists among the Pahutes with regard to the coming of the child; they recognize the approaching time for the addition to their household and tribe, and seek to make preparation for the advent of the young stranger; that is to say, they endeavor to make his journey easy and expeditious with the least possible pain to the mother. Their ideas are crude and fallacious, yet to them sufficiently convincing to be universally practised. They consider the sojourn of the off-

316

spring *in utero* as a voluntary matter, and after a given length of time, say nine moons or the lapse of certain seasons of the year, the child is to be starved out of its maternal quarters as a wood-chuck or other game is to be forced out of its hiding place; hence, for weeks before the expected event a fast begins with the mother, which becomes almost absolute as the time approaches, so that by the end of the allotted period of gestation the fetus will not only be ready, but anxious to come to the world in order to reach the supply of milk which the mother has now in waiting for the child starved in the womb. They of course act on the presumption that the child is nourished by ingestion from the mother. But another reason or object they have in view is, that this treatment, this fasting, reduces the maternal tissue over the genital organs and thus opens a wider door for the exit of the fetus. After this preparation, when labor has actually begun, they regard its phenomena as due to voluntary efforts on the part of the child to leave its inhospitable quarters for exterior life, and everything in their rude philosophy is done to facilitate and help the little fellow along on his journey.

LABOR.

Among primitive people, still natural in their habits and living under conditions which favor the healthy development of their physical organization, labor may be characterized as short and easy, accompanied by few accidents and followed by little or no prostration; the squaw of the Modoc Indians —a tribe which has been but little affected by the advance of civilization—suffers but an hour or even less in the agony of childbirth; the Sioux, the Kootenais, and the Santees are somewhat longer in labor, not, however, over two or three hours; two hours being about the average time among the North American Indians. The period of suffering is very much the same among the natives of Africa and of Southern India, the inhabitants of the Antilles and the Caribbees, of the Andaman and the Australian islands, and other savage people.

What little fear exists as to the occurrence of this event, which is so much dreaded by many of our delicately constituted ladies, may be judged from the instances of speedy and unexpected delivery so often related by those in contact with the Indians.   Dr. Faulkner, who spent some years among the Sioux tribes, tells me that he has known a squaw to go for a pack of wood in mid-winter, have a child while gone, wrap it up, place it on the wood and bring both to the lodge, miles distant, without injury.   Dr. Choquette says, that two or three years ago, an Indian party of Flat Heads and Kootenais, men, women, and children, set out for a hunting trip; on a severely cold winter's day, one of the women, allowing the party to proceed, dismounted from her horse, spread an old buffalo robe upon the snow, and gave birth to a child which was immediately followed by the placenta.   Having attended to everything as well as the circumstances permitted, she wrapped up the young one in a blanket, mounted her horse, and overtook the party before they had noticed her absence.

It seems to be an equally easy process among all people who live in a perfectly natural state.   As civilization is approached, the time of labor is more extended.   The Mexican Indians, half-civilized, require three to four hours for delivery, and the same is true for all such tribes as are in closer contact with the whites, as well as of other half-civilized people.   Accidents rarely occur; thus a physician tells me that during a residence of eight years among the Canadian Indians, he knew of no accident, and heard of no death in childbed.   Another professional brother, who lived four years with the Oregon Indians, was not aware of any irregularity occurring in that time, nor was he ever called upon to perform a more serious operation than the rupture of the membranes.

This may be accounted for by the active life which women lead among these people; all the work is done by them, so that the frame and the muscular system are developed, and the fetus, by constant motion, may be said to be shaken into that position in which it best adapts itself to the maternal parts, into the long diameter, and once in such a position it is held there by the firm walls of the maternal abdomen, and the birth becomes easy.   Moreover, they do not marry out of their own tribe or race, and the head of the child is adapted to the pelvis of the mother through which it is to pass.

As soon as there is any deviation from these natural conditions, trouble results.   Positive statements from several of the Indian tribes indisputably prove the truth of this rule; thus many of the Umpqua squaws die in childbed with half-breed children, whose large-sized heads do not permit of their exit. The Umpqua mother will be easily delivered of an offspring from an Umpqua father, but the head and body of a half-breed child is apt to be too large to pass through her pelvis. Unquestionably this is the case also among other savage tribes.

We can then readily account for the rapid and easy delivery of savage women who live in a natural state, and the rarity of accidents from these facts: First, they marry only their kind, and thus the proportions of the child are suited to the parts of the mother; secondly, their more healthy condition and vigorous frames; while, thirdly, from the active life they lead, head or breech presentations result. Should this latter fact not occur, the mother is generally doomed, or at best, the labor is extremely prolonged and fatiguing. If the child lie transversely in the pelvis, it cannot be born, and death follows.

The nearer civilization is approached, the more trying does the ordeal of childbirth become, as in the case of the Umpquas just cited. I am told that among the women of the Green Bay Indian Agency many deaths take place, and yet a physician states that he does not know of monstrosities or deformed pelves, but attributes the misfortune to malpositions; a greater number of half-breeds is to be found among them, and the resulting disparity between the child and its mother may be a cause of the trouble; again it may be the less active lives which they are supposed to lead, and the consequent cross-births. Dr. Williams has observed that the Pawnees are more exempt from accidents than the Menomonees, and inquires whether it is on account of the squatting posture assumed by the Pawnee women in labor; I should rather ascribe it to the more active life led by the Pawnees, and the less frequent intercourse of their squaws with the whites.

We see then certain differences and an increase of the difficulties of labor as civilization is neared. How different are the conditions upon which I have laid stress as existing among savage tribes, from those which we find in our centres of luxury! People intermarry regardless of difference in race or frame of body, and the consequence is the frequent disproportion between the head of the child and the pelvis of the mother. In addition, the system suffers from the abuses of civilization, its dissipations, and the follies of fashion. On account of the idle life led, and the relaxed condition of the uterus and abdominal walls, there is a greater tendency to malpositions; additional difficulties are presented by the weakened organization, and the languid neurasthenic condition of the subjects in civilized communities. We do, however, sometimes find in our cities, more frequently in our rural districts, strong hardy women, who lead more active lives, and who pass through labor with an ease and rapidity much more like that displayed by their savage sisters.

I can hear but little of labor troubles from physicians who are in contact with our Indians, as they rarely have the opportunity of witnessing a confinement; it is only in the most desperate cases, and hardly then, that even the Agency Physician is called in, and Indians are extremely reticent upon such topics; but I should judge from the robust health and hardiness of their squaws that mishaps are few. The most serious accident which occurs is the shoulder presentation, and that must necessarily prove fatal. This rarity of accidents is most fortunate, since neither our own Indians nor other savage tribes have any means of meeting them, save incantations or the howling of the medicine men.

The Papagos and some other tribes seem to have a philosophical way of regarding accidents in labor; they think that the character of the fetus has a good deal to do in causing the obstruction, and the more severe the latter the worse the former; hence, they deem it better for mother, child, and tribe that the mother and child should perish, than that so villainous an offspring should be born and grow up to do injury to his people.

Rigidity of the perineum has been occasionally mentioned, and in a case of this kind among the Dakotas the attending squaw relieved her patient by inserting her open hands, placed palm to palm, within the vulva, and making forcible dilatation, an assistance which few other uneducated people seem to have the knowledge of rendering. No attention being paid to the perineum, rupture is probably frequent; I know this to be a fact only of the negroes of Loango, as the information gathered by travellers does not usually extend to these subjects.

The prolapse of an arm is managed, among the Nez-Percés, and undoubtedly among other tribes also, just as it is by some of our midwives, by pulling upon it, as they do upon any part which chances to present.

Prolapse of the uterus is not unusual in Mexico and quite frequent in the interior of Russia. The Sclavonians, for instance, who are not unlike some of our Indians, endeavor to shake the child out of the womb in cases of prolonged labor; the natural consequence is that both the child and placenta drop out, to be followed not unfrequently either by prolapse or inversion of the uterus. In Russia, these accidents are so common that people are always prepared to correct them; the poor sufferer is at once brought into the bath-room and stretched upon a slanting board, the feet higher than the head; then the board with the patient upon it is successively raised and lowered in order to shake the uterus back into the pelvis, precisely as one would shake a pillow into its cover.

Hemorrhage, of which I do not often hear, is treated in some instances by sousing the patient into the nearest stream, or rather more tenderly by the Santees, where the attendant gives the patient a shower-bath by filling the mouth with water and blowing it over the abdomen with as much force as possible until the flow of blood ceases.

Whatever may be their social condition, primitive people preserve a certain superstition as regards woman and the functions peculiar to her sex. In many tribes it is customary to set apart a hut or lodge to which the woman is banished during the period of the menstrual flow; so also the child-bearing woman, as a rule, seeks a quiet nook away from the camp, or if the habits of the people are more sedentary, she is confined in a separate lodge a short distance from the one occupied by the family. Sometimes a house is erected for this special purpose, common to the entire village. Again, if better situated, she may have a separate room in her own house, sacred for these occasions.

On the Sandwich Islands, on the contrary, the confinement is more public and the performance is witnessed by all who happen to be about. The same lack of privacy prevails among the Mohammedans of India, who are as careless of the privacy of their confinements as they are of their copulations.

The wilder tribes of Southern India allow female relatives and friends to crowd around the woman, as do the Aborigines of the Andaman Islands. The Pahutes, the Brulé-Sioux, and the Umpquas conduct the labor in the family lodge, and the sympathizing as well as'the curious crowd around at will. A very good idea of such a scene is given me by Dr. Ed. V. Vollum, Surgeon U. S. A., who attended the wife of an Umpqua chief. He states that he found the patient lying in a lodge, rudely constructed of lumber and driftwood; the place was packed to suffocation with women and men ; the stifling odors that arose from their sweating bodies, combined with the smoke, made it impossible for him to remain in the apartment longer than a few moments at a time. The assembly was shouting and crying in the wildest manner, and crowding about the unfortunate sufferer, whose misery was greatly augmented by the apparent kindness of her friends. Not much better were the half-civilized Mexican inhabitants of Monte Rey in early days : but even in these cases where such publicity is permitted, men are, as a rule, excluded.

Commonly labor is conducted most privately and quietly ; the Indian squaw is wont to steal off into the woods for her confinement. Alone or accompanied by a female relative or friend she leaves the village, as she feels the approach of labor, to seek some retired spot; upon the banks of a stream is the favorite place the world over, the vicinity of water, moving water, if possible, is sought, so that the young mother can bathe herself and her child and return to the village cleansed and purified when all is over. This is true of the Sioux, the Comanches, the Tonkawas, the Nez-Percés, the Apaches, the Cheyennes, and other of our Indian tribes.

In winter, a temporary shelter is erected in the vicinity of the family lodge by those who make the solitude of the forest their lying-in chamber in milder weather.

The Chippewas, as well as the Winnebagos, also follow this custom. The natives of the Caucasus, the Dombars and other tribes of Southern India, those of Ceram, the inhabitants of Loango, of Old Calabar, and many of the African races, are delivered in this quiet way, and the women are not only kept apart from their husbands and the villagers during their confinement, but for weeks afterwards. The reason why we know so little of Indian labor is the great secrecy which they observe regarding such matters, and their extreme reluctance to speak to inquisitive whites of these subjects which are to them enshrouded in a veil of superstition and mystery.

Some of the Sioux tribes, the Blackfeet and the Uncpapas, are in the habit of arranging a separate lodge, generally a temporary one, for the occasion, as also do the Klamaths, the Utes, and others. The Comanches construct a shelter for parturient women a short distance outside of the camp and in the rear of the patient's family lodge. This is made of brush or bushes, six or seven feet high, stuck into the hard ground, the branches intertwining so as to form a circular shelter about eight feet in diameter, an entrance is provided by breaking the circle and overlapping the two unjoined ends. In

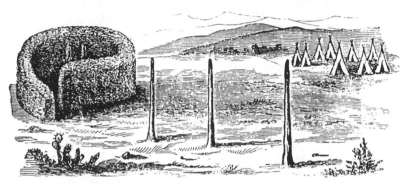

FIG. 1.—Temporary shelter for the lying-in woman, Comanches.

a line outside the entrance are placed three stakes made from the stems of small saplings with the bark left on; these are set ten paces apart and are four feet high. Inside the shelter are made two rectangular excavations in the soil, ten to eighteen inches in width, with a stake at the end of each. In one hole is placed a hot stone, in the other a little loose earth to receive any discharges from the bowels or the bladder. The ground is strewn with herbs. This is their usual mode of constructing a shelter when in camp, and at other seasons, when boughs fail them, pieces of cloth are used to cover up the gaps, or else the leafless brush is covered with skins; but on the march some natural protection is usually sought, or one is hastily extemporized out of robes with, perhaps, a lariat attached to the nearest tree for the woman to seize during the pains.

The Indians of the Uintah Valley Agency observe a similar custom. At the first indication of labor-pains, the parturient leaves the lodge occupied by her family, and a short distance from it erects for herself a small "*wick-e-up*," in which to remain during her confinement, first clearing the ground and making a slight excavation in which a fire is kindled; rocks are placed around the fire and heated, and a kettle of water is kept hot, from which copious draughts are frequently taken. The "*wick-e-up*" is made as close as possible, to prevent exposure to changes of temperature, and to promote free perspiration. Assistance is given by squaws living in the neighborhood, but no particular one is chosen, nor is any medicine-man called in to render aid. In Ceram, a temporary hut is hastily built in the woods, and in some parts of the interior of Russia a separate house is provided, as among our own Indians; such is also the custom of the Samojedn. The Gurians make use of a special room in the house; the apartment set aside for this purpose has no flooring, but the ground is plentifully strewn with hay, upon which the bed is made; above this a rope is fastened to the ceiling for the woman to grasp when in pain. The usual and favorite place of confinement for the Laps and other polar tribes is the bath-room.

As the place of confinement varies, so does the couch upon which the labor occurs. Some care is devoted to its preparation by all people, even the Susruta, that ancient system of midwifery, tells us that " the parturient should lie on her back upon a *carefully spread couch*, that a pillow should be given her, the thighs should be flexed, and that she should be delivered by four *aged and knowing midwives*, whose nails were well trimmed."

The women of ancient Greece were delivered upon stools; the large arm-chair is still at home in the East, while in Syria a *rocking* obstetrical chair is used. The Kootenais employ a box covered with buffalo robes; the Sandwich Islanders, a stone; and certain of the tribes of Finns and Mongols, as well as many of our Caucasian race, look upon the lap of the husband as the best obstetrical couch. Many of our Indians use nothing but the bare ground, others a buffalo robe or old blanket spread upon the floor of the *tepee*, or else some dried grass and weeds; in one way or other, however, they make a soft and comfortable couch upon the ground. A common method is to place a layer of earth beneath the buffalo robe upon which they are confined. Thus F. F. Gerard tells me that the Rees, the Gros-Ventres, and the Mandans, lay a large piece of skin on the ground, over which is strewn a layer of earth three to four inches deep, and upon this is spread the blanket or skin on which the parturient kneels.

The Japanese make their preparations for the coming event in the seventh month, so as to be sure of being in time. The bed which they then provide consists of a mat of straw about three feet square, on which is spread a layer of cotton or cloth. This simple arrangement upon which the patient is to be delivered is then set aside to be available at any emergency.

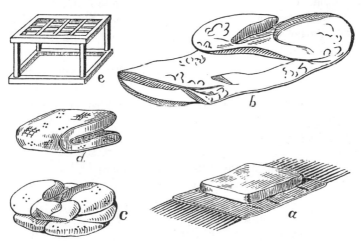

Fig. 2.—Japanese lying-in couch and supports used in childbed.

The above figure represents this mat, together with the mattrass upon which it is laid, and the cushions used to support the back during the puerperal state. I need enter no further into this subject, as I have frequently referred to it, and have treated of it fully in my paper on Posture.

With regard to the *assistants* who aid the parturient woman, there is some difference in the customs of the various races. In many cases she has no help of any kind. As a rule, the assistants, if any, are females, relatives, or neighbors, and the aid they give the sufferer is about the same as that which is too commonly obtained by her more civilized sisters, the world over, often worse than none at all. Occasionally they have professional midwives, whose qualifications depend chiefly upon their age or the number of children they have borne. In case that the patient is a lady of quality, the wife perhaps of a chief, or if the labor prove a very difficult one, the prophet or medicine man is summoned. The physician is mistrusted and is only consulted in the most desperate cases ; the medicine man is aware that the forceps of his white brother are more efficacious than the rattling of the tum-tum, and, actuated by that same professional jealousy which is occasionally observed in more civilized communities, he uses his influence to malign the stranger, and glorify himself.

In Siam and in Ceram, in parts of Africa and South America, among the Indians of Canada and some of our own—the Tonkawas, the Cheyennes and allied tribes, the Arrapahoes, and the Cattaraugus, there is no class corresponding to our midwives, and the patient has no help whatsoever ; but usually relatives and friends aid each other, or there is some assistance rendered by the habitual old woman. This is true of the savage tribes of the vast Russian empire ; each village or settlement has an old crone who possesses the power of second sight, and by this gift and other similar means drives away disease ; but above all haunts the lying-in room, where she causes much harm to both mother and child by her rude and ill-timed manipulations. Other tribes have their particular old women, who, for various reasons, are supposed to be specially skilled. Thus the Navajos and the Nez-Percés have their *sages femmes*, and in Mexico there are midwives who are acquainted with medicinal herbs and their properties. The Indians of the Quapaw Agency, those in some parts of Mexico, and many of the Pueblos have women who make this a specialty. So also the Clatsops, the Klamath, the Rees, the Gros-Ventres, and the Mandans.

Whenever a midwife or some other old woman assists the progress of labor, one or more younger women are always on hand to perform the actual work, whilst the midwife sits in front of her charge to receive the child. In Syria, the assistant is an old woman who learned her trade by practising with her mother who was a midwife before her; it is necessary for a woman there to practise for a long time before she thoroughly gains the confidence of the people. We find midwives also in Japan, in parts of India, where in ancient times only women assisted the parturient, whilst in ancient Egypt difficult cases were attended by surgeons specially skilled in midwifery, as it will be remembered that they had their specialists as well as we of the present day. Susruta speaks of *midwives* attending his patient, and the mention of midwives in Exodus i. 19 implies that these good women were as unskilful thirty-five centuries ago as they can still be found at the present day. From all that we have seen it appears that the *Yi* of India, the *Dye* of Syria, the herb-knowing hag of Mexico, and the midwife of the Bible are very much the same in their habits, their qualifications, and their knowledge. It is the same habitual old woman who figures in all countries and at all times, and with whose peculiar qualifications we are quite familiar. In cases where the midwife is at a loss, the aid of the medicine man is sought. The Baschkirs rely upon their "devil-seer" who discovers the presence of the evil spirit and drives him away if rewarded by the present of a sum of money or a fat sheep. Among others a priest is called who hastily mumbles a few verses of the Koran, spits into the patient's face, and leaves the rest to nature.

The *assistance* which is rendered to the parturient woman is very simple and consists entirely of external manipulations, support of the patient in whatever position she may be confined, together with compression of the abdomen for the purpose of expressing the child: in addition to this, the incantations of the medicine men as well as other means, by which they endeavor to act upon the imagination of the patient, must not be forgotten. How little actual help the lying-in woman receives, and how limited is their knowledge of correcting malposition or other of the accidents of labor, will be readily perceived if we state that but few of those primitive people, whose habits we have so far considered, ever manipulate within the vagina. I have positive statements to this effect from the Indians of the Pacific coast, the Umpquas, the Pueblos, as well as the natives of Mexico. The introduction of the hand into the vagina or into the uterus for any definite purpose is a manipulation unknown to the natives of other countries as well. At east I never see it referred to unless it be in a few instances for the purpose of distending the perineum or of removing the placenta from the vagina, which must remain if retained *in utero.* The midwife or older woman in attendance, as we have seen, usually receives the child, whilst the younger women support the patient, steadying the pelvis, resting her head and shoulders, and holding her arms and legs according to the position which she assumes. The younger women also compress the abdomen and rub the body wherever directed. The most reasonable of all their means of assisting the patient in her labor is the steady compression of the abdomen and the following down of the child in its descent. This is a feature common to the red, yellow, and black races, be it by compression of the fundus, by the encircling arms of the husband upon whose lap the patient rests; be it by the hands of one of the female assistants sometimes from behind, sometimes from the front; or by a broad cloth or binder (California Indians and the natives of Southern India) which an assistant tightens during each pain—a treatment which has not yet lost the favor of obstetricians and was once quite popular. There are some who still place a towel about the abdomen of their patients, thinking to assist the descent of the child by the pressure exercised; it serves both to correct the direction of the child's descent and to hasten its passage. In its extreme and worst feature we see this method of treatment exemplified by the Siamese who seek to force the expulsion of the fetus in difficult cases by permitting the attendant to trample upon the abdomen of the patient who is lying prone upon her back.

[To be continued.]

PREGNANCY, PARTURITION, AND CHILDBED AMONG PRIMITIVE PEOPLE.

BY

GEORGE J. ENGELMANN, M.D.,

St. Louis.

[Continued from p. 618.]

ALL primitive people resort to expression in one way or another. The Finns, in tedious cases, compress the abdomen by a belt or binder of some kind or by holding the patient up, suspended, and shaking her as they would a pillow out of its case—a proceeding which is more efficient than mild, and serves as a last resort to the natives of Mexico as well as other far distant people. In Syria, some effort is made to support the perineum in the same manner as is usual with us. In Mexico, as I have already said, they seek to overcome the tension by the introduction of the hands, and in India the parts are carefully anointed, as it is done by some of our Western tribes. The description of an Indian labor, as given me by Dr. McCoy from his experience at the Nisqually agency, will give an excellent idea of the assistance which is tendered the Indian woman in her confinement. "The midwives, of whom there are two in attendance, call upon the Great Spirit for help in a muttering tone, and in the same tones name over the parts immediately connected with the parturient effort, and often all the joints and limbs of the body. By applying their hands to the abdominal walls they try to ascertain the position of the fetus *in utero* and usually to correct malpresentation. They use oil to anoint the parts, and just before the expulsion of the child give medicines to increase the pains."

Somewhat similar was the experience of Dr. Shortt among

the natives of Southern India. He says: "When the woman is taken with labor pains, her relatives and family friends come in and crowd around the sufferer, who is directed to walk about. The midwife, an old woman of experience, rubs her with oil and bathes her back, loins, and lower extremities in warm water; if the pains are false, the woman may partake of food, but after the commencement of labor nothing is given. She is made to sit with her legs extended, one assistant supporting her back, whilst the nurse shampoos back and loins, and her friends keep up a constant noise by talking. Prior to the rupture of the membranes, the nurse places a bag filled with ashes under the perineum as a support and to prevent the clothes being stained. The pelvis and abdomen are rubbed with a limpid oil and shaken several times to promote delivery. The membranes are not ruptured; this is left to nature; when the head protrudes the nurse supports it with her hands and directs the woman to lie on her back."

Little is known to these people of the assistance given by the abdominal muscles, a help which has been recognized even in ancient times and so judiciously advocated by Susruta, who limits the efforts of the patient to the expulsive pains and advises more or less use of the abdominal muscles according to the progress made by the head of the child. The influence of the emotions is, however, thoroughly recognized, as is evident by the incantations to which the prophets of the tribe resort. In Russia, in India, and America, a sudden shock is often made use of and proves a wonderful help in hastening the expulsion of the child; it is appreciated as such by the Kalmucks who always have a number of men, with their guns in readiness, waiting near the bed of the patient; as soon as the midwife perceives the head distending the perineum she signals the men who fire simultaneously, thinking to assist nature by the sudden fright which the noise must cause. A similar practice is occasionally resorted to among the Comanches, and Dr. Forwood, who attended a Comanche squaw in a difficult labor, told me that at a former confinement of the same patient, a practical application had been made of the effect of fright. She was brought out on the plain and *Eissehaby*, a noted warrior, mounted on his fleetest steed, with all his war paint and equipments on, charged down upon her at full speed, turning aside only at the last moment when she expected to be pierced through the body and trampled under foot.   This terrible ordeal is said to have been followed by the immediate expulsion of the child.

Besides the incantations which are customary as a last resort in difficult cases, there are a great many ridiculous superstitions in regard to labor, and much nonsense is practised with the view of making labor easy.   Thus in the middle ages the stars were consulted.   Some of the most northern of the Russian tribes think to make labor easy by obliging the parturient to give the names of such men, besides her husband, with whom she has cohabited, and he, by a messenger, informs the midwife of his own misdeeds in that direction.   Should the labor prove a difficult one, notwithstanding this important proceeding, it is ascribed to a false statement on the part of husband or wife. The Finns kill a chicken and hold the animal struggling in the agony of death before the pudenda of the mother.   Another custom of theirs is to ply the husband with beer, mixed with *Ledum palustre*, upon the eve of his wedding day, in order to produce deep sleep, during which the wife crawls through between the husband's legs without his noticing it.   But no more of this.   All of these various superstitions are equally as efficacious as the incantations of the Klamath squaw who tells the child, as she anxiously watches the progress of the labor, that a rattlesnake was coming to bite it, if it does not hurry into the world and leave its present abode.

Although most savage tribes have roots and herbs to which they resort in various diseases, they rarely seem to make use of them during labor.   We have just seen that the Indians of Washington Territory give some medicine just before the expulsion of the child, and that *Uva ursi* is used by others.   The tribes of Russia use a decoction of *Artemesia vulgaris* to increase the pain ; in the same way *Achillea millefolium* is used, and this latter is universally resorted to in all uterine troubles. In the government Riäsan, *Comarum palustre* is used.   The Esthonians give the patient a decoction of valerian with beer. Those who have no medicines, or cannot afford them, in the interior of Russia, let the patient blow with all her force into an empty bottle, or place a vessel or pot, like a surgical cup, upon the abdomen, or they make the poor woman swallow some ashes or a few lice in place of other medicine.

We have seen that the Indians of the Uinta Valley Agency drink a good deal of hot water during labor. The Crow Indians of Montana drink tea made of various roots and leaves, the kind preferred being made from the root of a plant called *E-say*, said to resemble the tobacco plant, with a root about as large as a turnip. Small quantities of whiskey are also frequently given during labor, and so much importance is attached to this that any price will be paid for a pint or two which is frequently carried about for months before it is to be used. The Winnebagos and Chippewas give the patient, just before the delivery of the child, a drink from a root steeped in hot water which is supposed to relax the system and make delivery quick and easy. The Indians of the Skokomish agency use a tea made from the leaves of *Uva ursi* which they believe from their own experience to possess oxytocic properties. In India, it is considered very dangerous for the patient to drink water during labor. In ancient Mexico, a decoction of the root of a plant called *civapacthi*, which possessed some oxytocic properties, was given, but if the pains were too severe, a small piece of the tail of an opossum, carefully rubbed down in water, had to be taken. However ridiculous this may seem, it is not more so than a prescription given by the court physician in Siam to a lady of high rank at the time of her confinement: "Rub together shavings of sapan wood, rhinoceros blood, tiger's milk (a fresh deposit found on certain leaves in the forest), and cast-off skins of spiders." The Sandwich Islanders drink freely, before confinement, from a mucilage prepared from the inner bark of the halo or hibiscus tree. Susruta advises the parturient to drink quantities of sour rice gruel. In southern India, it is still customary to take some food in the early stages of labor, but as soon as the pains distinctly set in, no more is permitted. Where labor is so short, there is little opportunity to take food, hence little can be said of the customs of primitive people during labor in this respect.

Whatever villanous decoctions the lying-in woman may be obliged to take, her labor, as we have seen, is, as a rule, an easy one, and if we consider in connection with this the stoic character of the Indian, we will not be astonished that during the throes of labor the mother is usually dumb and patient, and willing that the child should inflict any pain to accomplish the delivery. Although comparatively quiet, at the recurrence of each pain the parturient woman will frequently utter a plaintive cry, and in this she differs somewhat from her white sister; the latter will most frequently announce the occurrence of pain by a sound which by the old women has been determined "grunt," the former. gives vent to a low plaintive cry, best expressed perhaps, by the words "wail" or "whine." But sometimes the Indian squaw gets noisy and restless in her suffering, and a description which is given of a laboring woman in the days of the ancient Hebrews, some thirty-five centuries ago, appears much more natural to us and is much more in accord with the sufferings which we suppose a woman to undergo. It is said of the parturient that "she trembles and writhes in her pain" (1 Sam. iv. 19). Her face is all aglow, she sees and hears nothing in her anxiety, especially the primipara cries out aloud and says, with extended hands, "Woe unto me, for my soul succumbs to the murderers" (Gen. iii. 16). And for men there seems to be no greater threat than "the heroes of Moab will upon that day show a bravery equal to that of a woman in labor pains" [1] (Jer. xlviii. 41; xlix. 22).

CHILD BED.

As I have treated fully of the third stage of labor in my last paper, I shall in no way here refer to it, but will at once pass to the consideration of the puerperal stage, and as so little attention is paid to the treatment of the patient during that period, I shall confine myself to the *treatment immediately after delivery*, as she is then for a few moments still under the control of the midwife or attendant, and something is always done before she is permitted to go to her home or her place of retirement through the period of uncleanliness that follows.

Among the Apaches, it is deemed very essential that, as soon as the placenta is expelled, the woman should be kept on her feet, walking about for half an hour or more, so as to favor a free discharge of all retained blood and prevent its coagulation in the womb. The same custom is observed among the Da-

[1] Kotelman: Die Geburtshülfe bei den alten Hebräern.

kotas, among the Flat-Heads, Pend-d'oreilles, Kootenais, and among other of the Indians of the Pacific coast, and wherever it is not especially mentioned I should suppose that the custom was at least unconsciously observed, because it is rarely the case that the Indian squaw remains abed after her confinement; she certainly moves about sufficiently to accomplish the end desired, even if it is not done with the purpose definitely in view. It will be remembered that upon the banks of a stream was the place usually sought by the laboring woman among primitive people the world over for her solitary confinement; delivered of her child she bathes in the cleansing waters—this is done by most of our Indians, by some of the natives of Africa, the inhabitants of Ceram, the still savage tribe of the Yurakere, by the natives of Bolivia, the Sandwich Islands, the Antilles, and of India. It is everywhere the same; the mother, usually with her babe in her arms, plunges into the stream to cleanse herself; or, if the labor is conducted by a midwife, she leads the patient to the water where she is washed *secundem artem*, redressed, and then allowed to return to her place of seclusion or to her home, and very frequently to work, according to the varying customs among different tribes.

Among many of the tribes of the Sclavonians, several buckets of warm water are poured over the patient's abdomen; the Klamaths steam themselves—a custom which they continue for several days after delivery. The Pahutes also continue their ablutions frequently for days after confinement, mother and father both indulging in frequent washings in imitation of some original first parents, whom tradition informs them were very cleanly. The Siamese cleanse themselves with still greater thoroughness, but with fire instead of water; "with the expulsion of the child begins a month of penance for the mother—exposure to true purgatorial fires. It is ingrown into the native female mind in Siam that the most direful consequences to both mother and child will ensue, unless for thirty days after the birth of her first child—a period diminished five days at each subsequent birth —she exposes her naked abdomen and back to the heat of a blazing fire, not two feet distant from her, kept up incessantly day and night. They think the due quantity, quality, and duration of the lochial discharge depends on their exposure to the fire. And this is done in the following way: A fire-place is brought in or extemporized on the floor of the lying-in chamber, by having a flat box or a simple rectangular framework of planks or trunks of banana trees, some three feet by four, filled in with earth to the depth of six inches. On this the fire is built with sticks of wood nearly or quite as large as one's wrists. By the side of this oblong frame, and in contact with it, raised to a level with the fire, a piece of board six or seven feet in length is placed, and on this a coarse mat spread; upon this, or on the bare plank itself the unfortunate woman lies quite nude, save with a narrow strip of cloth about her hips; with nothing else to secure her from a fire hot enough to roast a duck. Then, acting as her own turnspit, she exposes front and back to this excessive heat—an experience not to be coveted in any land, but in that burning clime of perpetual summer a fiery trial indeed. The husband or nurse is ever hard by, like her evil genius, to stir up and replenish the fire by night and by day. True, if it blazes up too fiercely for flesh and blood to endure, there is at hand a basin containing water and a small mop with which to sprinkle it on the flames and keep them in check; hot water alone is allowed to quench the patient's thirst. Those whom lack of merit causes to die in childbirth are buried, not cremated as is the rule with nearly all others who die in Siam. It is a custom almost universal on the entire peninsula of Indo-China and Bangkok; not only the Siamese, but the Laos, Burmese, Malays, and others practise it. The women of the Combodians improve upon the experience of those of other nationalities, for they place their couch of repose, the bench of bamboo slats on which they lie, not alongside of, but actually directly over the fire, so that the smoke and heat ascending do their full work, and they see their thirty days and nights drag slowly along, broiling on this Montezuma bed of misery. The Mohammedan Malays are as observant of this custom as are the Buddhist Siamese, so that it does not seem to be of religious origin. Sir John Bowing suggests there may be some vague idea of pacification or purification connected with it (certainly purification). There is one compensation to offset the mischievous consequences of this practice: it makes the woman of that land escape the evils that result in other countries so often from resuming household duties too soon after the birth of the child. The Siamese mother is guaranteed by this custom one month at least the fullest liberty and undisturbed rest by her own fireside."[1]

The *Binder*, which is now gradually passing away among civilized people, has its representative among some of the savage races: the squaw belt is used among most of the Sioux tribes, and is applied by them during confinement, either before the expulsion of the child or before the expulsion of the placenta, and is worn until the next day. It is a leather belt about four inches wide with three buckles. The Kiowas, Comanches and Wichitas use a broad bandage of buckskin, ornamented with beads, which they buckle tightly around the abdomen of the mother immediately after the completion of labor, and this bandage is thus worn for about a month. Some of the Sioux tribes use a broader belt, with a compress underneath, which is worn for a length of time. The Klatsops also make use of a squaw belt, retaining it as long as convenient to the wearer. Of some of our Indians, especially the Yumas, I am expressly told that they wear no bandage; and in old Calabar a handkerchief simply is tied around the abdomen and twisted so as to make it more like a cincture than a bandage; it is placed right over the hard contracting womb. In Syria the regular broad bandage is worn.

With regard to the *time of the puerperium*, or the time of rest which is given the woman in childbed, there is a greater variation among the customs of the different tribes and people than in almost any other feature of that great physiological function of woman. Some observe no period of rest, but resume their ordinary occupation as soon as they have had their plunge in the water after the birth of the child. But among many people there is a certain time of rest and isolation which is governed more particularly by their religious beliefs of their uncleanliness; and very likely some wise law-giver infused this idea into the unwritten laws of the people, with the view of necessitating a period of rest for the young mother. We find this custom as far back as we have record, and it seems that in the period of seven and of thirty days the two periods of

[1] Notes on Obstetric Practices in Siam. Samuel R. House, M.D., Archives of Medicine, June, 1879.

childbed are exemplified, first that of the *lochia rubra*, and secondly that of the *lochia alba*. With regard to the first period the puerpera should be as unclean during the time of the bloody flow as she is during the menstrual flow, and this period after the birth of a male child is fixed at seven days, but after the birth of a female at two weeks.[1]

Similar beliefs existed among many ancient people: in Athens the puerpera was considered unclean, and whoever touched her was forbidden to visit an altar; even the midwife who was present at the confinement was obliged to perform a religious cleansing of her hands at the feast of the Amphidromies, when the new-born child was carried about the family altar. When the Isle of Delos was to be made a sacred island, it was forbidden that a confinement should take place within its shores.

It is evident enough why the ancient Israelites considered the puerpera unclean during the first days after childbirth, but it seems difficult to explain why this uncleanliness should have lasted seven days after the birth of a male and fourteen after that of a female child. Kotelman believes that it was because the female sex was considered the weaker, the most despised, and the one which would cause the most uncleanliness. It is remarkable that among the Greeks the same idea was prevalent.

In the second period, during the white flow, the puerpera was obliged to remain at home for thirty-three days for a boy and sixty-six days for a girl baby, but was no longer considered unclean. We have already seen that some of our Indians seek to cleanse and purify themselves by frequent steaming, others by washing, and the Siamese by a purification of fire through a period of thirty days, which is diminished by five days for each succeeding child. According to other statements, and possibly in other parts of Siam, seven days of this fiery ordeal suffice to purify the unfortunate woman. Among the Kalmucks, a woman is regarded as unclean for three weeks after delivery, but never is she permitted to remain on her bed longer than seven days. The northern tribes of Russia, the Samojedes and others, consider the puerpera unclean for several months after confinement; her husband is very careful not to

[1] Kotelman: The Ancient Hebrews.

approach her, and she remains in her hut isolated, often very badly taken care of, so much so that mother and child may succumb to this neglect; only after the expiration of two months is she herself, and the tent in which the confinement took place, thoroughly smoked, and from that time on considered as clean. Ten days is the period of uncleanliness among the tribes of Alaska. In Egypt, those who are in easy circumstances remain abed for three to six days, but poor women resume their ordinary occupations, if not severe, in a day or two; in Syria, a rest of about six days in bed is permitted. In Japan, the puerpera is not placed in the usual recumbent position, but sits propped up by pillows, the mat upon which she was confined being left in place. In this upright position the woman remains for about three days, when gradually the prop behind is removed, till finally she is lying with her head on a high pillow, and at the end of three weeks she gets up and the customary congratulatory feast is given to the relations of the family. Another authority states that the patient retains the recumbent position until the twenty-first day, and then, if all has gone well, takes a bath and resumes her duties. The Yenadies of Southern India ordain a period of isolation of ten days, after which the mother returns to her household and its duties. The same is true of the Vedas, also of Southern India; the first five days after confinement are spent by the puerpera in a hut within call of the *Konan*, together with mother and sister or assistants; on the sixth day, she is moved to a shelter nearer to the *Konan*, in which she remains isolated for another five days. After the tenth day she washes with warm water and turmeric, anointing herself with oil; washing is continued for one month, when she resumes work. Dr. Shortt makes a similar report of other tribes of Southern India; he says that the woman lives in strict seclusion in a small lodge ten or twelve paces from the family home for thirty days after childbirth, frequently washing; before joining the others she has to wash all her clothes and undergo a general purification.

The Wakamba of Africa put their parturient to work four to six days after confinement. The Wazegua alone permit the woman to rest abed for fourteen days. Most of these tribes also purify by washing with hot water. The Abyssin-

55

ians and the Somali use slack lime. The women of the Was-waheli sometimes insert the juice of a lemon into the vagina to hasten contraction. The Wakamba ordain a coitus about the third day, and after this the puerpera is considered clean. Among some of the African tribes the women carry an ebony staff for forty days after confinement, for the purpose of keep-ing off the devil.

The North American Indians seem to be less careful of their women. I am positively informed of the Sioux, the Santees, the Apaches, the Indians of the Neah-Bay Agency, as well as the natives of Ceram and of the Antilles, and the Yuricaria of Bolivia, that they practically observe no period of childbed, but go to work upon the same day or the day after that of their confinement. Other of our Indian tribes observe a cer-tain period of rest; those of the Uinta valley take up their abode in the "*wick-e-up*" in which they are confined, and return to the lodge occupied by the family after from two to four weeks, and during this period they are considered to a certain extent unclean. The women of the Laguna Pueblo remain unwashed and in bed for four days; very early on the fifth the puerpera is washed and dressed under the super-intendence of a *Sheaine* or priest, who walks out, followed by the women, to see the sun rise and to render thanks for her safe delivery. As she walks after the *Sheaine* she throws corn blossoms into the air and blows them around as an offering of thanks. Thirty days after the child is born, the woman is clean and her husband returns to her, but some prefer to wait thirty-six, and others forty days. A good many of these Indians, however, have abandoned the fifth-day su-perstition, the sun worship, and are cleaned or washed at once and get up as soon as they feel able to go about their work. The native Mexican woman remains abed three days; on the third day she gets up and for the first time since her confine-ment changes her clothing. The lochial discharge is usually abundant and continues for a long time, seldom less than forty days. At any rate it is only after a period of forty days that the woman ventures to bathe herself. After that she drinks freely of a decoction of some native plant for the purpose of increasing the discharge and bringing it to a speedy close.

Very little or no attention is paid to the *food which women receive after childbirth*, yet some tribes make a reasonable change in their diet. The Kalmucks feed the puerpera mainly on broth during the first days, giving her but very little mutton, the quantity of meat being gradually increased. Among other of the Russian tribes, as I have already stated, the isolation of the patient is so complete that she is but scantily nourished and glad to get anything she can, and often, together with her offspring, suffers actual want. In Syria, mutton or chicken broth is given on the first and second days, then carminative drinks, cinnamon tea and so on, for six days, after which the quantity of food is gradually increased. In Old Calabar, the patient is allowed a pot full of chop, which her husband has prepared during the labor, to be given her, and she is expected to eat a quantity of it immediately after confinement. In southern India, the natives seem to pay greater attention to the diet of the puerperal woman than in almost any other country. Certain of the native tribes live for three days after delivery on the tender leaf bud or cabbage of a kind of date palm, *Phœnix sylvestris*, after which rice or other food, to which they are accustomed, is partaken of. The Domber give her plain rice on the first day, and on the second *chillie powder* and *curry-pillay* is mixed with the rice. Among the Kanikars the puerpera receives as a tonic for the first day a *kari* (ragout) seasoned with turmeric pepper and tamarind.

The negroes of Africa, as a rule, make very little change. The Waswaheli and Nyassa give the puerpera food highly seasoned with Cayenne pepper and other spices. The Wakamba, like the natives of the Andaman islands, make almost no change. The same I may say of our own Indians, with the exception of the Yumas, of whom I see it stated that the puerpera and the murderer are treated to the same diet; neither are allowed to eat either meat or salt for one month, for the purpose of purification. The Basuthos treat the patient cruelly in refusing her water for three days after confinement, the idea being probably the fear of too great a quantity of milk oppressing the breast. The Loango woman drinks quantities of hot water for several months in order to increase the flow of milk, and she also washes herself with a decoction of the leaves of *Ricinus communis*. With leaves of the same plant steeped in water, the genitals are rubbed and cleansed until the secretion ceases. The young mother, moreover, takes a great many baths in some secluded spot in a slight excavation made in the ground and laid out with mats, where cold and hot water is alternately poured over her and the body is kneaded, rubbed, and anointed.

Of the *medicines* used in the puerperal condition, I can only learn that in Mexico teas from native herbs are given to increase the discharge of the lochia; the same is accomplished in southern India by the use of saffron and *neem* leaves. In Syria, carminative drinks are given. In Siam, hot water has eased the thirst produced by the parching fire; whilst in Africa it is given to increase the flow of milk. Among the natives of Russia many of the stronger and more aromatic herbs are used in the various diseases, and many methods of treatment are resorted to in mammary affections, which seem to be very common in the puerperal state, as the remedies are so numerous. I will mention but one, on account of its peculiarity. In case of hardening of the breast, the patient places herself in front of the heated stove in order to warm the diseased part as thoroughly as possible. In the mean time some other person heats a woollen sock, which has been moistened with the urine of the patient, places it as hot as it can be borne upon her breast and attempts to keep the breast as well as the sock hot and moistened with urine; then some iron utensil, a knife or horse-shoe, chilled in ice, is placed upon the affected breast. The hotter and more moist the breast is, and the colder the iron, the more certainly will the cure be effected. I will not refer to any of the *ceremonies* which are here and there observed, either upon the birth of the child, especially if a male, or upon the return of the mother from her isolated state, when cleansed and purified, to her home and her family, but will simply call attention to a remarkable feature common to the natives of the coast of Borneo and to some of our Indians. For instance, among the land Dayokas of Borneo the husband is always treated badly after the birth of the child, when he is dieted on rice and salt, and for a few days forbidden to bathe or show his face out of doors; whilst among some of our Indian tribes the father, after calling his relations and friends together and having a feast of boiled dog and other Indian delicacies spread for them, goes off and *cachés* himself until the child is a week old. This practice, however, is only observed by the young men who are so ashamed of the occurrence that they go to some friend and stay until they summon sufficient courage to come back, when the wife presents the child for the first time to its father. The management of the puerperal stage by the Indians of the Pacific coast has been so well described by Dr. J. Fields, formerly of the Grand Ronde Agency, Oregon, that I will quote verbatim that part of his letter referring to this subject. He says:

" The treatment resorted to is not alike in all the tribes; some with whom I have come in contact require the woman to keep on her feet the greater part of the day, taking short walks around the camp and resting only when she becomes very weary; as a support she uses a staff, an instrument through the aid of which relief comes, as the body is frequently bent forward which brings the abdominal walls immediately over the uterus against the upper end of the stick, on which she also holds her hand, as a man walks with a cane; for a period of three or four days the woman continues the prescribed walks, with an occasional hour in a reclining posture to rest her feet; then she is considered well. The object of this, as old women of the tribe informed me, is to facilitate the flow of the lochia; they think that should the woman lie in bed the blood would accumulate in the abdominal cavity and she must die.

From all I can learn about the practice of the Indians here before the white men came among them, their procedure in the after-treatment was solely for the purpose of encouraging a free flow of the lochia, and I hear of no death from hemorrhage.

Those tribes of Indians on the Pacific coast who follow a different course of treatment, place the woman on a bed as soon after delivery as possible, securely wrap her in a blanket or some covering, and place her near the fire, where she is kept in a closely wrapped condition to escape taking cold and having fever; here she is kept for four or five days, when she at once takes charge of the babe and resumes all the duties that fall to the lot of an Indian woman.

During two and a half years' life among the Indians I neither saw nor heard of a case of puerperal fever, puerperal eclampsia, or any diseases peculiar to lying-in women. Neither did a death in labor come under my observation; few women have any mammary trouble, notwithstanding their being exposed to the same cause that is a prolific source of mammary complication among white women."

Management of the Child.

The management of the new-born child is so intimately connected with the treatment of the mother in the puerperal state that the subject would not seem complete without a brief consideration of the treatment of the babe. Although the savage mother is not wanting in love for her offspring, the treatment of the child from the very first moment is one well suited to fit it for the hardships of its future life. Even among those people where kindness is shown the little stranger, where he is well cared for, and not left to starve in isolation with the mother, as among some of the Russian tribes, he receives at once a hint of the exposure to which he may be subjected in the future. As an ancient chronicle and "Early History of Virginia" says, in speaking of the original inhabitants of that country: "The manner in which they treat their young children is very strange, for instead of keeping them warm at their first entry into the world, and wrapping them up in I don't know how many cloths, according to our fond custom, the first thing they do is to dip the child over head and ears in cold water, and then to bind it naked to a convenient board, having a hole fitly placed for evacuation, but they always put cotton wool or other soft things for the body to rest on between the child and the board. In this posture they keep it several months, till the bones begin to harden, the joints to knit, and the limbs to grow strong. Then they loosen it from the board, and suffer it to crawl about, except when they are feeding or playing with it. While the child is thus on the board, they either lay it flat on its back, set it leaning on one end, or hang it up by a string fastened to the upper end of the board, the child and board being all the while carried about together. As our women undress their children to clean and wash their linen, so they do theirs to wash and grease them. The method the women have of carrying their children after they are suffered to crawl about is very particular. They carry them at their backs in summer, taking one leg of the child under their arm, and the counter-arm of the child in their hand over the shoulder, the other leg hangs down, and the child all the while holding fast with its other hand. But in winter they carry them in the hollow of their *match-coat* at their back, leaving nothing but the child's head out." The child is tucked away in an equally peculiar manner by some of the Polar tribes of Russia; until it begins to crawl it is placed in a fur sack, and carried by a strap about the mother's forehead. Later it is sewed up in a fur garment of one piece; for the sake of cleanliness a doorway is left in the posterior portion, which is opened from time to time as necessity demands, but the garment is not once removed or changed until outgrown by the child.

Among the Sioux, Crows, Creeks, and other of our Indians, the mother plunges into the stream with her child immediately after delivery, or, if no running water is at hand, at least dips the child in cold water as soon as it is born; salt water is used by some people who live upon the sea shore, also by the Kalmucks, who wrap the child in furs as soon as it has had a salt-water bath. A cold-water bath seems to be the customary initiation of the new-born child into the troubles of this world; it is the case among most of the Negro tribes, among the people of Bolivia, of Ceram, and of the Andaman Islands, and in some parts of India; in others, in Southern India, for instance, the child is washed in tepid water; so also in Syria, and, as a rule, by those people who are advanced in civilization.

Usually the child is bathed immediately after delivery, but in Southern Arabia at least two hours are permitted to pass by, during which the child is wrapped in soft warm cloths, then it is washed and anointed. This is also the custom of numerous African tribes, some waiting for several hours, others performing the ceremony at once; some use fat, others, such as the Wakamba, Somal, Wanika, and other tribes use fresh butter. The Masai and the Waswaheli throw a slightly acid and astringent powder, made from the fruit of the *adansonia* tree; over the child, to facilitate cleansing, just as we use oil or fat. The Cheyennes and Arapahoes envelop the child as soon as it is born in dry horse manure, and do not wash it for several days. The Umpquas wrap it in dirty rags, and also put it away without washing.   In India, in Africa, and among the American Indians, there are many tribes who bathe their children for at least one year.   In Syria, in India, and in Africa, there are many who anoint the children regularly, often after every bath, and great attention is paid to the kneading and stretching of the limbs and joints, with the view of making the child straight and strong, and stimulating the healthy development of the muscles.   Some strap the child or have various methods of bundling it, so as to carry it conveniently.   Some, like the Chinooks, of Oregon, compress the head to shape it in a peculiar way.   This method of kneading and stretching the child is well described in a paper on the inhabitants of the Andaman Islands (*Zeitschft. für Ethnologie*, 1877, p. 51).   There it is usually done by the father, who warms the palm of his right hand, presses firmly upon the temples and upon the base of the nose, whilst the left hand fixes the lower jaw; then the wrists and elbows and the septum of the nose are compressed between the thumb and index finger, and so on quite a number of manipulations are performed.

It is interesting to see that the same variations exist in regard to their customs as to the *time of applying the child to the breast* which we find among civilized people.   Thus among the Kanikars and several other tribes of Southern India the child is applied at once to the breast, as is done by some of our Indians.   In Alaska it is customary to suckle the child as soon as it has vomited for the first time; among the Kalmucks the new-born is given a piece of raw mutton to suck, and is not permitted to take the breast for several days.   Upon the Andaman Islands it is customary for any neighbor or friend who is suckling to nurse the new-born child for a day or two until its mother's milk appears.   In Southern India, the child is fed on boiled honey until the third day, and not until then is the mother allowed to suckle it.   In Transvaal, a soft mush is fed to the child for the first three days, and in Loango the same custom prevails, and the people seem to know the qualities of colostrum, at least they make a difference between the milk of the first days and that which afterwards serves for the nourishment of the child.   The negroes of Loango hold a suckling child just as the Caucasian mother does, and it seems that the breast is only given at certain times.

As regards the period of suckling, the time seems to vary greatly, yet it is governed by about the same circumstances among all primitive people as it is among our Indians. As a rule, the child is nursed as long as the mother's milk lasts, or until another conception takes place; at all events, the children are nursed unreasonably long. Thus the Kanikars suckle the child for three to five years; the inhabitants of the Sierra Leone often until the child can walk; those of Australia, from one to three years, according to circumstances; the Alaskans, from ten to thirty months; the Tartars and Esthonians, for a very long period, not only limited as it is among our Indians by another conception, but they suckle the child until the next confinement forces them to make room for a younger offspring. The Arabians seem to nurse for a period of perhaps two years; the Waswaheli, from one to two years; in the eastern portions of Africa, it is the custom to nurse as long as the mother's milk will last, and often during the next pregnancy. A child which is nursed during such a period is called an external twin.

For the purpose of *weaning* the child, it is customary in Southern Arabia to smear myrrh or asafetida upon the nipple. The Somal use the fresh juice of aloe leaves for the same purpose, and in Zanzibar, cayenne pepper or the gum of the aloe is applied. In case that the breasts are inflamed during the process of weaning, the natives of Southern Arabia press out the accumulated milk and cover the breasts with a poultice of soft mud or clay.

I have already remarked that insufficient or inferior *food* is frequently a source of injury to the puerperal woman when isolated during her period of uncleanliness, as it is often the cause of sickness and death of the child. This is especially the case among some of the Russian tribes. Convulsions occur frequently among the children who are partially fed with heavy bread which has been first chewed by the mother; then berries of various kinds are given the infants, not even always ripe; they are kept in a filthy condition, and take frequent colds by the use of the steam baths so common among those people. Coarse food and constitutional syphilis are the causes of early death among many of the Tartars. In Alaska, the fat of some sea animal is the first food which is given the infant. The

Masai and several other tribes of Africans put a little fresh butter, which is especially prepared for this purpose, into the child's mouth after the second day. Among the Wakikuyu the child, after the tenth day, receives chewed bananas, which have been mixed with the saliva of the mother, in addition to the butter. The Wakamba give the infant, very soon after birth, a little mush, and the Somal make them take a little of the juice of the myrrh daily after the sixth month has been reached. In case of the death of the mother, the Wakikuyu and Waswaheli raise the child upon goat's milk; other tribes employ nurses, others feed the child upon mush and other food common among them. The Kossacks think wine a necessary addition to the food, even of suckling infants. In Siam, honey and rice-water is given from the first days, and the soft pulp of the banana is crammed into the little mouth. Dr. Shortt tells us that, in Southern India, the child is fed on boiled honey after the third day, when the mother is allowed to suckle it, and if the external parts are cold, five drops of the *milk hedge* (*Euphorbia Firucalli*) are given it. On the third day, it is rubbed with sweet oil, bathed in warm water, and half a pie-weight of garlic, one-quarter pie-weight of black pepper heated in a kin-weight of castor oil is given, and repeated every second day. Some give castor oil every morning for the first, once a day for the second, and every other day for the third month. From the third day the mother suckles the child; if unable to do so, it is brought up on goats', cows', or asses' milk.

The Villees, another of the tribes of Southern India (Transacts. London Ethnolog. Soc., 1865, III.), give the child for the first two or three days a preparation of black pepper, neem bark, jaggery, garlic and onions, several pots full of which are made at once and slowly dished out. In Old Calabar, the child is first rubbed over with fine sand, then with soap and water; the acid juice of an *Ammomum* is squeezed into its mouth, and a supply of tepid water follows, and for the first three days, during which it is not allowed to suck, it gets nothing but water, and later, although the mother has an abundance of milk and the child is well able to suck, a large quantity of water is given at least once a day. Every morning whilst the child is washed, water is thrown into its mouth continually for several minutes, the child gasping and struggling. This, they say, is done to distend the abdomen and make it capacious to take plenty of food, to hasten growth. If the mother is away, the child is kept quiet by filling with water, and they deem this cheap liquid very useful in this respect; although too much water is rarely taken, it may prove injurious, and possibly the enlarged spleen, which is very common among children in this country, and not among adults, may be traced to the over-dose of water.

The Kanikars begin to give rice-water the third month. The child which is nursed from three to five years, gradually, from the third month on, receives other food, but it is not until its seventh year that it eats with the rest of the family. The Vedas simply suffer the child to die if the mother's milk does not suffice, as no other woman dare nurse it, and cow's milk rarely succeeds. After the daily bath, the babe is anointed with oil and turmeric, and rubbed and kneaded in accordance with certain rules, as we have related of other tribes.

Just as adults are treated with the herbs of the country in their various diseases, so the children are made to put up with them. Teething is furthered in Russia by the use of the fresh juice of the lemon sweetened with sugar, or the gums of the child are smeared with the blood which comes from the comb of a black rooster which has been repeatedly scratched and irritated with a comb. In case of restlessness, a decoction of poppy seed is given the child after it has been carried to the ordinary roosting-place of the chickens and kept there for a while. In case of convulsions, a decoction of *Gentiana pneumonanthe* or the root of *Valeriana phec* is used. The powder of *Origanum*, starch, or lint is applied in case of soreness of the skin, and there are many other equally efficacious remedies in use, many of them most amusing and of extreme interest to the ethnologist, but beyond this of little or no value.

SUPERSTITIONS IN OBSTETRICS.*

By STUART B. BLAKELY, M.D.,

BINGHAMTON, N. Y.

SEX is a fundamental instinct of the human race. Pregnancy, childbirth and the puerperium wear thin the veneer of civilization. The remarkable processes, dangers and results of these periods of woman's life must have been a profound mystery and a source of perpetual wonder to the untutored mind of savage man, as it is to our own to-day. Theories, explanations and beliefs were inevitable. In addition, the care of women in pregnancy and childbirth has always been for the most part in the hands of other women, as a sex conservative and tenacious of belief, clinging to form and tradition, and as midwives generally untrained, ignorant and superstitious. It is therefore not surprising that in the practice of obstetrics one hears, if one but ask and listen, so many echoes of the race's dim and pagan past, down the long road of woman's memory.

The present study is not an attempt to collect a large number of obstetric superstitions, nor an effort to explain or classify even all those mentioned. The examples quoted have been gathered during the past five years in an average industrial American city. In them the ignorant and foreign born have no monopoly. The origin of some is complex, even utterly obscure. Many illustrate the tenacious grip of the strange and the bizarre. The great majority clearly demonstrate that man's modes of thought and his primitive beliefs survive religions and civilizations. The vast mass of womankind to-day, though more or less clearly realizing that these tales and practices of her savage ancestors are neither civilized nor Christian, nevertheless, half ashamed and half defiant, fears and believes them in the depths of her woman's soul.

The two great sources of obstetric superstitions are ancient magic and primitive ideas about women. Ancient magic was based on a mistaken conception of the association of ideas. It reasoned (1) that like produces like, that things that

* Read at the Annual Meeting of the Medical Society of the State of New York, at Brooklyn, May 5, 1921.

resemble each other are the same; this is imitative magic: (2) that things can retain and transmit properties of other things with which they have once been in contact or a part, and can act on each other at a distance; this is a contagious magic. Both have a positive and a negative aspect. By precepts, charms and sorcery a desired result could be produced; by prohibitions and taboos an undesirable result could be avoided. Frazer, in the "Golden Bough," shows how worldwide, deep and unchanging has been and is this mode of thought. Force was all pervading. Good and evil were treated as material things, little differentiated. Magic, primarily, had nothing to do with spirits, though later inextricably involved. It probably antedated religion, which it has fought, permeated and become subject to. Many magic practices survive in ritual and rite. The ancient struggle for souls between the forces of good and evil relives in the baptism of the new-born. The water, so applied as to run off some portion of the infant's body, carries with it the uncleanness of original sin, as though it were a material thing. It is a sacred symbol, but nevertheless, a conception of ancient magic.

To ancient man woman was a strange and mystic being. She differed from the dominant male in many ways, notably in her sexual physiology. She discharged blood from her body, gave birth to babies and produced milk. All this was mysterious and incomprehensible, therefore dangerous and to be feared. Primitive woman was subject to many taboos, especially at her times of special function, when she was believed to be particularly subject to outside forces of good and evil, chiefly the latter against which the restrictions were defensive. Her discharge of blood represented accumulated uncleanness, which idea is in our theory that menstruation prepares the uterus for pregnancy. Menstrual blood was both polluted and polluting, and the fear of its deleterious effects has been and is still worldwide. It is still believed that a menstruating woman can spoil dairy products and cause flowers to fade. It was not so long ago that a nurse was barred from the operating room during her periods. Many of us dislike to operate on a menstruating woman, though the procedure be not gynecological. Primitive woman was also isolated and secluded after childbirth because she was unclean, therefore a danger to others, and also because she herself was in danger at that time. To-day the drawn curtains, the darkened room and the banishment of visitors, particularly children, is but the survival of that taboo. The harmful effect of light on the baby's eyes and the excitement as causing nervousness and fever are surely later ideas. Before she could mingle again in society this contagion of uncleanness must by one of many methods be removed. From this pagan thought arose the practice of the churching of women, now somewhat fallen into disuse.

The restrictions laid on the pregnant woman, during the most momentous period of her life, are almost unlimited in number, in the last analysis mainly defensive in character, protective to the mother and her conception. Weighing the mother will make the baby daring. Bathing will cause the child to die of drowning. Eating too many apples causes kidney trouble. Too much meat toughens the cord and makes the child's bones harder. Coitus during pregnancy will make a blind, sick or dead child—recalling the old idea of the inherent danger of sexual intercourse. The admonition not to attend a christening is a very complicated taboo. The chief evils to be prevented are (1) accidents of labor, particularly the cord around the neck and adherent placenta; (2) injuries to the unborn child resulting in abortion or deformity. The occurrence of the cord around the neck, popularly considered to be of grave moment, is favored by the mother putting her arms above the head or by reaching up, thereby making the cord longer; by walking under anything, usually a clothesline; by hanging anything around the neck, like a sewing thread or a string of beads. Lack of exercise, lying long in one position, fastening anything sharp to the dress, or the sewing of anything on the person will cause adherent placenta. These two groups of superstitions are taboos of almost pure imitative magic.

It is true that a severe physical or psychic shock can cause abortion. Sexual immorality during pregnancy is put into this class. Many pregnant women refuse to take any drug whatsoever, fearing miscarriage. Dental work during pregnancy is widely taboo, as causing abortion, harelip, or maldevelopment of the child's teeth. It is even claimed to be illegal.

The whole subject of fetal malformations is adequately and interestingly discussed by Ballantyne in his "Antenatal Pathology." The ancient explanations of their cause have practically disappeared save the one of mental origin. There is probably no more common obstetric superstition today than that the fetus can be "marked," in mind or body, for good or (usually) evil, by a mental impression of the mother at the moment of conception or during pregnancy. This idea, worldwide among all peoples of all times, has gathered about it a considerable literature, has been the theme of many books and is held by intelligent laity and even some physicians. The cases of "markings" reported and seriously believed in are multitudinous. We can only touch briefly on the subject.

It is held that the "mark" is caused by a thought or emotion of the mother, either originating in her own mind or produced by a physical impression received through the senses. Voluntary mental concentration or allowing the mind to dwell on some object or subject may give the child a physical mark, or direct its later mental activities along the same line. Unsatisfied longings, usually for foods, may "mark" the baby with an imprint of the thing longed for, or convey to it either the same longing (so that it will cry till satisfied) or an idiosyncrasy against the food in question. Cf. the practice of giving the baby a bit of the food that eaten by the nursing mother disagrees with the baby through the milk.

The "marks" by physical impressions are caused by seeing or by being touched by unusual or disagreeable inanimate or animate things, especially the latter. These physical experiences are usually sudden, violent or fright producing. The sight of injured, crippled, deformed or peculiarly acting animals or men is particularly dangerous. The sight or touch of anything dead carries with it also the ancient contagion of death. Color and, to a less degree form, play important roles. Cf. nevi or birthmarks from fire, iodine, lightning and blood (magically very potent), and pigmented moles from berries, leaves and mice. The location of the "mark" on the baby usually corresponds either with the location of the mark on the object seen, or with the spot of the mother's body to which the object was applied or touched by her in her fright. To prevent "marking" the mother should avoid any possible exciting cause, particularly any expression of sympathy or interest, and avoid touching herself when frightened. To recall the fact that she is pregnant seems to act as a powerful protective charm.

There seems to be two basic elements in this complex superstition—magic and the scapegoat. Magically, as we have seen, things can act on each other at a distance and produce results like unto themselves. The woman and her conception were considered to be extremely susceptible to evil influences, and the relation between the two was thought to be very close. We know that the fetus is only a parasite, having no direct blood or nerve connection with its host. It has been aptly asked how can images of things be transmitted by a column of liquid in a tube. We also know that development is so rapid that gross malformations are precluded after about the 10th week of pregnancy. It is interesting to note that it is sometimes claimed that the baby cannot be "marked" after life is felt. The other element in the superstition is the ancient idea of the scapegoat to which may be shifted blame and responsibility. Thus fetal deformities were explained and excused. None deny that prenatal influences are important and far-reaching, but they are chemical and subtle. It seems scarcely necessary to defend the statement that "marking" by a mother of her unborn child in the ordinary sense is an impossibility, and that the whole idea is a fabric of superstition.

The application of oil to the abdomen during pregnancy is widely practiced, for it is claimed to strengthen the muscles and make an easier labor. Oils for this purpose are advertised to-day. It is probably ancient magic—as the abdomen is made slippery so will be the birth canal at labor. It may also be associated with the idea of correcting malpositions by external manipulations. Ignorant midwives often advise pregnancy to cure retroversion, and claim to be able to diagnose pregnancy by looking into the eye—the latter a very ancient belief. Many of the signs used to diagnose sex before birth were in use centuries ago in many lands. It will be a boy if more pain is felt on the right side (in ancient thought the more important sex came from the right ovary or tesis, the right being the stronger, holier and luckier side) ; if it is carried far forward; if life is felt early and if the child is lively (ancient idea that males developed faster) ; if the mother has a bad color; if she has much heartburn—also a strong, hairy child, if she goes over term. The converse means a girl, though there is no general agreement and even much confusion and contradiction.

There are few survivals of the former belief in a close relationship between the father and his unborn child. He occasionally suffers with nausea and vomiting, and second to the mother is most apt to "mark" the child by untoward acts. True labor is supposed to start exactly two weeks after the false or "wild" pains, and its onset is influenced or precipitated by changes of the moon. The young woman who returns to her maternal home at the approach of labor simply follows an ancient and widespread custom of womankind.

The ancient lightening of labor by supernatural or other aid has few survivals. The husband's presence is sometimes considered helpful. The French midwife is still sage femme, or woman magician. The Mother of Heaven is often supplicated. The warning not to cry out with the pains probably rests on the idea that cries at such times attract the unwelcome attentions of evil spirits. Old women sometimes object to any knots in the woman's garments or to the braiding of her hair, for the imitative magic of anything tight, knotted or closed hinders the opening of the cervix and birth canal. Likewise crossed legs in the labor room are generally taboo. Our pagan forebears believed it possible to coax the baby from its mother's womb. The writer has seen a foreign workman place a cracker soaked in some liquid on the bed between his wife's thighs in a difficult labor. A fellow physician, once condoling the writer on the loss of time at a long labor, jokingly remarked that he had not used the right "bait." One finds an occasional trace of the idea that the child, by pushing with its legs, helps in its own expulsion. The domineering, even vengeful, attitude of the women, even the maids, at a confinement toward the men recalls the old solidarity of the sexes, to which the midwife partly owes her origin and persistence. The lying-in room is commonly kept unsufferably hot.

The building of a fire was a very ancient method to ward off evil spirits. The modern celebration of the end of labor is mental rather than material.

Traces of two ancient and curious ideas about the human uterus persist. The uterus was a wandering animal, desirous of pregnancy, that could migrate to various parts of the woman's body causing distress and illness. The very ignorant even to-day frequently ascribe vague abdominal pains to this cause. Our "globus hystericus" locates it in the throat. It was also a devouring animal, apt to suck back into itself the newborn and the afterbirth. Occasionally still an old lady will hang on to the cord after the child's birth or place it between the mother's toes, so that "the afterbirth won't go back in her, get around her heart and kill her." However, this may be a survival of the belief that the products of conception, loath to leave the uterus, may creep back unless prevented.

The belief that a seven months' child is more apt to live than one born at eight months is a curiously persistent survival. Two very ancient beliefs are its plausible source. At the seventh month the child turned over, ready to be born—even struggled to do so; at the end of the eighth month it was not ready but even exhausted by its previous struggles. Also kindly Venus ruled the seventh month of intrauterine life, while Saturn's baneful influences dominated the eighth. Through all runs the magic thread of the uneven number seven.

The expulsion of the afterbirth is aided by sneezing, or by blowing salt through the hands or into a bottle. Not so physiological though magically correct is the wearing of the husband's hat for the purpose—for any part of a person's dress contains properties of the owner and the strength of the male sex may thus be impressed into service. The number of varices, or so-called "knots," in the cord of the first baby foretells how many other children the woman is to have. A child born with a caul, or the possessor of a piece thereof, especially if obtained by theft (which procedure in no way seems to prejudice the original owner) will be lucky, gifted with second sight and will not die of drowning, the last idea probably from the observation that the child survived though born with its face surrounded by fluid. The caul of a seventh son of a seventh son is of course exceptionally valuable.

In ancient belief the placenta was the child's twin, or contained part of its external soul. Its disposal was therefore magically important. Strangling by the afterbirth is an occasional explanation of a still birth. It is sometimes not buried for three days, as usual for the dead. It should be buried fetal surface upward with the cord coiled inside the membranes to prevent the child vomiting. It must be buried deep, or the place covered with stones, lest dogs dig it up and eat it, thus injuring the child or drying up the mother's milk. It must not be buried directly in a beaten path, lest a menstruating woman contaminate the spot and make the child sick. The use of placental soup to lessen afterpains and increase the secretion of milk is recognized by the recently proposed use of placental extract for the latter purpose.

The existing superstitious practices of the puerperium deal with the prevention of fever, the production of milk and the care of the breasts, and recall the ancient fear of the lochia and the surrounding forces of evil. The recently delivered woman should be kept warm and in no manner come into contact with anything cold. She should be kept awake; she should lie in one fixed position; her bedding and clothing should not be changed; she should not be bathed; her hair should not be combed—all for a varying number of hours or days postpartum. The mystic numbers 3, 7, 9, and 40 are much in evidence. Cf. also 7x40 days as the duration of pregnancy. On the ninth day "everything goes back with a click." If her hair is dressed the combings must be carefully disposed of, preferably by burning, never being allowed to drop on the floor for some one might cast their shadow on them or get possession of them in some other way. Hair and nails, removed from our bodies, are in the magic sense still part of us, containing portions of our souls. Their disposal is therefore important for possession by an enemy exposes their former owner to the operations of evil magic. Food taboos postpartum are numerous, though generally vague and foolish restrictions to prevent fever, improve the flow of milk or prevent harmful effects through the milk on the nursing child. Cold foods and drinks are tabooed by imitative magic. By the same reasoning milk is highly regarded as a galactogogue. The so-called "acid" foods are considered harmful through some action on the milk. There is a general unwillingness to nurse another's child, or to mix two milks. The methods used to dry up the milk are legion. A comb, stroked downward over the breasts, prevents "caking" by "keeping the muscles straight." Sometimes its mere presence suffices. It was an ancient conception that the sweetest part of the blood, namely the milk, flowed to the uterus to nourish the child during pregnancy, and postpartum to the breasts for the same purpose. If fever supervened it might be diverted to other parts of the body. This idea of milk metastases is preserved in the term "milk leg" which is still believed to be so caused. The former theories of lochial anomalies have been abandoned. Some Syrians admit no unmarried visitors for seven days, but a soiled diaper and the cord stump placed over the door of the lying-in room prevent such persons harming the child. The seclusion and purification of women after childbirth has already been mentioned.

We dimly strive to reincarnate our ancestors when we name children after them, and have an uncanny feeling when we recognize in feature or trait of character the "spitting image" of some one long dead and gone. When a baby smiles he is dreaming of the angels. His later babblings are their speech. Twins always excite interest, and the close relationship is thought to persist between them through life. A baby born prematurely will sleep continuously till the estimated date of its birth arrives. The cause and cure of navel hernia has several superstitions. The value of a scorched cloth, especially linen, as a cord dressing is a remarkable observation antedating asepsis, but the principle involved is often ignored. The careful burning of the stump to insure good healing of the navel is pure ancient magic. A raisin, applied to the unhealed stump is also used to insure a like result. On analysis this is fair sense, for the sugar is antiseptic and the tannin astringent. A nut or a bit of wax (this takes longer) on the unhealed stump draws out the "hairs," preventing later rheumatism, and develops the chest. The dried stump with ligature, preserved as amulet, is given to the child when he goes to school at the age of seven. If he succeeds in untying the knot he will be strong and wise. Binding a baby straight will, of course, make it grow straight. There is no sound reason for laying the newborn on the right side, either to favor the closure of the foramen ovale or to prevent pressure of the heavy liver on other abdominal organs. Jaundice is treated by decoctions of various herbs, usually yellow in color. It may be prevented by the mother not turning her back on the baby, and cured by allowing it to look into the holy communion cup. Cutting an infant's finger nails either stunts its growth by making it so much shorter, or a thief by allowing his fingers to grow longer. The old fear of anything sharp, especially of iron, requires that they be bitten off. The hair should not be cut for a year, or longer if the child is weak, or until the trees are in full leaf, for in ancient thought the hair was the seat of strength, or the abode of the spirit of the head. The first haircutting often occasions tears, and a bit of this hair is to the mother a bit of her baby's soul. For sore eyes the magic fluids of mother's milk or urine may be employed. The drinking of urine by mother or child promotes its secretion. The local application of a soiled diaper cures thrush. Infantile eczema is caused by a pregnant mother or a menstruating nurse; it, as well as "scald head," should not be cured, for it is dangerous to "drive in" eczema. A child nurses the virtues and vices of its nurse, because the milk is a part of the person producing it. The presence of teeth at birth brings luck, if not divulged for seven years. If they appear before the fourth month, the mother will soon become pregnant; if first on the upper jaw, the child will die. Turning a baby end over end three times on three successive mornings will make it good-natured. Allowing it to lie too long in one position is apt to make it "liver-grown." It should be lifted or carried first up rather than down, so that by imitative magic it will rise in the world, and if in company with a book it will also be learned. Unclench the hands and rub salt in the palms for a convulsion. Vanity or death lie in a mirror during the first year of life. To measure it is to measure it for its coffin. Traces of the ancient idea that a person's name is an essential part of the personality are seen in the christening by which the little soul is fixed and removed from danger and in the institution of god-parents whose moral qualities, it is still felt, may pass to the child. At a circumcision one witnesses one of man's most ancient magic rites. Wean when the "signs" are in the knees or feet and never when the moon is high, and avoid weakmindedness. An analysis of the little nursery rhyme beginning "Monday's child is fair of face, Tuesday's child is full of grace" would be interesting.

Darker superstitions of witchcraft and the evil eye persist among the very ignorant. The breast secretion of the newborn is known as "witches' milk," for which massage is advised to break the "nipple strings." Witchcraft can make a woman bear only girls, dry up her milk and confine her to bed for years. Charms against such practices can still be bought. The idea that cats kill babies by sucking their breath probably originated in the belief that witches frequently took such form to steal children's souls. The child's clothes should not be hung out till it has been baptized. Envious, evil spirits may steal a baby's soul, substituting therefor another of less worth. Such a changeling or "devil baby" cries constantly, doesn't grow, is foolish and doesn't walk for seven years. Blasphemy, or ridicule of a holy thing or picture may be thus punished—though a comparatively late idea. These evil spirits are usually described as feminine (witches) most common in autumn, and occasionally visible. They were originally the haunting family dead, envious of the newborn soul. Marks with blessed chalk on door or window bar their entry. The sharpness of an iron knife in the cradle or the smell of a bit of garlic around the neck are defenses against them. In any event the newborn should not be left alone, which idea is suggested in the solicitious care given it, often to the neglect of the mother. If substitution has taken place putting the child into a hot oven may drive out the possession, and under no circumstances should a mother nurse a "devil baby." Baptism both prevents and cures.

The old woman, who in the same breath with which she praises a newborn baby adds a saving "God bless him," avoids by this magic formula even the appearance of casting the evil eye, that old superstition of envy. When we boast we still knock on wood. If a woman wants a baby too much she will never live to have one. Any one, even the mother herself and even unconsciously, but especially a stranger, can "overlook" an infant, causing it to wither and die. Washing the face with holy water or making over it the sign of the cross are preventatives. Among the Slovaks when a person, especially a stranger, enters a room where there is a newborn child, he commonly spits three times and looks up. This embodies three very ancient beliefs—the protective charm of human saliva, the fear of the evil practices of strangers, and imitative magic that the baby may grow up and not die. If a baby has been "overlooked" two orthodox magic methods to rid it of the contagion are in use to-day—cleansing by some magic fluid and holding in the smoke of some magic substance. Of magic fluids the most common ones are holy water and human urine, particularly that of the mother. Of magic substances burned in fumigation the writer has heard of three—piece of the clothing of the person suspected of casting the evil eye, oil-soaked rag blessed by a nulliparous woman, and seven pieces of straw together with seven stones from seven different streets.

This paper is not learned nor scientific. It has brought you no new methods of diagnosis or treatment. Its purpose has been to interest you, and to point out the prevalence of ancient thought and practices in obstetrics. It is not true of obstetrics alone. Close beneath our feet lies t' : solid stratum of paganism that reaches down to the veriest beginnings of mankind and covers all the earth. Its outcroppings among the culture and flowers of civilization is a disquieting discovery, almost surpassing belief. The mass of mankind still believes in the efficacy of magic and still respects taboos. At heart we are all still pagans.

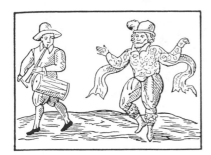

AFTER
OFFICE HOURS

THE BEHAVIORAL IMPLICATIONS OF
SOME OLD WIVES' TALES

LOUDELL F. SNOW, PhD, SHIRLEY M. JOHNSON, PhD,
AND HARRY E. MAYHEW, MD

A study was designed to gain information on the concerns, attitudes, beliefs, and knowledge that women have about reproduction to determine how these affect their health practices during pregnancy. A low-income multiethnic clinic population was studied in which the majority of the patients were in a high-risk category for pregnancy. They often failed to follow suggested regimens and/or engaged in negative health behaviors. Interviews with patients revealed that they too identified a number of risk factors in pregnancy, but that there was a disparity between their perceived risks and those of concern to the clinic staff. Many of the problems ascribed to patient noncompliance may be attributable to this differential perception of what constitutes a danger to pregnant women. In clinical settings where patients and professionals are divided by social class and cultural differences, it is suggested that physicians be aware of such beliefs so that patients may be reeducated to improve pregnancy outcomes.

From Michigan State University, East Lansing, Michigan.
Supported by funds from the Brush Foundation.
Submitted for publication September 16, 1977.
The illustration at the top of the page, Avicenna, Galenus, Hippocrates, is from an early medical book. Woodcut, 1511 (The Bettmann Archive).

A NUMBER of social and medical factors have been identified as contributing to poor pregnancy outcomes.[1-4] Medical risks include age of mother, parity, birth interval, history of miscarriage or neonatal death, or other medical conditions complicating pregnancies. Social risks include low income, single marital status, race, and the mother's education if less than high school. There is also evidence that a stressful life situation may increase the likelihood of pregnancy complications, particularly in the absence of a viable social support system.[5,6]

Adequate prenatal care is seen as essential in identifying and attempting to deal with these factors. One study has defined adequate as a) first prenatal visit within the first 11 completed weeks of pregnancy, b) nine or more prenatal visits, and c) delivery on private service rather than general or ward service.[7] Unfortunately, those women at highest risk generally receive the least prenatal care. The study presented here suggests that even when access to prenatal care is available the belief system of patients may influence the utilization of health facilities and compliance with suggested regimens.

MATERIALS AND METHODS

The research for this study was carried out in a public prenatal clinic in a mid-Michigan city, staffed by the faculty and residents of a family practice residency program. It was instituted at the request of the medical director of the clinic, who felt that cultural factors might underlie some existing problems of patient compliance. The clinic served a multiethnic, low-income, relatively poorly educated patient population. Routine communication problems were frequently exacerbated by a language barrier, as the clientele included Mexican-American migrant workers and the wives of foreign students at a nearby university.

The data were derived from responses to a 2-hour questionnaire administered to half of all patients arriving at the clinic for a first prenatal visit over a 3-month period (N = 31); study patients were paid a small fee for their participation. Information elicited covered demographic details, knowledge and beliefs on menstruation, venereal disease, childbearing, contraception, pregnancy, abortion, and menopause, and health care experiences. This information was entered into a computer programmed to handle open-ended multiresponse type information, and individual and summary data were tabulated and analyzed from the computer sheets. A bilingual interviewer talked with those patients who were not comfortable speaking English or who were unable to do so. Table 1 gives the sociodemographic profile of the women in the interview sample.

355

TABLE 1. SOCIODEMOGRAPHIC PROFILE OF CLINIC POPULATION (N = 31)

	Patients	
	Number	Percent
Married	18	58
Single, separated, or divorced	13	42
Educational level less than high school	14	45
High school	13	42
College–1 year	2	7
College degree	2	7
White	16	52
Black	6	19
Latin-American	8	26
American Indian	1	3
Speak languages other than English*	14	45
Incomes less than clinic determined poverty level'	26	84

* Languages spoken included Spanish, Ottawa, Chippewa, German, Dutch, Otetelo, French, and Arabic.
' The clinic used a sliding fee schedule based on income and dependents, eg, a family of three with an income of $6300 or less would be considered in poverty and pay no fees.

TABLE 2. MEDICAL RISKS AMONG CLINIC POPULATION (N = 31)

		Patients	
Risk	Category	Number	Percent
Unfavorable combination of age and parity⁴	All under 15 years of age 15–19 years; second pregnancy or higher 20–24 years; fourth pregnancy or higher 25–29 years; fifth pregnancy or higher 30–34 years; first pregnancy, sixth or higher 35–39 years; first pregnancy, fifth or higher All 40 years or more	16	52
Birth interval⁴	Less than 24 months since termination of last pregnancy	12	39
Medical history⁴	Previous relevant infant death, congenital defect, premature birth; obstetric complications, abortion; history of diabetes, cardiovascular, renal disease, or other medical condition increasing risk of pregnancy to mother or fetus	27	87

The 31 women had all come to the clinic believing that they were pregnant. They had had 57 previous pregnancies ($\bar{X}$ = 1.8) and had 36 living children. Twenty-seven of them were found to be pregnant, raising the total number of pregnancies to 84 ($\bar{X}$ = 2.7). Four women were not pregnant. However, 3 had amenorrhea for medical reasons other than pregnancy, and there was 1 patient with pseudocyesis. The majority of them were medically at risk for pregnancy (Table 2).

RESULTS

Although the majority of the women in the sample were in a high-risk category, there was little correlation between a poor past pregnancy history and early entry into the medical system for this pregnancy. Furthermore, there was a discrepancy between what they stated was desirable prenatal behavior and what they actually did. All, for example, said that prenatal care should be sought in the first trimester; in reality only 24% came in at that time. On the average, the women appeared for their first prenatal appointment when they were in their 21st week of gestation, the range of time varying from 10 to 35.5 weeks.

In part, this may be blamed on the difficulty of reaching the facility. The city had a poor public transportation system and the clinic lacked the funds to provide rides for women who needed them. Long periods of time in the waiting room before being seen probably also deterred some patients from coming to the clinic early in their pregnancies. The staff was forced to overschedule patients as, on any 1 day, an average of one-third to one-half the women did not keep their appointments.

For those who did, this meant sitting for a long time in a waiting room crowded with other pregnant women and small children; the clinic did not have space or funds for baby-sitting services. Such problems are common to many health facilities serving a low-income clientele.

This late entry into the health care system was seen by the clinic personnel as undesirable behavior, and, as so many of the women had histories of pregnancy complications, seemed difficult to understand. Responses to questioning, however, showed that the belief system of the women contributed to the problem. Their explanations for adverse symptoms and poor pregnancy outcomes were seldom related to what health professionals see as the causal factors. In some instances the clinic personnel identified risk factors not seen as such by the patients (Table 2). In others, both the health professionals and the patients agreed that some habits and practices should be changed or avoided by pregnant women, but with completely different explanations for this. The women also identified an entirely different set of risk factors which were largely unknown to those responsible for their care (Table 3). Similar findings have been reported in the few cultural studies of pregnancy and birth in the United States.[8-12] The authors are aware of no studies comparing the attitudes and beliefs about pregnancy of lower class women and their better educated and wealthier counterparts.

Factors Seen as Risks by Clinicians But Not by Patients

Although clinicians have precise definitions supported

356

TABLE 3. FOLK BELIEFS CONCERNING EFFECT OF MATERNAL BEHAVIOR ON FETUS

Maternal behavior	Believed outcome
Pregnant woman worked too hard or breathed paint fumes	Miscarriage
Pregnant woman lifted arms over head	Fetus strangled by cord
Pregnant woman slept too much and baby stuck to uterus	Difficult delivery
Pregnant woman cursed by enemy or punished for sin	Neonatal death
Pregnant woman craved food and touched self	Birthmark
Pregnant woman pitied or mocked retarded person; had unfulfilled desire	Retarded infant
Pregnant woman saw something frightening	Malformed infant
Pregnant woman went out during lunar eclipse without protection	Cleft palate or body part missing
Pregnant woman saw someone suffer seizure and pitied or mocked them	Infant suffers seizures

by the literature of what characteristics constitute risk factors for delivery, the patients did not share these views. For example, clinicians categorize patients younger than 19 and older than 30 years of age as being at higher risk at delivery than women in their twenties. However, when patients were questioned about childbearing during various stages of life, childbearing even in the menopausal years was not seen to be of any special medical concern for the mother or the child. Only half of the sample even knew it is possible for a woman to become pregnant during the change of life, and 87% did not know about the increased potential for fetal abnormalities at that time.

Clinicians would also categorize women who had a history of certain medical problems or who had had obstetric difficulties with a previous pregnancy as high risk patients, and would like them to come in for prenatal care early in their pregnancies. The behavior of these patients did not appear to demonstrate the same level of concern about these problems, and they did not seem to view early prenatal care as helpful.

Venereal disease is a medical risk in pregnancy although many of the patients did not see it as such. In fact, 16% did not believe that a fetus could be affected by a venereal disease in the mother. One woman said that this obviously could not be a problem since during pregnancy "... the uterus is closed and germs cannot enter." Although 90% of the women mentioned sexual contact as a possible mode of contracting such diseases it was by no means the only possibility mentioned. Thirty-five percent also believed that one can develop venereal disease by simply being dirty, not bathing frequently enough, failing to bathe after a menstrual period, or wearing dirty underclothing, and 16% felt you

can "pick it up" by using public toilets. Three women saw promiscuity as the cause: too many sex partners, none necessarily infected. This lack of awareness is of further concern because these women might not understand the necessity of laboratory examinations for venereal disease early in their pregnancies. Many were in fact appearing for medical care after syphilis might have effected some congenital problem.

Factors Seen as Risks by Both Clinicians and Patients

A number of practices are seen as potential risk factors by both the patients and the health personnel responsible for their care, but for quite different reasons. For example, modification in the use of tobacco and alcohol was seen as important by both groups. The clinic staff saw changes in smoking and drinking habits as important in fostering an optimal biochemical environment for the developing fetus. The women, however, were fearful of affecting the fetus by the old notion of "marking the child." They, too, were concerned about the fetal environment, viewing alcohol or tobacco smoke as substances reaching the child directly. Seventy-one percent of the patients stated that it is not a good idea for the pregnant woman to smoke, but only 2 patients mentioned a correlation between smoking and low birthweight. One woman stated that it would turn the baby black and several others feared that smoke could enter the baby's lungs to cause emphysema or bronchitis, "... the baby may inhale some smoke down there."

The women were less concerned about alcohol consumption, with 58% agreeing that it was acceptable in moderation. Too much alcohol was seen as being dangerous either directly—"Who wants a drunk baby?" or by affecting the coordination of the mother and causing her to fall down. One patient said whiskey might cause a pregnant woman to fall asleep on her stomach, thereby deforming the child's head. These latter concerns are based on a widespread fear that maternal overexertion or physical trauma can injure the infant; 87% of the sample believed that hard work on the part of the mother could result in a miscarriage.

Poor nutrition is another factor viewed as a potential risk by both the clinic staff and the patients, again for very different reasons. Physicians focus on providing nutrients necessary for the good health status of both the pregnant woman and her fetus. The women, on the other hand, worried again about marking the child, feeling that any food craving should be immediately satisfied if the baby is not to be marked in some way.[13] One patient reported that if a pregnant woman craves chicken and cannot have it, her baby may "... come looking like a chicken" or have chicken skin on its body.

Another thought that unsatisfied cravings might be responsible for mental retardation in a child, causing it to "... go around with its mouth hanging open all the time."

This emphasis on satisfying food cravings seems to be based on a notion that the unborn child is aware of its nutritional requirements and is thus signaling these to the mother; to ignore them is, therefore, to jeopardize the health of the child. One young woman, a vegetarian, declared that "you can feel what the baby needs ... ," going on to explain that a different group of foods should be eaten each month of pregnancy "... according to the baby's development." One month she "felt" that the baby needed iron and she ate mainly avocados and "sea vegetables;" she arrived for her first prenatal visit at 31 weeks' gestation, severely anemic. Another vegetarian patient felt that pregnant women should not eat eggs, meat, or fish as these are "dead" foods and cannot "regenerate" for the necessary fetal development.

The belief that the body needs what it craves was also used to justify pica by a third of the sample, who admitted to ingesting such items as clay, dirt, laundry starch, match boxes, the heads of matches, ice cubes, and baking powder. One woman viewed the eating of "healing earth" as bodily cleanser, "... a scrub brush through the organs." Another insisted that a physician had told her that she needed minerals and that she should eat dirt from her backyard with a spoon. Comments against pica, in fact, usually did not have to do with nutritional value but with overindulgence; several women said if you eat too much starch or clay, it is necessary to wash the excess off the baby at birth.

There were a number of misconceptions about diet and its effect on blood pressure. One woman thought that high blood pressure is caused by "... eating food with no salt in it." Several others adhered to folk beliefs concerning high and low blood pressure which have been reported among blacks and Southern whites and is of particular concern.[14] There is a terminologic confusion between a folk illness, "high blood," considered to be an excess of blood from eating too much meat, and high blood pressure. The folk treatment for "high blood" is to cut down on the amount of animal protein in the diet and to take in useless or potentially harmful substances thought to "cut" the blood and bring it down to a more acceptable volume. Such substances include vinegar, epsom salts, and the brine from pickles or olives. The pregnant woman who is told that her blood pressure is high may be using home remedies dangerous to her health completely unbeknown to the physician. "Low blood," on the other hand, is seen as being too little blood, or anemia, but is terminologically confused

with low blood pressure. It is believed to be brought about by poor diet or by taking medication for "high blood" too long. The woman who is told that her blood count is low and her blood pressure high may understandably think her doctor is a fool, as obviously one cannot have "high blood" and "low blood" simultaneously.

Other food avoidances of a cultural nature are common among Latin-American women who may classify bodily states, illnesses, foods, and medicines according to whether they are "hot" or "cold," believing that these must be kept in balance to maintain health.[15,16] Harwood has reported that Puerto Rican-American women view pregnancy as a "hot" state and may avoid iron and vitamin supplements which they also see as "hot," believing that they would throw the body out of balance and cause illness. [17] Our Mexican-American patients were concerned as well that "cold" foods might impede normal vaginal blood flow and they eliminated them from the diet during the menses and the 40-day postpartum period known as la dieta.[18] "Cold" foods include chiles, citrus fruits, tomatoes, and green leafy vegetables, all important vitamin sources in a traditional Latin diet already poor in vitamins.[19,20]

Factors Seen as Risks Only by Patients

Most of the patients also had a number of beliefs which caused anxiety in the perinatal period but which were not shared by the clinicians. Here "marking the child" is seen as resulting from strong emotional states on the part of the mother, divine punishment for behavioral lapses, the evil intentions of others, or simply the power of nature. According to these beliefs, in fact, virtually every time a pregnant woman ventures from home she places herself in a situation in which her unborn child might be permanently disfigured or even killed. No less than 77% of the patients interviewed believe that such marking is possible.

The Mexican-American patients shared a set of concerns which were unknown to the other women, although these are common in Latin-American cultures.[16, 17,21] In one instance, such a belief is at complete variance with what they are told is beneficial by the health professionals, ie, an increased amount of rest for the pregnant woman—in Latin folklore the pregnant woman should stay active and not sleep or rest too much for fear the baby will "stick to the uterus" and make delivery difficult or impossible. They also feared the danger seen as inherent in a lunar eclipse, believing that if a pregnant woman goes out unprotected at such a time, her baby will be born with a cleft palate, with a body part missing, or dead. She is believed protected from such an eventuality by wearing a key tied around the waist so that the metal touches the belly. One staff member at the clinic had noticed this practice but thought that it was simply an extra doorkey worn there for safekeeping. The still birth of a child born to a clinic patient the year before the study was attributed to the failure to wear the key, and the family not only mourned the loss of the infant but blamed the young mother for her folly.

The majority of the patients were also concerned with the potential ill effect on the fetus of any strong emotional state on the part of the mother: fear, hate, jealousy, anger, sorrow, pity—all are dangerous if allowed to become excessive. Fear was mentioned most often: if the mother sees something that frightens her, the baby may be born resembling whatever she saw. The mother-to-be should, therefore, avoid horror movies lest the infant resemble a monster; she should not go to the zoo lest she be startled and the baby be born looking like a monkey; if she were to be frightened by a cat, the baby might have cat hair on its face, and so on. One woman reported that her mother had been frightened by a fish so that her sister ". . . has two holes in the roof of her mouth and she can swim like a fish." Another attributed her first child's blue eyes to a frightening movie in which she saw a murder victim's ". . . blue eyes opened wide." One can avoid a horror movie, of course, but not all the problems of daily life—several patients mentioned the especially ill effect of the sight of blood and were concerned lest they see any sort of accident.

Another very powerful theme often expressed was that of punishment for sin. Should a woman gossip about someone the baby might resemble that person; should she laugh at a cripple or make fun of a retarded person God might afflict her infant with the same problem to teach her a lesson. What is seen as sinful differs from group to group, of course, and belief in such punishment serves to inhibit certain types of behavior.[22] Kay's Mexican-American informants reported that God might mark a child if the parents failed to attend mass.[16] Our data show that a child born to young Mexican-American parents the year before the study was not only dead but badly malformed. The family attributed this tragedy to the fact that the girl had been pregnant before marriage, a significant sin in Latin culture. The couple refused genetic counseling as they felt they understood the reason for the problem for which they had "paid" and their next child would be normal. Two of the patients in the sample also described deformity as part of a child's "karma," a punishment perhaps from a previous lifetime, or something to overcome in this life to purify the spirit.

Poor social relationships may also be translated into beliefs about poor pregnancy outcomes. Several black patients said that if someone really hated the mother,

they could put a curse on her to kill the child *in utero* or "mark it for death" later in life, a belief also reported by other researchers.[23-25] Family friction or an argument with neighbors might therefore enhance anxiety about the pregnancy.

Participation in the beliefs described above makes the unease so many of the women felt and freely verbalized understandable. Virtually anything the mother-to-be does during pregnancy has the potential for directly affecting the fetus—every emotion, every thought, every swallow of food may indelibly mark the unborn child. There is danger in the world of nature, in the patient's social network, in her relationship with God; she must be on guard every waking minute, monitoring her least thoughts and activities to insure that all is calm, temperate, and happy. Above all she must avoid excess and try not to crave a food, eat too much, drink or smoke too much, or, most important, allow her emotions to be aroused. It is small wonder, believing these risks likely, that so few of the women felt that early entry into the health care system would be particularly helpful in guaranteeing a safe pregnancy and normal delivery.

CONCLUSIONS

The belief system practiced by the patients in the prenatal clinic influenced their utilization of available health facilities and their acquiescence to suggested health regimens. Both the health practitioners and their patients shared a common goal, the birth of a healthy child to a healthy mother. The health practices thought necessary to achieve this goal, however, were not fully shared. Often behaviors which seemed perfectly reasonable to the patients were seen as evidence of hopeless noncompliance by the professional staff. In contrast, some instructions thought perfectly clear by the health care personnel were almost meaningless to their patients. Good health care delivery depends on meaningful communication between patient and practitioner. In a health care setting where social class and cultural background divide the two groups, health professionals must be aware of patients' folk beliefs to allow such communication to occur. Patient education can then be presented in a more meaningful manner. If obstetric risks can be lessened by increasing patient compliance with good health practices, physicians need to know why their patients are not complying, and patients need to know why they should.

REFERENCES

1. Lewis R, Charles M, Patwary KM: Relationships between birthweight and selected social, environmental and medical care factors. Am J Public Health 63:973–981, 1973
2. Lesinski J: High-risk pregnancy. Unresolved problems of screening, management, and prognosis. Obstet Gynecol 46:599–603, 1975

3. Dott AB, Fort AT: Medical and social factors affecting early teenage pregnancy. Am J Obstet Gynecol 125:532–536, 1976
4. Perkin GW: Assessment of reproductive risk in non-pregnant women. Am J Obstet 101:709–717, 1968
5. Nuckolls KB, Cassel J, Kaplan BH: Psychosocial assets, life crisis and the prognosis of pregnancy. Am J Epidemiol 95:431–441, 1972
6. Rabkin JG, Struening EL: Life events, stress, and illness. Science 194:1013–1020, 1976
7. Chase HC: A study of risks, medical care, and infant mortality. Am J Public Health (Suppl)63:103, 1973
8. Murphree AH: A functional analysis of Southern folk beliefs concerning birth. Am J Obstet Gynecol 102:125–134, 1968
9. Stekert E: Focus for conflict: Southern mountain medical beliefs in Detroit, The Urban Experience and Folk Tradition. Edited by A Paredes and E Stekert. Austin, University of Texas Press, 1971, pp 95–127
10. Frankel B: Childbirth in the Ghetto. San Francisco, R & E Research Associates, Inc, 1977
11. O'Grady IP: University of Arizona Tucson (Unpublished data)
12. Newman L: Floklore of pregnancy: Wives' tales in Contra Costa County, California. West Folklore 28:112–135, 1969
13. Snow LF, Johnson SM: Folklore, food, and the female reproductive cycle. Ecology of Food and Nutrition (In press)
14. Snow LF: "High blood" is not high blood pressure. Urban Health 5:3:54–55, 1976
15. Clark M: Health in the Mexican-American Culture. Second edition. Berkeley, University of California Press, 1970
16. Kay MA: Health and illness in a Mexican American barrio. Ethnic Medicine in the Southwest. Edited by EH Spicer. Tucson, University of Arizona Press, 1977, pp 96–164
17. Harwood A: The hot-cold theory of disease. Implications for treatment of Puerto Rican patients. JAMA 216:1153–1158, 1971
18. Snow LF, Johnson SM: Modern day menstrual folklore: Some clinical implications. JAMA 237:2736–2739
19. Cardenas J, Gibbs CE, Young EA: Nutritional beliefs and practices in primagravid Mexican-American women. J Am Diet Assoc 69:262–265, 1976
20. Hunt IF, Jacob M, Ostergard NJ, et al: Effects of nutrition education on the nutritional status of low income pregnant women. Am J Clin Nutr 19:675–684, 1976
21. Kelly I: Folk Practices in North Mexico. Austin, University of Texas Press, 1965
22. Hand WD: Deformity, disease and physical ailment as divine retribution, Studein zur Volkskulture, Sprache und Landesgeschichte. Edited by E Ennen, G Wiegelmann. Bonn, Ludwig Rohrscheid Verlag, 1972, pp 519–525
23. Clinicopathologic conference case presentation (BCH # 469861), Johns Hopkins Med J 120:186–199, 1967
24. Rocereto, LR: Root work and the root doctor. Nurs Forum 12:414–427, 1973
25. Cappanari SC, Rau B, Abram HS, et al: Voodoo in the general hospital. JAMA 232:938–940, 1975

Address reprint requests to
Loudell F. Snow, PhD
Department of Anthropology
Baker Hall
Michigan State University
East Lansing, MI 48824

Accepted for publication October 11, 1977.

732

360

ANNALS OF SCIENCE, 49 (1992), 63–85

'Out of Sight, Out of Mind?': The Daniel Turner–James Blondel Dispute Over the Power of the Maternal Imagination

PHILIP K. WILSON

The Wellcome Institute for the History of Medicine,
183 Euston Road, London NW1 2BN, U.K.

Received 29 April 1991

Summary

In the late 1720s, Daniel Turner and James Blondel engaged in a pamphlet dispute over the power of the maternal imagination. Turner accepted the long-standing belief that a pregnant woman's imagination could be transferred to her unborn child, imprinting the foetus with various marks and deformities. Blondel sought to refute this view on rational and anatomical grounds. Two issues repeatedly received these authors' attention: the identity of imagination, and its power in pregnant women; and the process of generation and foetal development. In their discussions of these issues, differences between the authors' acceptance of general medical theories and philosophies became apparent. Blondel invoked Newtonian matter theory, experimental philosophy, and iatro-mechanism, while Turner adhered more to the authority of the Ancients and advocated a more direct role for the Creator as an alternative to mechanism in explaining natural phenomena. Additionally, the authors held differing views of what they regarded as experience. The widespread contemporary interest in their dispute suggests that Turner and Blondel raised the phenomenon of the maternal imagination from an issue of folk belief to a concern of eighteenth-century medicine.

Contents

1. Introduction

In November 1726, Mary Toft became the 'general Talk of the Town' in London for, it was rumoured, having been delivered of sixteen rabbits over a course of months. These claims provoked responses from premier London physicians, including Sir Richard Manningham and James Douglas; surgeons William Cheselden, Thomas Braithwaite, and Phillipus van Limborck; and man-midwives William Giffard and John Maubray. Sergeant Surgeon Claudius Amyand, together with Cyriacus Ahlers and Nathanael St Andre, surgeons to George I, also became involved. As recorded by some of these figures, Toft was removed from her home in Godalming, Surrey, and taken to Guildford and eventually to London. In London, the Duke of Richmond, the Duke of Montague, Lord Baltimore, and Samuel Molyneaux, a natural philosopher and private secretary to the Prince of Wales, took personal interest in Toft's claims.

0003-3790/92 $3·00 © 1992 Taylor & Francis Ltd.

Controversy over the 'rabbit breeder' extended to the monarch being provided with an anatomical demonstration of the 'facts' on Saturday, 26 November 1726. Within a fortnight, Toft confessed a fraud.[1]

At least fifteen pamphlets and songs appeared at the time satirizing what was portrayed as a mass delusion. Many of these depicted Toft's surgical and medical attendants as gullible and credulous. The medical attendants were also parodied in engravings, including one by Hogarth, and in a Drury Lane play. Toft was vilified as a cheat for securing animal parts and leading her attendants to believe she had delivered the animals naturally. She had long accounted for the rabbits by explaining that while thinking she was with child, she was startled by a rabbit while working in the fields. Immediately she desired the rabbit for a meal, but was unable to catch the animal. Her cravings were further increased by a dream about rabbits, yet her longings remained unfulfilled. However, few of the popularized versions of Toft's case gave her longing more than casual notice.

In May 1727, a pamphlet entitled *The Strength of Imagination in Pregnant Women Examined* appeared in London. The anonymous author (James Blondel) identified himself as a member of London's College of Physicians and claimed to have written the work in response to the delusion created by the 'Cheat at Godalming'.[2] However, another member of the College, Daniel Turner, deemed *The Strength* to be an attack on a chapter, 'Spots and Marks of a Diverse Resemblance Imprest upon the Skin of the Foetus, by the Force of the Mother's Fancy' in his book on skin disease first published in 1714.[3] In September 1729, Turner responded to Blondel's pamphlet with *An Answer to a Pamphlet on the Powers of Imagination in Pregnant women*. Later that year, Blondel issued a second work, *The Power of the Mother's Imagination over the Foetus Examined*, in which he identified himself. This work prompted Turner's final reply, *The Force of the Mother's Imagination upon the Foetus in Utero still further Considered* (1730).[4]

Toft's case was not the first to incite controversy over whether a pregnant woman's emotions, cravings, or imaginings could mark or deform her foetus. Some of the earliest examples citing the possible consequences of an expectant mother's imagination are

[1] L. Lewis Wall reviewed this incredible case in 'The Strange Case of Mary Toft (Who was delivered of sixteen rabbits and a Tabby cat in 1726)', *Medical Heritage*, 1 (1985), 199–212. An earlier work, not cited by Wall, by S. A. Seligman 'Mary Toft—The Rabbit Breeder', *Medical History*, 5 (1961), 349–60, recounted the adventure in a similar way. See also Lord Onslow's letter to Sir Hans Sloane, cited in the *British Medical Journal*, 25 July 1896, p. 206. The broader political and social components of this case have yet to be delineated.

[2] Hereafter, James Blondel's *The Strength of Imagination in Pregnant Women examined* (London, 1727) will be referred to as *The Strength*. His comment regarding the Toft case appeared in *Power of the Mother's Imagination over the foetus examined* (London, 1729), p. ii. Hereafter, *The Power*.

[3] The twelfth chapter of Turner's *De Morbis Cutaneis. A Treatise of Diseases incident to the Skin* (London, 1714). Turner appears to have used the terms fancy and imagination synonymously and interchangeably in his writings on the maternal imagination. According to his preface Turner received an *imprimatur* from the College of Physicians of London for this work in 1712, and had it published two years later by Rebecca Bonwicke. Hereafter, this work will be referred to as 'Spots and Marks'.

[4] Hereafter, *The Force*.

found in Greek writings; others in the Bible.[5] Although convictions about the power of the maternal imagination can be found primarily in folk belief, many medical, religious and philosophical authorities also supported this view.[6] It can also be found in many popular writings.[7]

By the early eighteenth century, several medical authors had expressed incredulity that children's physical markings, resembling such things as fish scales or limbs deformed in the shape of bear's claws, were the results of the mother's wayward imagination, fright, or cravings.[8] Yet, as numerous citations suggest, it was the dispute in the late 1720s between Turner and Blondel which drew unprecedented attention to this issue.

In this paper, I will examine the arguments presented by Turner and Blondel, and discuss probable reasons for their differences. Two primary points of their disagreement; the identity of the imagination, and the process of generation will be analysed. Then, the authors' endeavour to gain public appeal will be examined. Finally, I discuss the response which this dispute provoked in the periodical literature, and in English and Continental commentaries which appeared later in the century.

2. Turner and Blondel on the mother's imagination

James Blondel presented the whole issue of the power of the mother's imagination as a 'vulgar error', scorning the credulity of the medical practitioners involved in the Toft case.[9] Nothing 'can be more scandalous', he exclaimed, 'than to suppose, that those Whom God Almighty has endow'd,... with so many charms... [and] an extraordinary Love and Tenderness for the Children... [are made to] bread [*sic*]

---

[5] One case, purportedly from ancient times, involved a child of 'Ethiopian Complexion' who was delivered to white parents. Physicians and philosophers explained the child's colour as the result of the mother's 'Intent viewing' of a picture of an Ethiopian that hung in her bedchamber throughout her pregnancy. Many authors, including Daniel Turner, attributed this case to Hippocrates. M. D. Reeve, in a recent work covering much of the Renaissance literature on 'Conceptions', *Proceedings of the Cambridge Philosophical Society*, No. 215, n.s., No. 35 (1989), 93, has shown that this case did not originate with Hippocrates; rather its misattribution to the father of medicine can be traced to *De viribus imaginationis*, the 1608 writing of Thomas Fienus. I am indebted to Amal Abou-Aly for this reference. James Blondel, Turner's opponent also argued that no such case existed in the Hippocratic Corpus. Yet, a similar case which Reeve described as the 'Andromeda effect' appeared in *Aethiopica*, a work of Heliodorus. Discussion of the Biblical passage will follow.

[6] Such authorities as Galen, Michel de Montaigne, and René Descartes addressed the power of the mother's imagination. J. W. Ballantine's comprehensive search of the medical and philosophical literature from antiquity through the early twentieth century for reference to this maternal power remains the most complete bibliographic source to date. See the section on maternal impressions, the general nineteenth-century term describing the effects of the mother's imagination in his *Manual of Antenatal Pathology and Hygiene*, vol. 2: *The Embryo* (Edinburgh, 1904), pp. 105–28. Many of the works published since 1904 are included in the bibliography of my thesis '"Out of Sight, Out of Mind?": The Daniel Turner–James Blondel Debate over Maternal Impressions' (M. A. Thesis, The Johns Hopkins University, 1987), pp. 83–95.

[7] The widespread appeal of popular medical writings such as Robert Burton's *Anatomy of Melancholy* and *Aristotle's Masterpiece* may have helped perpetuate a belief in the power of the mother's imagination. Janet Blackman discussed the popularity of the latter in 'Popular Theories of Generation: The Evolution of Aristotle's Works, the Study of an Anachronism', in *Health Care and Popular Medicine in Nineteenth Century England*, edited by J. Woodward and D. Richards (New York, 1977), pp. 56–88.

[8] For example, Johann Conrad Brunner, in 1683, criticized Johann Conrad Peyer's belief that maternal influences were capable of marking the foetus. See F. J. Cole, *Early Theories of Sexual Generation* (Oxford, 1930), pp. 57–8, 61. Francesco Maria Nigrisoli also argued against the common belief in the power of the maternal imagination in his *Considerazioni Intorno alla generazione de' viventi* (Ferrara, 1712), p. 5.

[9] Blondel, *The Strength*, title page. Blondel's use of 'vulgar' in the sense of the common people is similar to Thomas Browne's discussion of such errors in his *Pseudodoxia Epidemica: or, Enquiries into Vulgar and Common Errors* (London, 1646). Browne did not, however, include the power of the mother's imagination as an erroneous belief.

Monsters by the Wantonness of their Imagination'.[10] In order to disprove this 'vulgar error', he set out an argument based 'partly by Reason, and partly by Anatomy'. Blondel acknowledged that circumstances such as falls, accidents, irregular diet, dancing, running, riding, excess laughter, and frequent sneezing had caused some mothers to damage the 'Prosperity of the *Foetus*' and miscarry.[11] Sudden surprise, or strongly expressed anger or grief were also, on occasion, capable of producing similar results.[12] Yet, he noted most women experience various emotions of longings at some time during their pregnancy without producing marked children. Furthermore, many mothers of marked or deformed children claimed to have endured an entirely peaceful pregnancy. Blondel therefore concluded that the imaginationists' claim was based on recognizing some irregularity of the child after birth (*ad hoc, ergo propter hoc*). He further noted the imaginationists' inconsistency in attributing the same defect to opposing causes. For example, he surmised that if a pregnant woman either longed for or had 'a great Aversion' to mussels, she was 'reputed to run a vast Risque' of delivering a child marked with a resemblance of that shell fish somewhere on the body.[13]

Blondel provided alternative explanations of ape-like, frog-faced, and bear-clawed children. For instance, he recounted a tale, which he attributed to Nicolas Malebranche, in which a child was born with bones 'broken, in the same Places where Malefactors are broke[n upon the rack]'. Unlike Malebranche, who attributed the cause of this condition to an expectant mother having witnessed such an event, Blondel argued that 'Tis very probable, this young Man...[was] troubled with the Rickets, [such that] the Bones of the *Carpus* and *Tarsus* had never come to their full Perfection [*in utero*], but did remain *Cartilaginous*, [so that] the Ligaments...relaxed, and the Articulations...[appeared] loose...upon the least Touch'.[14] Blondel also re-examined a biblical example which had been frequently used to prove the power of imagination. Genesis 30: 25–39 recounts Jacob's revenge against Laban. Laban, who had offered Jacob all the mottled offspring from his flock removed all the sheep with spots and speckles, provoking Jacob to devise a plan to produce mottled sheep. Jacob stripped the bark from some branches, giving them a ring-streaked appearance, and placed them by a water trough. He planned that when the ewes, in heat, came to drink, they would see the streaked branches and be inclined to produce marked offspring. Blondel claimed that this tale exemplified an 'Axiom of Logick' which stated that an argument which proved too much, proved nothing.[15] Blondel further argued that the 'Diviners' (i.e., translators) during the reign of James I had been 'guided more by their Prejudices, than by the Original [Hebrew]'. Preferring, he said, the pristine over 'all the Commentators in the World', Blondel identified the inconsistencies

[10] Ibid., preface.

[11] Ibid., p. 10.

[12] Ibid.

[13] Ibid., p. 14: J. Du Plessis described and illustrated the contemporary case of a child born 'in all respects like a Lobster' due to its mother's longing when unable to pay the 'Exorbitant Price' for the shellfish in Leadenhall market. See his *A Short History of Human Prodigious & Monstrous Births of Dwarfs, Sleepers, Giants, Strong Men, Hermaphrodites, Numerous Births, and Extream Old Age &c.*, British Library, Sloane MS 5246, stencilled p. 13.

[14] Ibid., pp. 28–29. As later described, Blondel was a Huguenot. Following the principles of his faith, Blondel would likely have opposed Malebranche's attempt to reconcile Cartesian physics and philosophy to the Catholic doctrine. See T. L. Hankins, 'The Influence of Malebranche on the Science of Mechanics during the Eighteenth Century', *Journal of the History of Ideas*, 28 (1967), 193.

[15] Ibid., p. 34.

between the 'Authorized' version and his own translation.[16] He surmised that the ewes in 'that hot Country' had learned a 'Trick...in Expectation of their Victuals', so that they 'could have no water, except [when] they drank it, where the party-coloured Rods [i.e., dappled branches] were placed'. Although this colour may have become 'very pleasant to them', their offspring resulted only from their 'natural...Inclination towards the speckled Rams [in] preference to the others'.[17]

Blondel credited other imaginationists' fables to the 'Ignorant People's' lack of judgement, the 'tale-monger's...Enthusiasm and Bigotry', and the attempts of 'Cruel Mothers' to move 'Charity and Benevolence' in order that they might live 'lazy and indolent' lives.[18] As evidence for his view, Blondel urged his readers to consider why it was that 'Irregularities...occasioned by the Strength of Imagination...appear more on the Body of Beggars, than...[on] any other people?'[19] He also claimed that the only reason so many midwives and physicians supported the imaginationists' view was to cover up mistakes made during the childbirths they attended.[20]

Blondel argued that the irregularities seen on children appeared 'over and over again' in such a similar pattern that they could be compiled into a 'catalogue' of four classes.[21] First were marks caused by variation in the number and combination of body 'Particles'. For example, blemishes could be accounted for by the superficial blood vessels appearing through the surface of the skin, when the blood was more 'rarified' in summer, as opposed to winter when it was more 'concentrated'. Second, distempers could arise from obstructions *in utero*. For instance, hydrocephalus, in which obstructions could 'turn' humours to favour the brain over another part of the body. Third, if the growth of foetal parts was disproportionately interrupted by an 'Obstruction of some vessels', 'Nutrition' of dependent parts could stop, thereby hindering development. This situation, he claimed, accounted for abnormal protrusion of the viscera. Finally, any extreme force or violence on the body of the uterus could create such a convulsion that 'two or three *Ova*...[were] intermixed...to make an odd and monstrous Combination'.[22]

In 1729, Turner responded to Blondel's *Strength* with *A Defence*, repeating much of the argument contained in his original 'Spots and Marks' first published in 1714. In this earlier work, Turner had described the 'great Influence' which passions such as joy,

---

[16] Blondel's preference of a strict scriptural interpretation rather than supposition is indicative of the sustained influence of Frederick Spanheim, his Leiden Professor of Theology. See F. L. R. Sassen's 'The Intellectual Climate in Leiden in Boerhaave's Time', in *Boerhaave and his Times* edited by G. Lindeboom (Leiden, 1970), pp. 2–3. Blondel's appreciation of his instructor is identifiable by the dedication of his medical thesis, *Disputatio Medica Inauguralis de Crisibus* (Leiden, 1692), to Spanheim.

[17] Ibid., p. 21. According to the biographical entry in Ollivier and Raige-Delorme Dezeimeris's *Dictionnaire Historique de la Médecine* (Paris, 1828), I, p. 418, Blondel was well versed in the Dead Languages, particularly Hebrew, and he wrote a large number of theological works. Reeve (footnote 5), 97, claimed some aspects of Blondel's account were 'more accurate than any I have found in the commentaries'. Samuel Kottek, in his 'La Force de L'Imagination chez les femmes enceintes. 'A propos d'un texte biblique apporté par J. Blondel en illustration à ce théme controversé', *Revue D'Historie de la Medécine Hébraique*, 27 (1974), 43–48 elaborates on Blondel's Biblical citations.

[18] Blondel, *The Strength*, pp. 20, 22.

[19] Ibid., p. 21. He further recommended such deceitful vagrants to be tried by the 'Coventry Act'. Although J. Du Plessis (footnote 13), 52, described how deformed children were often left to beg on the streets, he also tells of one poor London couple who got a 'Hansom Lively Hod [sic]' from showing, for money, the lifeless skeleton the wife reputedly delivered.

[20] Ibid., p. 14.

[21] Ibid., p. 95.

[22] All of these examples were drawn from Blondel's *The Strength*, pp. 94–106.

anger, sorrow, and fear had over the 'Blood and nervous Fluid, or animal Spirits, and consequently [over] the whole body'.[23] Like the passions, Turner described how the imagination could induce 'great [physical] Changes and Alterations'. In this case work, written for a surgical audience, Turner included forty case histories drawn from classical and contemporary sources, in which markings, deformities, or diseases were attributed to the 'Fancy' or 'Force' of the imagination.[24] Of the cases, thirty-six specifically pertained to pregnancy. For example, one attributed a girl's extreme hairiness to her mother's 'unhappy ruminating' over a picture of the hirsute St John the Baptist.[25] Another case described a cat-headed girl who was delivered from a mother who had been frightened during her pregnancy by a cat jumping into her bed.[26] A third, which had occurred in London, involved the child of Sir 'J.B.' whose 'Lady [then with child, was] frightened at the unexpected View of a Beggar's stump Arm upon her Coach Door'. Following this incident, Lady B. was 'brought to Bed of a Child ... wanting one of its hands'.[27] Other deformed children were presented as evidence of the potential for maternally marking a foetus. Turner also repeated accounts of variegated markings (*Naevi sive Maculae Maternae*) on infants, which arose from a pregnant woman's craving for various fruits or longing for red wine. Although Turner claimed to have included such cases in a chapter of a treatise on skin diseases simply 'For the Reader's Diversion', he also introduced similar cases which he claimed to have attended himself.

In his work on *Diseases Incident to the Skin*, Turner, an experienced surgeon,[28] guided his readers through the treatment of many external disorders.[29] On the treatment of 'fruit-shaped excrescences' which arose from the maternal imagination, Turner instructed his readers that it was 'necessary to consider the Part on which they are seated, to what Parts adjoining, and with what communicating: What vessels they may be fed by: What Compass they take, [and] how deep they enter'.[30] Once this was determined, the growths could then be tied off at their stalk or 'pedicule' and cut away, but only during 'the Season when they look palest, lie flattest and softest, and are least troublesome'.[31] He argued that these tubercles and spots, 'like the Fruits they resemble,

---

[23] Turner, 'Spots and Marks', p. 105. For example, he described that when people experience sorrow, 'their Spirits move slow and dull, both in the Brain and into the *Praecordia* [around the heart], hence from their languid Influx, the Circuit of the Blood is retarded through the Ventricles', ibid., p. 104.

[24] Turner's examples were drawn from such classical authorities as Aristotle, Pliny, and Soranus, together with more contemporary sources including Ambroise Paré, Thomas Bartholin, Joannes Schenkius, and Robert Boyle.

[25] Turner, 'Spots and Marks', p. 114. This case was also included in the works of Schenkius and Pare.

[26] Ibid., attributed to Bartholin.

[27] Ibid., p. 116. 'J'B.' was most likely the MP, Sir James Bateman (1660–1718), from Soho Square, London.

[28] In a later publication, Turner detailed several hundred cases which he attended as a London surgical practitioner roughly between 1694 and 1711. Turner's view of London surgical practice as a corrupt trade, dominated by untrained and unskilled pretenders is documented in his *Apologia Chyurgica: A Vindication of the Noble Art of Surgery* (London, 1695) and *The Present State of Chyrurgery* (London, 1703). I am producing a biography of Turner as part of my dissertation.

[29] Perusal of surgical texts from this period suggests that surgical practitioners were employed to treat skin disorders and venereal disease, incise and dress boils and swellings, reduce fractured bones and dislocated joints, 'couch' cataracts, extract teeth, repair ruptures and fistulae, amputate limbs, and 'cut' for bladder stone. Turner claimed that a surgeon was 'the most proper Person to be consulted' for disorders requiring 'Manual Operation' in the preface to his *Syphilis. A practical Dissertation on the Venereal Disease* (London, 1724). Attempts by officials of the Barber-Surgeons Company of London to expand their realm of care legally has been documented in many traditional surgical histories, for example, Cecil Wall, *The History of the Surgeons Company, 1745–1800* (London, 1937), pp. 25–6.

[30] Turner, 'Spots and Marks', p. 122.

[31] Ibid.

have their Times of bloom, ripening and languishing, tho' never quite dying or falling off [by] themselves'.[32] Illustrating the treatments he proposed, Turner presented three cases in which he had achieved success. He described how he had surgically removed from three children facial markings which were shaped like a raspberry, a currant and a shrimp. Turner reported the mothers' testimony that these markings had all resulted from unfulfilled longings which they had experienced during pregnancy.

Discussion of monstrous births of all sorts were common in London, and Londoners had a taste for accounts of human monstrosities.[33] Members of all classes regularly gathered at 'raree' shows to see freaks of nature.[34] The social elite frequently sponsored private exhibitions of nature's aberrations, while the intellectual elite discussed the origins of monsters before such bodies as the Royal Society.[35] Although many natural philosophers had turned their attention to analysing the underlying forces and powers of natural phenomena such as gravity, light, meteors, and earthquakes; marvels, miracles, and magic apparently still remained 'in vogue' among London's populace.[36] Given this setting, it is perhaps not too surprising that Turner's discussion in 'Spots and Marks' seems scarcely to have been noticed when first published in 1714.[37]

The issue of folk beliefs about pregnancy only appears to have been seriously raised after the Toft case. Unlike contemporary disputes within the College of Physicians which were often intraprofessional and divided along political lines,[38] the Toft case involved professional and public beliefs. Physicians and surgeons were scorned by fellow practitioners for having been duped by a country woman's tale about her pregnancy. This was the context in which Blondel sought to expel from physic what he saw as a folk-belief.

Blondel had become a licentiate of the College of Physicians in 1711. Reportedly born in Paris in 1665, Blondel studied medicine at the University of Leiden, receiving

---

[32] Ibid.

[33] C. J. S. Thompson, in *The Mystery and Lore of Monsters* (New York, 1968), p. 63, claimed that London was the Mecca for every variety of monster, and Colin Clair, in *Human Curiosities* (London, 1968), p. 93, stated that by the early 1700s, inhabitants of this city had acquired a taste for monsters that reached 'the proportions of a disease'.

[34] Richard Altrick, in his delightful *The Shows of London* (Cambridge, Massachusetts, 1978) provides many well-documented accounts, see especially pp. 36, 42, and 49.

[35] From Robert Boyle's description of a monstrous calf in the first issue of the *Philosophical Transactions* in 1665/6, through the first third of the eighteenth century, monsters were frequently reported to the Royal Society. Katherine Park and Lorraine J. Daston discuss several of these reports in 'Unnatural Conceptions: The Study of Monsters in Sixteenth- and Seventeenth-Century France and England', *Past & Present*, 92 (1981), 46–51.

[36] See Blondel, *The Strength*, p. 3. John Maubray claimed that the birth of monsters 'signify and portend something *extraordinary* or more than NATURAL to us *Mortals*' in his popular *The Female Physician, The Whole Art of New Improv'd Midwifery* (London, 1724), p. 372. See also Daniel Defoe's popular *A System of Magick* (London, 1727). Although Keith Thomas concluded that traditional belief in magic had significantly declined by the end of the seventeenth century, he noted that remnants of these beliefs continued to linger in the eighteenth century. See his *Religion and the Decline of Magic* (London, 1971), especially pp. 633, 656–68.

[37] The lack of references to this chapter before 1727 is corroborated by Turner's view that until 1727 his work 'never gave offence, at least that I have heard'. See Turner's 'An Answer to a Pamphlet on the Power of Imagination in Pregnant Women', also printed under the title *A Defence of the XIIth Chapter of the First Part of a Treatise De Morbis Cutaneis* affixed to Turner's *Discourse Concering Gleets* (London, 1729), p. 3. The latter publication was available for my use. Henceforth, *A Defence*. Turner's opponent, James Blondel, also claimed that he was the 'First, who has ever writ on this Side of the Question'. See his *The Power*, 143.

[38] See A. Wilson, 'The Politics of Medical Improvement in Early Hanoverian London', in *The Medical Enlightenment of the Eighteenth Century*, edited by A. Cunningham and R. French (London, 1990), pp. 4–39.

his medical degree in 1692.[39] Iatro-mechanical theories, like those taught in Leiden and later espoused by many London physicians,[40] are evident in Blondel's writings. Little else, however, is known about his life other than his Huguenot affiliations.[41]

Turner's writings are more self-revealing than those of Blondel. Turner was a High-Churchman and ardent supporter of Tory ideals. His professed intolerance of separatists from the Anglican Church would likely have set him against the dissenting Huguenots.[42] Moreover, as he ranked staunch Whigs, including Richard Mead, William Cockburn, and Nicholas Robinson, among his adversaries, the Huguenots' support of Whig ideas may have fuelled Turner's antagonism to Blondel.[43] However, Turner's writings were also directed against fellow Jacobites such as Archibald Pitcairne, James Keill, John Freind, and Joshua Ward, suggesting that his criticisms were based on more than recognizable partisan politics. Turner castigated medical writers who 'dogmatically' proclaimed that medicine should be based on particular theories or hypotheses. He was opposed to the iatro-mechanical theories common among contemporary 'Newtonian' physicians. His disagreement with Blondel's iatro-mechanical arguments is central to their entire dispute.

Similar in format to Newton's *Principia*, Blondel's work began with a set of propositions.[44] He argued that once these propositions were 'all put together', they would 'amount...to a full *Demonstration* of his thesis'.[45] In his *Defence*, Turner selectively criticized Blondel's 'hypothetical' deductions. He claimed that Blondel's propositions were 'no more to the Matter in hand, than if you had told us, that if we take three or four Strands of equal length, and lay them in the proper Position, they will make either a *Triangle* or a *Quadrangle*; but if any one of the three or... four be longer or shorter than the rest..., neither [figure]... will be *equilateral*, and so deduced this

---

[39] Standard biographical entries state that he was born in Paris in 1665, and that his father, a French legal counsellor, desired a similar career for his son. The most informative sources for Blondel that I have found are N. F. J. Eloy, *Dictionnaire Historique de la Médecine* (London, 1778), I, p. 360; Dezeimeris (footnote 17), 418; A. Rees, *The Cyclopedia or Universal Dictionary of Arts, Sciences, and Literature* (London, 1819), IV, section BLO; and *Dictionary of National Biography*. Although I found few records of his medical education in Leiden, he was presumably exposed to the same teaching as his classmate, Herman Boerhaave. See Lindeboom's *Herman Boerhaave, the Man and his Work* (London, 1968), especially pp. 23–30, and also Sassen (footnote 16), 1–16.

[40] Anita Guerrini has studied Newton's influence on contemporary medical writing. See, for example, her 'Archibald Pitcairne and Newtonian Medicine', *Medical History*, 31 (1987), 70–83, and 'Isaac Newton, George Cheyne and the "Principia Medicinae"', in *The Medical Revolution of the Seventeenth Century*, edited by R. French and A. Wear (Cambridge, 1989), pp. 222–45.

[41] Dezeimeris (footnote 17), 418. Neither university nor municipal archives in Oxford substantiate speculations that he practised there. The Huguenots continued to gain numerical and political strength in early-eighteenth-century London. Since the 1689 Toleration Act of William and Mary, Huguenot assemblages as organized factions of protestant dissent received increasing support from the English. See R. D. Gywnn, *Huguenot Heritage: The History and Contribution of the Huguenots in Britain* (London, 1985). Blondel was 'certified' as a member of the French Church on Threadneedle Street in 1700, and resided in one of the large Huguenot areas of 'Northeastern' London. *Livre des Temiograges, 1669–1719 De L' Englise de Threadneedle Street* transcribed and edited by W. Minet and S. Minet (London, 1909), p. 24. Blondel was also recorded in *The Registers of the French Church, Threadneedle Street, London*, edited by T. C. Colyer-Fergusson (Aberdeen, 1906), pp. 208, 221, and in *Letters of Denization and Acts of Naturalization for Aliens in England and Ireland, 1603–1700*, edited by W. A. Shaw (Lymington, 1911), p. 193.

[42] Turner's religious convictions are most explicit in the preface and 'Espostulatory Epistle' of his 'Religio Medici Reformata. Or, Private Devotion in 2 Parts'. British Library, MS 14404.

[43] Gwynn, *Huguenot Heritage* (footnote 41), 110–43.

[44] See Appendix 1. Although somewhat different in content from the principles predicating the *Principia*, Blondel's propositions were used as the foundation of his argument in a way markedly similar to Newton's.

[45] Blondel, *The Strength*, p. 4.

Ergo, that *the Mother's Imagination can not mark the Body of her Infant'*.[46] Turner explained that no hypotheses were needed to account for the consequences of the maternal imagination other than that 'our Maker [had] placed such a relation between certain Causes and their Effects'.[47]

Blondel, on the other hand, represented the imaginationists' belief as irrational and mathematically unsound. He postulated that for every 100 000 pregnant women, at least 25 000 of them were 'exposed to the Danger and Fury of Imagination'. Yet, only 300 children would appear 'stampt with any tokens' of their mother's imagination. Of these 300 children, he estimated that one half were born to women who were unexposed to wayward thoughts during their pregnancies. From these approximations, Blondel calculated the numerical odds against an effect of the force of imagination were 24 850 : 150 (or 166 : 1).[48]

Turner responded to these criticisms with *The Force*. He rejected Blondel's arithmetical argument as mere 'guess Work, or frivilous Supposition', reaffirming that even if the 'smallest Number [of people]...carry the most indubitable Marks or *Signatures*...they may well be the Objects of our Admiration, and justify the Power...[of] the *Mother's Imagination'*.[49] He hoped that his readers would accept the '*Facts* [of the mother's imagination] we see before our Eyes, altho we cannot [wholly] account for their *Modus*', rather that to 'absolutely...deny them, or pretend to account for them by some mere *Hypothesis'*.[50]

3. Identity of the imagination and its power

Historians, philosophers, literary critics, and psychiatrists agree that the imagination intrigued 'Enlightened' English authors, but there was no consistent philosophical basis to its invocation.[51] For instance, Joseph Addison popularized Lockian ideas when describing the 'Pleasures of Imagination' in eleven consecutive issues of *The Spectator* in June–July 1712. Robert James's *Medical Dictionary* on the other hand described the imagination using Aristotelian terminology, as did *Chamber's Cyclopedia*.[52] Remnants of Cartesian views can be found in some contemporary medical

---

[46] Turner, *A Defence*, pp. 88–9. This is perhaps the most distinct example of Turner's criticism of the mathematical way of argument as purported by many iatro-mechanical, as well as iatro-mathematical physicians.

[47] Ibid., p. 69.

[48] Blondel, *The Power*, p. 21.

[49] Turner, *The Force*, p. 22.

[50] Ibid., p. 8.

[51] G. S. Rousseau, 'Science and the Discovery of the Imagination in Enlightened England', *Eighteenth Century Studies*, 3 (1969), 108–9; M. Nicolson, 'The Scientific Background of Swift's "Voyage to Laputa"', reprinted in her *Science and the Imagination* (Hamden, Connecticut, 1976), pp. 110–54; and L. King, *The Philosophy of Medicine: The Early Eighteenth Century* (Cambridge, Massachusetts, 1978), pp. 152–81. J. J. MacIntosh provided a prelude to this era in 'Perception and Imagination in Descartes, Boyle, and Hooke', *Canadian Journal of Philosophy*, 3 (1983), 327–57. Additionally, the philosophical usage of imagination over several centuries has been addressed by J. Engel, *The Creative Imagination: Enlightenment to Romanticism* (Cambridge, Massachusetts, 1981). For variations of the early descriptions of imagination, see C. E. MacMahon, 'The Role of Imagination in the Disease Process: Pre-Cartesian History', *Physiological Medicine*, 6 (1976), 179–84, and C. E. McMahon and J. L. Hastrup, 'The Role of Imagination in the Disease Process: Post-Cartesian History', *Journal of Behavioral Medicine*, 3 (1980), 205–17. 'The Imagination and Psychological Healing' has recently been addressed by S. W. Jackson in *Journal of the History of Behavioral Sciences*, 26 (1990), 345–58.

[52] Philip Shorr noted that many marvels, including children born alive without heads, were discussed in *Chamber's Cyclopedia*. Yet, he added, 'in all fairness to the cyclopedist', that some of the more questionable ancient marvels had been omitted. *Science and Superstition in the Eighteenth Century: A study of the treatment of science in two Encyclopedias of 1725–1750* (New York, 1932), p. 110.

writings on imagination, but most authors incorporated Newtonian ideas and terminology into their works. The most explicit example of Newtonian borrowing seems to have been that of the self-proclaimed London physician Thomas Morgan who, in 1725, defined the passions, including the imagination, according to a Newtonian equation of a force equal to the product of nerves (body) and the animal spirits (acceleration).[53] As the titles of Turner's and Blondel's writings suggest, the idea of 'Force' or 'Power' of the imagination was also a key issue in their discussions.[54]

Turner and other imaginationists claimed that imagination acted similarly to the passions. Blondel denied this. He began his discussion of this issue in *The Strength* by proclaiming his intention 'to determine What is Passion, and how, and where it affects the Body'.[55] He explicitly borrowed the Lockian definition that Passion 'In Respect of an intellectual Being, is a modification of Thoughts; in respect to a corporeal Being, [a modification of] Motion'.[56] Blondel used this definition to distinguish between passions which affect the mind and those which affect the body. Although both Turner and Blondel claimed that some passions could produce bodily effects, Blondel specified that the action of the imagination was confined to the mind. Blondel then sought to establish the conditions by which the passions were capable of producing physical effects. He claimed that strong mental attention to a particular object, whether with 'Desire' or in 'Abhorrence', was incapable of producing any change in the body since the blood or spirit flow remained localized within the brain. Any impassioned longings or cravings during pregnancy were, he argued, like the imagination and other 'intellectual' thoughts, 'Scene[s]...confined within the Mother's mind'.[57] The corporeal self, he claimed, could only undergo a physical response to a violent passion which was mentally sensed as a 'sudden change'. Fright, for instance, could, he argued, 'violently' accelerate the flow of blood and spirits throughout the body. This altered flow, he continued, resulted from the 'Mind' detecting a distinct change, i.e., making a judgement, between an 'Object, which we are used to, and an extraordinary one'.[58]

Employing Lockian ideas, Blondel refused to accept that the comparative judgement of objects and events was an innate 'species' of understanding. Instead, he argued that some 'Ratiocination' was required for making such judgements. Foetuses, so he claimed, were in a 'Limited' developmental state, and unable to reason logically. They were both 'unacquainted with...objects that disturb the Mother' and incapable of making any 'Reflexions' on them. Consequently, even if a pregnant women experienced a violent passion, her foetus was unable to 'sense' any change, and therefore it was protected from harm.[59] This view had an anatomical corollary (see below).

---

[53] T. Morgan, *Philosophical Principles of Physick* (London, 1725), pp. 365–95, as cited by Rousseau (footnote 51), 124. See also Morgan's *Mechanical Practice of Physick* (London, 1735), pp. 220–1.

[54] Turner's use of 'Power' of Imagination in 'Spots and Marks' and *The Force* in his 1730 work implied, as will be discussed, an immaterial impetus, whereas the implications of Blondel's use of the terms 'Strength' and 'Power' remains uncertain. Such terms were consistent with his adherence to 'Newtonian' doctrine, but given Blondel's displayed talent as both a scholar and wit, he may have used these terms as a parody on Turner's titles. As such, it supports Simon Schaffer's claim that a Newtonian language was often used 'for specific pugnacious purposes'. See 'Newtonianism', in *Companion to the History of Modern Science* edited by R. Olby, G. N. Cantor, J. R. R. Christie, and M. J. S. Hodge (London, 1990), p. 617.

[55] Blondel, *The Strength*, p. 52.

[56] Blondel included this as his fourth proposition listed at the beginning of *The Strength*.

[57] Blondel, *The Strength*, p. 54.

[58] Blondel, *The Power*, p. 101.

[59] Blondel, *The Strength*, pp. 51, 94.

Unlike Blondel, Turner claimed that the imagination could produce both mental and corporeal effects. His view of the imagination as a 'Faculty of the sensitive [not rational] Soul', together with his mechanical explanation of its actions, explicitly followed the expositions of Thomas Willis.[60] In his account of the working imagination Turner identified the *Image* of the thing desired or 'fear'd, being constantly represented to the mind' as the *'formal Cause'* of imagination. He also noted that when an individual was 'excited at the Appearance of the Object', his 'Appetite' was stirred so as to incite 'local Motion' of the 'Blood and nervous Fluid' in 'some Part of the Brain'.[61] Having generated such a 'power', the images or 'Species' which had been sensed and impressed 'upon the outward Organs', were, 'by a most quick Irradiation of the nervous Fluid [,] delineated inwards... apprehending all the... corporeal Things according to their external Appearance'. To explain the specific process in which a likeness of the image was produced on the foetus, Turner drew upon the Galenical writings of Thomas Fienus. In his *De viribus Imaginationis* (1608), Fienus had explained that the imagination induced 'real changes' in the body solely by stirring up the emotions. Such rarefied emotions were 'transformed' from the mother's body to the foetus via humours and spirits. Fienus argued that in the foetus, the impressed immaterial 'species' from the mother's imagination became expressed as a result of the imagination's conformative power. Turner, like Fienus, argued that only the malleable foetus, and not the adult mother, was susceptible to any impressed 'species' from the imagination.[62]

Many early-eighteenth-century medical theories had been formulated in the light of mechanistic philosophy. British medical writers including Archibald Pitcairne, James Keill, James Jurin, William Cockburn, George Cheyne, Stephen Hales, and Henry Pemberton used mechanically based deductive arguments in their explanations of animal oeconomy and physic. For example, they explained consumption, jaundice, and fevers, in terms of forces, powers, and causes adopted from natural philosophical writings.[63] Newton was their model and the exchange of theories between the Royal Society and the College of Physicians was fostered in having men like Hans Sloane and James Jurin as leading figures of both groups. Furthermore, many members of these groups shared antiquarian and literary connections, political and religious allegiances, and, for some, royal privileges, as well. Although rival factions had formed within the

[60] See R. G. Frank, 'Thomas Willis and His Circle: Brain and Mind in Seventeenth-Century Medicine', in *The Languages of Psyche: Mind and Brain in Enlightenment Thought*, edited by G. S. Rousseau (Berkeley, California, 1990), pp. 107–46. A. Meyer and R. Heirons previously elaborated 'On Thomas Willis's Concepts of Neurophysiology' in *Medical History*, 9 (1965), 1–15, 142–55. See also W. F. Bynum, 'The Anatomical Method, Natural Theology and the Functions of the Brain', *Isis*, 64 (1973), 445–68.

[61] Turner, 'Spots and Marks', pp. 106–7.

[62] Ibid., beginning on p. 120. Thomas Fienus described this particular action of the imagination in *De viribus Imaginationis* (Louvain, 1608). Turner also drew upon Fienus's account, implicating the role of imagination in 'producing almost every kind of disease', namely, squinting, stuttering, small pox, and the plague (p. 110). For a further outline, translation, and description of Fienus's writing, see L. J. Rather, 'Thomas Fienus' (1567–1631) Dialectical Investigation of the Imagination as Cause and Cure of Bodily Disease', *Bulletin of the History of Medicine*, 41 (1967), 349–67. Earlier descriptions of powers of the imagination are discussed in M. W. Bundy, *The Theory of Imagination in Classical and Medieval Thought* (Urbana, Illinois, 1927).

[63] Newton's influence on fever discourse is found in the works of Archibald Pitcairne, Richard Mead, George Cheyne, and John Freind. See for example W. Coleman, 'Mechanistic Philosophy and Hypothetical Physiology', *Texas Quarterly*, 10 (1967), 263; R. J. J. Martin, 'Explaining John Freind's *History of Physick*', *Studies in History and Philosophy of Science*, 19 (1988), 406; and Guerrini (footnote 40), 227–8.

College of Physicians of London and the Royal Society during the 1720s, physicians who might have been described as rational, empirical, mathematical, or experimental nearly all invoked Newton in their writings.[64]

Blondel, who had attended Pitcairne's lectures at Leiden, used a deductive Newtonian approach to sustain his hypotheses regarding the maternal imagination. As his first proposition illustrates, Blondel claimed all life was reducible to atoms. He further argued that the interactions of the atoms were 'deduc[ible] from the Laws of Motion'.[65] This reductionist argument echoed that of other iatro-mechanists who removed or displaced God from a central position in their depictions of natural phenomena. Peter Earle described this view in his reconstruction of the world of Blondel's contemporary, Daniel Defoe: 'God had created Nature; but now Nature had taken over from her creator and God himself was obliged to conform to the natural laws of His own creation'.[66] The basis of this 'natural religion' was reason.

Like Blondel, Turner also described the imagination as being 'transacted by mechanick Laws'.[67] However, Turner appears to have accepted these mechanical analogies only to a point, beyond which he resorted to nature as the explanation or cause of action. Underlying his mechanistic terminology, Turner accounted for the actions of the imagination as derived from a hidden, vital, spiritual, unknowable ultimate 'Cause' which, he claimed, had been provided by the Creator. For example, Turner described how intermeshed between the 'sensitive Soul and nervous Fluids' there were 'Springs and Wheels' which, by the intervention of '*Nature*', open 'little Doors of the Nerves, and conduct... certain Spirits to [them]'.[68] It has been argued that by the end of the 1720s, following Newton's death, the mechanical explanations of invisible actions were gradually giving way to more 'quasi-vitalistic' theories.[69] Turner possibly drew on this vitalist outlook when arguing that humans were guided as Nature dictated. He claimed that Nature's role in internal physical workings was akin to the force underlying the 'effects of the Magnet'.[70] It was this same immaterial force, he argued, which drew the mother's imagination to the foetus.[71] Turner's emphasis on an

---

[64] See Guerrini (footnote 40) and *idem*, 'James Keill, George Cheyne, and Newtonian Physiology, 1690–1740', *Journal of the History of Biology*, 18 (1985), 247–66; and T. M. Brown, 'Medicine in the Shadow of the *Principia*', *Journal of the History of Ideas*, 41 (1987), 629–48.

[65] Blondel, *The Power*, p. x. For a recent, concise survey of atomism see M. Tamny, 'Atomism and the Mechanical Philosophy', in *Companion to the History of Science*, edited by R. Olby, G. N. Cantor, J. R. R. Christie, and M. J. S. Hodge (London, 1990), pp. 597–609.

[66] P. Earle, *The World of Defoe* (London, 1976), p. 35. He comments on the common belief in the power of the mother's imagination in p. 207.

[67] Turner, 'Spots and Marks', pp. 53–4.

[68] Ibid.

[69] Guerrini, 'James Keill, George Cheyne, and Newtonian Physiology' (footnote 64), 248–9. M. Brown claimed that Turner, an 'articulate skeptic [of materialism]' in the junior ranks of the College during the 1710s' had already adopted mechanical explanations which incorporated an understanding of the essential vital element within his writing. See his 'From Mechanism to Vitalism in Eighteenth-Century English Physiology', *Journal of the History of Biology*, 7 (1974), 200, footnote 72. Opposition to mechanism in both early- and late-eighteenth-century contexts needs to be more fully explored.

[70] Turner, *A Defence*, p. 133. Turner did not mention this reference to the attractive force of the magnet in 1714, but added it to his 1729 treatise. Over this timespan, the study of attraction had gained the status of an independent field of study in natural philosophy. Nicholas Robinson, perhaps London's most staunch Newtonian physician, claimed, in 1725, that one problem unsolved by attractive particles was the influence of the mind on the body. As cited by Guerrini (footnote 40), 242.

[71] Turner, 'Spots and Marks', p. 154.

underlying immaterial substance, existing in both the mind and the body, was in distinct contrast to Blondel's mind–body dualism.[72]

Turner and Blondel also disagreed over who was reliable as an authority. Turner's reliance on Fienus's and Willis's descriptions of the imagination exemplify his appreciation of earlier authoritative doctrine. Such appreciation is also seen in the numerous case histories he selected from ancient or classical writings. Blondel ridiculed the imaginationists' use of 'ancient' authority, noting that they were 'obliged' to place their arguments in 'old Antiquity or in remote Places' since outrageous examples were not to be found in modern literature.[73]

Although distinguishing Turner's adherence to traditional doctrine from Blondel's espousal of Newtonian science allows some differentiation between the two physicians, it would be inaccurate to designate this dispute as a controversy between the Ancients and the Moderns.[74] For Turner also used terminology and 'quasi-vitalist' ideas consistent with contemporary modern medical writers. Moreover, he challenged the use of mathematical or hypothetical reasoning as evidence. Such a challenge, particularly when emphasizing the role of observation, was, as Theodore Brown has shown, beginning to gain much support from leading modern figures of the College of Physicians by the mid-1720s.[75]

The role of observation brings forth another crucial distinction between Turner and Blondel; their use of the term 'experiment' as opposed to 'experience'. Blondel used experiment to mean demonstrable evidence or proof suggesting a Newtonian borrowing. He claimed to accept 'nothing but what is certain and known, or demonstrable by Experiments'.[76] This was in contrast to imaginationists' accounts which, he said, were based on 'Quibbles and Puns, Suppositions and *Canterbury Stories*'.[77]

Turner appears not to have distinguished between the evidence offered by 'experiment' or 'experience'. For example, he described each of his case histories as an 'experiment' and collectively referred to them as 'experience'.[78] Relatedly, Turner represented these collective cases as multiple verifications of the 'truth'. The 'greatest part' of the cases, taken from Hippocrates, Galen, Malebranche, Fienus, Boyle, and other authorities, had been 'undeniably attested and unquestionably recorded'.[79] The earliest reported cases were validated by similar accounts observed and recorded by

---

[72] Material/immaterial distinctions in early modern philosophy and psychology have recently been re-examined in E. Michael and F. S. Michael, 'Two Early Modern Concepts of Mind: Reflecting Substance vs. Thinking Substance', *Journal of the History of Philosophy*, 27 (1989), especially 39–43; and E. Michael and F. S. Michael, 'Corporeal Ideas in Seventeenth-Century Psychology', *Journal of the History of Ideas*, 50 (1989), especially 44–8.

[73] Blondel, *The Power*, p. 21.

[74] Joseph M. Levine, in his reappraisal of the debate between the Ancients and the Moderns beyond that of R. F. Jones, qualified the eighteenth-century supporters of the ancients as selectors, borrowing only the passages they found most useful from ancient doctrine and ignoring the rest. Moreover, he argued that the essence of the battle was a question of history, i.e., the 'meaning and Use of the past' and the 'method of apprehending it'. See 'Ancients and Moderns Reconsidered', *Eighteenth Century Studies*, 15 (1981), 78, 84. The ancients/moderns question was brought to public attention in London literature of late 1726 with the publication of *Gulliver's Travels*. The work added support to those who preferred the ancients for, as G. S. Rousseau argued, it illustrated the modern's 'craze over absurd scientific effort'. See Rousseau's 'Science', in *The Context of English Literature: The Eighteenth Century*, edited by P. Rogers (London, 1978), p. 161.

[75] Brown (footnote 69), 188–92.

[76] Blondel, *The Strength*, p. 37.

[77] Blondel, *The Power*, p. v.

[78] Turner, *The Force*, p. 137.

[79] Turner, *A Defence*, p. 111.

later authorities. Turner argued that these men, like gentlemen of his own time, were to be taken on the 'credit' of their word.[80] Should we, he enquired, 'discredit all ancient History...[regardless of] how well or sufficiently...[cases were] attested at the times they fell out, and credit nothing we have not seen, or cannot warrant from the Testimony of the our own Senses'?[81] He added that if the conjoined twins who were recently paraded around London would have been 'presented one hundred Years past, it...[would] have been reckoned by Dr. B[londel] as a Fiction'.[82]

Turner's apparent indiscriminate use of these two terms also distinguishes what he and his opponent accepted as proof. Blondel defined experience as the 'Knowledge of a Matter of Fact' drawn from 'a sufficient Number of Observation[s]'. To qualify as valid, he claimed that such observations should relate to 'several Branches of the Fact in question'. Additionally, they should be 'clear, and intelligible, and grounded upon the Testimony of our Senses, and not depending upon occult Qualities, Suppositions, Conjectures, Hear-says, and Casualities'. For example, he argued that no credence should be given to reports from Bartholin, whose writings he characterized as a 'Net [catching] any Thing communicated...good or. bad, without any Distinction'.[83] Instead, the observations should be 'Uniform, and not contradictory', and procured 'in such a Number, as to over-ballance [sic] all Objections, or Counter-Observations, by a vast Disproportion'. Testimony from 'Hear-say,...[i.e.] second or third Hand' was 'to be received with a great deal of Caution'. Blondel claimed that the cases from Heliodorus, whom Turner had cited, were an admixture of 'Fable[s]' and fact, aimed only to 'beautify his work'.[84] Instead, Blondel urged his readers to set each of the case histories within the period in which they were written. Credit given to witnesses unknown to the observer should diminish 'In Proportion of the Distance of Places and Times' of the occurrence. Blondel directed that witnesses should be 'true, honest, and without any Interest to cheat'. Additionally, they must be 'Judicious' and 'neither credulous, nor prepossest [sic], nor too hasty' in their judgement. Finally, 'Witnesses are not to be trusted, if it be discovered that, at any Time, they have been found to be false'.[85] By following such guidelines, Blondel assured his readers that their 'impartial judge[ment]' would find them concurring with his arguments regarding the power of the maternal imagination.

4. Generation and foetal development

Although Turner organized his writings around the mother's imagination, Blondel argued that generation was the central issue.[86] Historians of reproduction have represented preformationism as the predominant generation theory of the 1720s.[87]

---

[80] Ibid., p. 70.
[81] Turner, *The Force*, p. 45.
[82] Ibid., p. 59.
[83] Blondel, *The Power*, p. 42.
[84] Ibid., p. 39.
[85] Ibid., pp. 6–7.
[86] Blondel repeatedly turned the course of the argument to foetal development and generation. Additionally, his citations are primarily verifications of his views on these topics.
[87] Cole (footnote 8), 53. William Harvey's epigenetic theory, which had gained many intellectual disciples in England lost support to the preformation theory, first proposed by Jan Swammerdam. E. Gaskings, *Investigations into Generation, 1651–1828* (London, 1967), p. 30. For a discussion of the rise of preformations, see S. A. Roe, *Matter, Life, and Generation: 18th Century Embryology and the Haller-Wolff Debate* (Cambridge, 1981), especially pp. 2–9. See also, D. C. Foulke, 'Mechanical and 'Organical' Models in Seventeenth-Century Explanations of Biological Reproduction', *Science in Context*, 3 (1989), 365–81.

This theory proposed that the embryo was existent in a fully preformed, yet miniature state prior to conception. Arguments arose between preformationists over whether the preformed entity existed in the ovum (ovists) or in the sperm (animalculists).[88]

Blondel was a preformationist, and claimed that ovism and animalculism both held 'a great Deal of Truth...*partly* grounded upon many undisputable Experiments'. Citing the disparate experimental findings of Regnier de Graff, and Antony van Leeuwenhoek, Blondel noted that he could 'reconcile' their conclusions about formation.[89] Specifically, he claimed that 'they all agree...that the Parts of the *Foetus* are existent somewhere before conception'.[90] Blondel also employed the *emboitment* theory.[91] This stated that the embryonic forms of all living beings had been in existence since the beginning of time. Smaller and smaller forms of each species were encased or embodied within the generative seed *ad infinitum*. Development occurred by an increase in the size of a pre-existent embryo. Blondel argued for the consistency of preformation with mechanism and design.[92] He placed the active role of the Creator back to the 'Beginning of the World'; the time, he claimed, when the 'Rudiments of all Plants and Animals' were formed.[93] Providence had guided generation along a determined path since then. Following this path was consistent with Blondel's view of uniformity in Nature and it allowed him to disavow that a creative or vital force was necessary to explain each individual creation. Instead, the events of conception were dependent on general providence. Blondel expanded the emboitment argument to support his proposition that 'conception is independent of the mother's will'. He claimed that just as a women cannot, by her fancy or imagination, promote or delay conception, withhold nourishment from her embryo, or select the sex, number, colour, size, strength, or resemblance of her child, 'it is not within her power to disfigure it either'.[94]

Turner rejected preformationism. He claimed that both the ovist and the animalcular theories of generation were 'unsatisfactory' and 'ambiguously...concluded'.[95] To highlight such ambiguity, Turner argued that neither animalculists nor ovists had fully accounted for the presence of mixed generations. He noted that, regardless of whether the male or the female was thought to provide the essential seed, neither theory could account for mixed breeds such as mules. Therefore, generation must be, Turner claimed, the result of contributions from both

---

[88] Jacques Roger's broad characterization of embryology in the seventeenth and eighteenth centuries is summarized in F. B. Churchill's 'The History of Embryology as Intellectual History', *Journal of the History of Biology*, 3 (1970), 157. L. W. B. Brockliss provides an illuminating account of contemporary French embryological ideas in 'The Embryological Revolution in the France of Louis XIV: the Dominance of Ideology', in *The Human Embryo: Aristotle and the Arabic and European Tradition*, edited by G. R. Dunstan (Exeter, 1990), pp. 158–86.

[89] Blondel, *The Power*, p. 109.

[90] Ibid., p. 46.

[91] *Emboitment*, first proposed by Swammerdam and Malebranche in 1669, is lucidly discussed by P. Bowler in 'Preformation and Pre-existence in the Seventeenth Century: A Brief Analysis', *Journal of the History of Biology*, 4 (1971), especially 221–2, 237–43.

[92] Blondel did not develop his argument to the religious extremes of Malebranche and Swammerdam who extended their account of *emboitment* to explain the doctrine of original sin (ibid., p. 238).

[93] Blondel, *The Power*, p. 141.

[94] Blondel, *The Strength*, p. 48.

[95] Turner, *The Force*, pp. 100, 102.

male and female seed.[96] This argument was akin to that used to support epigenesis in the preceding century.[97]

Turner, however, was not supportive of materialist epigenesis. Rather, he explicitly adopted the argument of his contemporary, James Drake. Drake, a London physician and Tory pamphleteer, refused to accept preformationism on the grounds of a lack of human evidence.[98] To account for individual variation, and deformities, Drake invoked the mother's wayward imagination and the 'Plastick Power' of nature. This power had been described in various ways by seventeenth-century British luminaries including Ralph Cudworth, Matthew Hale, Henry More, Robert Boyle, George Rust, and William Harvey.[99] Its use appears to have declined by the 1720s, but both Turner and Drake continued to rely on it in their explanations of foetal development.[100] Turner argued that merely acknowledging 'the general Providence... of that Being which created [nature]', as Blondel had done, showed insufficient reverence to the Creator.[101] Indeed, he claimed that most attempts to explain situations by general providence failed to demonstrate life's total dependence on God. Humans were, as Turner noted in his private devotional, 'only passive' beings, dependent on individual guidance by the Creator's 'Invisible hands'.[102] This presence was, Turner argued, especially necessary at the beginning of life. For, it was at this time that the 'Plastick Power' of nature first intervenes, and the Creator moulds the 'Dough' or 'Paste' into human form.[103] Although Turner argued that these actions of the 'plastick power' established God's presence, he claimed they revealed nothing about the true operations of nature. The underlying forces and powers of Nature were, he said, known 'only to the Creator', and remained 'impenetrable' to human understanding. In this sense, he allowed that God was the 'only mathematical physician', and that man was not 'enlight'd to see through the end of all' living things; to discover the Creator's Wisdom, Power and Goodness' until his 'Entrance into the [Heavenly] Sanctuary'.[104] On these grounds he concluded that the ovists' and animalculists' attempts to explain the operations of generation were futile.

In addition to their differences over theories of generation and the role of the Creator, Turner and Blondel also disagreed over the anatomical relationship between the mother and the foetus. Turner argued, adopting the London anatomist William

---

[96] Ibid., p. 90. Turner had not reintroduced this classical notion, but rather re-emphasized this argument which may be found in many other contemporary accounts. Specifically, he cited Sir John Floyer's report in the Royal Society's *Philosophical Transactions*.

[97] T. M. Brown has claimed that Drake's generation arguments were directed against the preformationist theory of the Newtonian mathematico-physician, Archibald Pitcairne. See 'The Mechanical Philosophy and the 'Animal Oeconomy': A Study of the Development of English Physiology in the Seventeenth Century and Early Eighteenth Century' (Ph.D. Dissertation, Princeton University, 1968), p. 269.

[98] Drake had argued that the 'Existence of a form'd Animal in the *Ovum* has never been prov'd, but suppos'd only from Analogy... to the Seed of Plants'. Additionally, he claimed that animalcules 'may only be Particles of a mixt Fluid in motion'. See his *Anthropologia Nova; or, a New System of Anatomy* (London, 1707), 1, 352.

[99] W. B. Hunter, 'The Seventeenth Century Doctrine of Plastic Nature', *Harvard Theological Review*, 43 (1950), 197–213. He noted that this theory had provided 'a convenient explanation for the production of monsters', p. 209.

[100] Turner *The Force*, p. 103.

[101] Turner (footnote 42), p. 3.

[102] Ibid., p. 6. Passive obedience was also the dictate of High Anglican endurance to the threats against Stuart succession.

[103] Turner, *A Defence*, pp. 97–8.

[104] Other than in his private devotional, Turner's published views on the role of the Creator are found in his *Discourse Concerning Fevers* (London, 2nd edition, 1736), preface and especially pp. 90–4.

Cowper's description, that blood circulated between the mother and the foetus and that this blood flow was developed during the early stage of pregnancy.[105] Blondel, however, argued that since 'before Pregnancy, the [mother's] Veins and Arteries of the *Uterus* are all matched together', one simply does not find '*idle* uterine Vessels, to joyn with those of the *Placenta*' during pregnancy.[106] He concluded that the placenta was solely of foetal origin, and was in no way connected to the uterus. Allowing that the uterus was merely an elastic container in which the developing foetus took 'Lodging for a short time',[107] he postulated that no connecting circulation to the foetus was necessary. Turner, denying Blondel's claim, invoked the opinion of contemporaries, including James Keill, James Drake, and John Freind, that foetal nourishment was entirely dependent on designed and interconnected circulations.[108]

Blondel replied with further 'evidence' supporting his argument. He explained that the vessels seen as tortuously winding around the uterus had been laid out and adapted to 'check the Violence of the Blood' that reached the area.[109] Nature, had taken 'great Care...[to] preserve the *Ovum* against the *Impetus* of the Blood and of the Spirits'.[110] This arrangement of vessels, he claimed, provided additional proof that independent circulations existed. Were it not so designed, Blondel argued, birth itself would present such an 'eminent Danger, because so much Blood...would discharge in a short Time' that the mother's life would be in jeopardy.[111] Blondel added a list of quantitative proofs, noting that there was 'not...an equal Number of Pulsations' between 'the Mother's Pulse, and...the Umbilical String'.[112] Thus, having combined rational, anatomical, and experimental evidence, Blondel claimed to have 'proved' that no blood circulated between the mother and the foetus. He presented a similar argument against any nervous connection, and concluded that no pathway existed through which any maternal passions could be transported to the foetus. Turner responded to Blondel's claims with contrary evidence. He reported that an acquaintance in London 'who has a large Share in the Practice of Deliveries', informed him that 'very little variation' existed between the maternal and foetal pulses.[113] However, even if variations were found in individual cases, Turner reminded readers that it was 'well known' that the pulse is, at times, 'different...[between the] two Wrists'.[114] At a time when, according to one historian, enthusiasm and philosophical predilection were the criteria which readers used to distinguish among theories of generation, Turner's and Blondel's dispute can be seen as more than an argument between a rationalist and an empiricist.[115] Their disagreements often originated from their different choices and interpretations of evidence, particularly as to whether that evidence was derived from experiment or from

[105] William Cowper, *The Anatomy of Humane Bodies* (Oxford, 1698), see Table 54 and its explanation. Cowper described this blood flow as bidirectional.
[106] Blondel, *The Power*, p. 123.
[107] Blondel, *The Strength*, p. 47.
[108] Turner, *The Force*, pp. 105–10, 112–15.
[109] Blondel, *The Strength*, p. 121.
[110] Ibid., p. 114. Furthermore, Blondel argued, following William Harvey's claim, that since the 'most violent of all' passions, that of coitus, did not cause the ovary to swell or alter the generative process in any way, any lesser passion would not be transmissible either.
[111] Ibid., p. 124.
[112] Ibid., p. 123.
[113] Turner, *A Defence*, p. 153.
[114] Ibid., p. 154.
[115] C. W. Bodemer, 'Embryological Thought in Seventeenth Century England', in *Medical Investigation in Seventeenth Century England* (Los Angeles, 1968), p. 3.

personal experience.[116] This difference underlying Blondel's and Turner's use of evidence significantly altered their explanations of similar case histories for their readers.

5. Appeal to the public

Unlike the discussions and demonstrations in the closed meeting halls of the Royal Society and the College of Physicians, Blondel and Turner staged their dispute in public. Such polemical pamphlet warring was not uncommon in early-eighteenth-century London.[117] Unlike lengthy books, pamphlets were quicker to print, lighter to distribute, cheaper to purchase, and easier to digest in a short period; all of which allowed authors to reach a wider audience. Turner and Blondel reserved the final judgement of their dispute for their readers.[118] Like contemporary advertisements for specific remedies, their pamphlets aimed to persuade the public. However, Turner and Blondel waged their war over medical beliefs and philosophies rather than a particular type of treatment or practice.[119]

Although the care of pregnant women might be considered a matter of their dispute, both authors offered similar practical recommendations. Turner cautioned women to remain calm during their pregnancies; urging them to resist cravings for particular food or drinks and to avoid any environment in which they might become frightened.[120] Blondel also attempted to calm expectant mothers, urging them to 'bear those Sights' commonly believed to produce marks and deformities on their children with 'Christian Pity and Compassion', rather than with 'Fear and Apprehension'.[121]

In their arguments concerning the power of the maternal imagination and the process of generation, Turner and Blondel endeavoured to establish a 'particular

[116] Joseph Needham made this claim in 'Limiting Factors in the Advancement of Science as Observed in the History of Embryology', *Yale Journal of Biology and Medicine*, 8 (1935), 15. Although Blondel specified reason as one component of his argument and Turner gathered empirical detail, a lack of a clear distinction between the two protagonists supports Andrew Wear's recent claim that rationalist/empiricist divisions more likely represent an historical categorization than an historical fact. See A. Wear, 'Medical Practice in late Seventeenth- and Early Eighteenth-Century England: Continuity and Change', in *The Medical Revolution of the Seventeenth Century*, edited by R. French and A. Wear (Cambridge, 1989), p. 304. Indeed, Turner praised London surgeon Richard Blundell for having 'Declined Mathematical Argumentation...[and] invoke[d], rather a rational Empiricism'. See the dedication in Turner's *Syphilis* (London, 1717).

[117] See D. Harley, 'Honor and Property: the Structure of Professional Disputes in Eighteenth-Century English Medicine', in *The Medical Enlightenment of the Eighteenth Century*, edited by A. Cunningham and R. French (Cambridge, 1990), pp. 138–64. Adrian Wilson (footnote 38), 7, 8, also discusses the uses of pamphlets as '*appeals* for public support'. Hillel Schwartz described a contemporary appeal for a wide audience by religious groups in his *The French Prophets: The History of a Millenarian Group in Eighteenth-Century England* (Berkeley, California, 1980).

[118] N. D. Jewson first discussed the public's role in determining the care and medicines they received in 'Medical Knowledge and the Patronage System in Eighteenth-Century England', *Sociology*, 8 (1974), 369–85. Roy Porter has also argued that part of a physician's success at this time depended upon 'public favour', and has documented how physician's arguments were addressed to the public. See 'Laymen, Doctors, and Medical Knowledge in the Eighteenth Century: the Evidence of the *Gentleman's Magazine*' in *Patients and Practitioners*, edited by R. Porter (Cambridge, 1985), p. 311; and D. Porter and R. Porter, *Patient's Progress: Doctor and Doctoring in Eighteenth-Century England* (Cambridge, 1989), p. 102. Marina Benjamin has also discussed the role of the patient as judge in 'Medicine, Morality and the Politics of Berkeley's Tar-Water' in *The Medical Enlightenment of the Eighteenth Century*, edited by A. Cunningham and R. French (Cambridge, 1990), especially pp. 176–80.

[119] Medical practitioners regularly confronted 'quack' remedies in attempts to dispel any mystery about 'miraculous' curative powers that the remedies were claimed to have held. See for example, Francis Doherty, 'The Anodyne Necklace: A Quack Remedy and its Promotion', *Medical History*, 34 (1990), 268–93.

[120] Turner, *The Force*, p. 137.

[121] Blondel, *The Strength*, p. 58.

reading of nature and its behaviour'.[122] To do so they employed rhetorical devices common in contemporary pamphleteering. For example, Blondel depicted his position as if he were 'at the Bar pleading... [his] Cause' for judge and jury.[123] While at first he claimed to have 'thought it unreasonable, unjust, and *contrary* to the Laws of War, to single Dr. *Turner* in a Crowd of *Tale-mongers*, and to fire upon him separately', he later exposed Turner to the public as 'the Aggressor'.[124] Furthermore, Blondel represented his opponent's criticisms as a personal 'Injustice'. Turner, Blondel claimed, does 'seldom quote me right, he alters my Words, or intermixes some of his own, and yet he has the Confidence to print the Whole in *Italick*'. Such tactics, Blondel added, proved Turner's work to be a 'gross Imposition upon the Publick'.[125] This portrayal of Turner as a devious or dishonest rhetorician held particular significance given that the public were designated as the ultimate arbiters of their dispute.

Turner also appealed to the public, and used legal accusations which gave his argument the sense of a need for adjudication. 'Judge B___l' had not proved what he had intended in this 'Trial'. Instead, Turner claimed, Blondel had only succeeded in misleading the reading public [his jury] by 'banter[ing them] out of their senses'.[126] Turner reassured his readers that despite Blondel's excellence in pamphlet soldiery, his 'Gunnery' had been received as 'nothing but mere *Flash*, and *empty Bounce*'.[127]

In his quest for public support, Turner devoted particular attention to Blondel's explication of the Biblical passage on Jacob's sheep. This 'Textuary', Turner argued, exemplified how Blondel could alter a 'plain, natural, and genuine Construction' into one which, 'for the most [part was] confus'd, perplex'd and unintellible [*sic*]'.[128] Turner denounced Blondel's translation calling it 'irrelevant', and claimed it was typical of the way Blondel misrepresented the entire maternal imagination issue. 'What [a] pitiful *spoiling* of a *Text*', Turner observed, 'What a jumbled Story furnished out of two as plain Versus [as] are to be met with in the sacred *Pandects!*'.[129] Thus, appealing to fellow Anglicans and other religious readers, Turner represented Blondel as sacrilegious for having tampered with the word of God.

The arguments and aims of Turner and Blondel are similar to those in contemporary political pamphlets. *Fog's Weekly Journal* of 1729 claimed that political pamphlets were written either to 'disabuse the Publick in Respect to some false notions with which the People by the *Articles* of designing men may be posses'd', or to serve 'some *Parts*, *Faction*, or particular Set of Men, in which case... [the pamphleteer had] a Tendency towards... deceiving and imposing upon Mankind'. The *Journal* claimed that, in the first case, authors generally relied on 'undeniable Facts, and plain Reason, for the Support of Truth'. While in the second, one finds 'Supposition, Conjectures, long Arguments grounded upon Facts which cannot be prov'd, and which perhaps many *know to be false*'. To 'silence the Opposition', the anonymous author claimed, 'it is Ten to One' that the pamphleteer calls 'God to witness'.[130]

---

[122] *The Uses of Experiment: Studies in the Natural Sciences*, edited by David Gooding, Trevor Pinch, and Simon Schaffer (Cambridge, 1989), p. 5.

[123] Blondel, *The Power*, p. iii. Legal terminology comprised much of the pamphlet warring of the day. Yet, Blondel may have been familiar with such terminology for some biographical sources claim his father was a French legal counsellor.

[124] Ibid., p. ii.

[125] Ibid., p. iii.

[126] Turner, *The Force*, p. 4.

[127] Ibid., pp. 57, 79.

[128] Ibid., p. 126.

[129] Ibid., p. 129.

[130] *Fog's Weekly Journal*, Saturday, 30 August 1729.

6. Aftermath of the battle

The extent to which the public exercised any adjudicatory role is unknown. In part, this stems from our lack of understanding 'who read whom' during this period.[131] Turner's and Blondel's use of pamphlets, however, appears to have effectively advertised their names and medical campaigns which, despite the personal slanders, perpetuated the reputation of both authors. Although the readership remains unknown, sources suggest that 'Dr. Blondel's dispute with Dr. Turner made no small noise'.[132] 'N.M.', a Grub Street journalist, represented their dispute as causing such a commotion that he urged 'Waste-paper merchant', James Jones, to 'speedily interpose, and reconcile [these authors]...who have poured out such a profusion of learning and logic,...that it is feared, they will soon intirely [sic] exhaust, not only the argument, but themselves'.[133]

The responses from the public and from fellow professionals which this dispute continued to provoke demonstrated that, unlike the Toft case, there was no immediate resolution of the imagination issue. Both Turner's and Blondel's arguments continued to gain support for a number of years. For example, one London treatise of 1772 supporting Blondel's claims, stated that if mental longings were actually conveyed from the mother to the foetus, children's deformities would have been much more varied. Since women think so often about their clothing, the author argued, the imprinted markings on their children should 'depend on the reigning fashion'.[134] The London physician John Mauclerc helped sustain Blondel's argument for more than a decade after Blondel's death.[135] Following Blondel, Isaac Bellet also claimed to have 'proved, by incontestable arguments, drawn from both reason and experience that it is a ridiculous prejudice to suppose it possible for a pregnant woman to mark her child' via her imagination.[136]

Turner's argument also received support. A report in *Gentleman's Magazine* of 1735 claimed it uncanny that the mother of a young boy whose skin annually turned to a dusky yellow colour and was subsequently shed 'can't remember any Fright' during her pregnancy.[137] As with other similar reports in the periodical, this case history was abridged from the *Philosophical Transactions*.[138] Besides natural philosophical

---

[131] This lack of understanding is also central to difficulties in determining what knowledge became 'popularized' during this time. See Philip K. Wilson, 'Acquiring Surgical Know-How: Occupational and Lay Instruction in Early Eighteenth-Century London', in *The Popularization of Medicine 1650–1850*, edited by R. Porter (London, 1992), pp. 42–71.

[132] John Henry Mauclerc, *The Power of Imagination in Pregnant Women Discussed* (London, 1740), and idem, *Dr. Blondel Confuted: or, the Ladies Vindicated with Regard to the Power of Imagination in Pregnant Women* (London, 1747).

[133] *Memoirs of the Society of Grubstreet* (London, 1737), p. 546.

[134] Giovanni Fortunato Bianchini, *An Essay on the Force of Imagination in Pregnant Women. Addressed to the Ladies* (London, 1772), p. 16.

[135] Blondel died on 4 October 1734, and was buried 'Privately and with as little Ceremony as...possible' at Stepney Causeway, near the London environs in which he had practised for many years. Public Record Office, Chancery Lane, Prob. 11/667.

[136] [Isaac Bellet], *Letters on the Force of Imagination in Pregnant Women* (London, 1765), subtitle. Blondel's influence was previously shown in the 1745 French version of this work, *Lettres sur le Pouvoir de l'Imagination des Femmes Enceintes*.

[137] *Gentleman's Magazine*, 4 (1735), 635–6. Turner died on 13 March 1740, having amassed considerable wealth, and was buried at the Church of St Andrew and St Mary in Watton-at-Stone, Hertfordshire. For more than twenty years, his practice had been based at his Devonshire Square residence in London. Public Record Office, Chancery Lane, Prob. 11/709.

[138] The Royal Society interest is also seen in Dr Superville's refutations of Blondel's claims in *Philosophical Transactions* 41 (1744 from 1740 proceedings), 306.

writings and the popular press, extraordinary childbirths attributed to a mother's wayward imagination also featured in the popular tales of Martinus Scriblerus, Peregrine Pickle, and Tristram Shandy.[139]

The imagination remained a controversial subject in medical, scientific, and literary writings throughout the eighteenth century. Consider, for example, the attempts of two widely recognized authors to quantify the force and intensity of imagination. David Hartley described the relationship between maternal longings and his own doctrine of vibrations and associations in his *Observations on Man* (1749).[140] James Long also discussed connections between images and actions in his *Inquiry into the Origin of Human Appetites and Affections* (1747).[141]

Reproductive generation, the other major component of the Turner–Blondel dispute, also remained both a controversial and popular area of investigation. Disputes over preformationism became increasingly pronounced later in the century,[142] when new experimental evidence was adduced in favour of epigenesis.[143] In the light of this experimentation, some physicians and natural philosophers re-examined the question of whether the mother's imagination could affect embryological development.[144] Although few specifically referred to Turner and Blondel, they continued to address concerns about a generation similar to those which had been raised in Turner's and Blondel's dispute.

Turner's and Blondel's influence spread beyond London. Turner's *De Morbis Cutaneis*, including 'Spots and Marks', was translated into French (1743) and German (1766). Blondel's 1729 pamphlet was printed in French (1737), Dutch (1737), German (1756), and Italian (1760).[145] The citation of these works in Continental disputes over

---

[139] Additional cases of extraordinary childbirth from this period are discussed in G. S. Rousseau's 'Pineapples, Pregnancy, Pica, and *Peregrine Pickle*', in *Tobias Smollett: Bicentennial Essays*, edited by G. S. Rousseau and P. G. Bouce (New York, 1971), pp. 93–4.

[140] David Hartley, *Observations on Man*, part 1 (London, 1749). Hartley's elucidations of vibrations and mental phenomena are more fully addressed in T. Mischel's '"Emotion" and "Motivation" in the Development of English Psychology: D. Hartley, James Mill, A. Bain', *Journal of the History of Behavioral Sciences*, 2 (1966), 124–9.

[141] James Long, *An Inquiry into the Origin of Human Appetites and Affections* (London, 1747). For further discussion, see C. McMahon's 'Images as Motives and Motivators: A Historical Perspective', *American Journal of Psychology*, 86 (1973), 472.

[142] For example, the Haller-Wolff debate as analysed by Roe (footnote 87).

[143] Cole (footnote 8), 53. Yet ovists continued to battle animalculists. The evidence which ovists Albrecht von Haller, Charles Bonnet, and Lazzaro Spallanzani gathered showed that the female was chiefly responsible for *in utero* development. It was used, by some, in support of the impressionists' argument.

[144] For example, it has been claimed that William Hunter questioned each pregnant woman in a 'large' London lying-in-hospital whether anything had 'specially affected' her mind during pregnancy, and he recorded the answers. After many year of collecting this information, Hunter had not found 'one instance' suggesting a relation between the woman's answer and any 'abnormal structure' on the child when delivered. John Brown, 'Notes and Observations on Maternal Impressions' (M.D. Thesis, Glasgow, 1887–1888), p. 3. Hunter scholars, however, have not uncovered any evidence that such experimentation occurred. (As related in Wellcome Institute Inquiry RQ No. 817b, 6 December 1983.)

[145] Daniel Turner, *Traité des Maladies de la Peau en General, avec un Court Appendix sur l'Efficacité des Remedes Topiques dans les Maladies Internes, & leur Maniere d'Agir sur le Corps Humain* (Paris, 1743), and D. Turner, *Abhandlung von den Krankheiten der Haut: Nebst einem Kurzen Anhang von den Ausserlichen Mitteln, und der Art, wie sie Wirken* (Altenburg, 1766). James Blondel, *Dissertation Physique sur la Force de l'Imagination des Femmes Enceintes sur le Fetus*, translated by Albert Brun (Leyden, 1737), J. Blondel, *Natuurkundige Verhandeling. Wegens het Vermoogen der Inbeelding van Zwangere Vrouwen op Haar Vrucht*, translated by Jan van der Hulst (Rotterdam, 1737), J. Blondel, *Drey Merkw Urdige Physikalische Abhandlungen von der Einbildungskraft der Schwangern Weiber, und Derselben Wirkung auf ihre Leibesfrucht* (Strasbourg, 1756), and J. Blondel, *Dissertazione della Forza dell' Immaginazione delle Donne Gravide Sovra il Feto* (Ferrara, 1760).

the power of imagination attest to their international appeal.[146] Lengthy quotations from the Turner–Blondel dispute also appeared as one of the remarkable, newsworthy, international events reported in the widely published letters of *The Jewish Spy*.[147] Many European authorities expressed interest in the power of the maternal imagination. Buffon, for example, used an argument similar to Blondel's, denying that the transfer of the mother's imagination to the foetus was possible since no maternal–foetal vascular connections existed.[148] Albrecht von Haller discussed the role of the invisible mechanisms, including the imagination, in his writings on sensibility and irritability. Since the eighteenth century, many writers have cited the Turner–Blondel dispute in their histories of embryology and sexuality, discussions of human variation, beauty marks, general literary criticism, anthropologies of the body, and most recently, as evidence for reincarnation.[149] However, although Whiggish historical accounts have praised Blondel as victorious, and designated Turner as 'credulous', re-examination of the debate shows, from a contemporary perspective, the partiality of such judgements.[150]

Acknowledgements

Research for this work was partially supported by an Owsei Temkin scholarship (Johns Hopkins Institute, Baltimore) and a Wellcome Trust studentship (Wellcome Institute, London). I gratefully appreciate the insightful comments of Harold Cook, Christopher Lawrence, Roy Porter, Antonio Poza, Akihito Suzuki, Andrew Wear, Janice Wilson, and Alexander Zahar, on earlier drafts of this paper. I should also like to thank two anonymous referees.

[146] N. Lemery, and J. B. Winslow, *Memories Academie Royale des Sciences* 33 (1733), 38 (1738), and 40 (1740). Ignazio Vari, *Discussione 'Ragionamento del Sig. Dottore Ignazio Vari…al Sig. Dottor Lucio Bonaccioli'* in Blondel, *Dissertazione della Forza dell' Imaginazione* (footnote 145), 175–212.

[147] A letter from Aaron Monceca to Isaac Onis quoted at length from the Turner–Blondel dispute in Jean. Babtiste de Boyer, Marquis d'Argens, *The Jewish Spy*, IV, letter 69, (Dublin, 1753), 95–109.

[148] George Louis Leclerc Buffon, *Oeuvres completes de Buffon*, edited by M. Flourens (Paris, 1853–1855), I, pp. 642–7, cited by King (footnote 51), 174.

[149] In addition to the works of Blackman, King, Park and Daston, and Rousseau already cited, Blondel and Turner also appear in the chapter entitled 'Rabbits and Quacks' of Harvey Graham's (pseud.), *Eternal Eve* (Altrincham, 1950), pp. 345–6. Numerous midwifery texts of the nineteenth century also referred to the debate, see for example Michael Ryan, *Manual of Midwifery* (Burlington, 1835), pp. 64–73. In another context, see P.-G. Bouce's 'Imagination, Pregnant Women, and Monsters in Eighteenth Century England and France', in *Sexual Underworlds of the Enlightenment*, edited by G. Rousseau and R. Porter (Manchester, 1988), especially pp. 89–94. Barbara Stafford discusses this debate in her chapter on 'Markings' in *Body Criticism: Imaging the Unseen in Enlightenment Art and Medicine* (Cambridge, Mass., 1991). Finally, Ian Stevenson delivered a lecture entitled 'The Mother's Possible Influence in Birthmarks in cases of the Reincarnation Type' on 22 January 1989 at 'Parapsychology: A State-of-the-Art Conference' in New York. One goal of my ongoing work on Turner is to re-examine this dispute in respect of his later expressed concern for 'disorders peculiar to women'.

[150] See, for example. L. J. A. Lowenthal, 'Daniel Turner and 'De Morbis Cutaneis'', *Archives of Dermatology*, 85 (1962), 517–23, R. J. Mann, 'Daniel Turner, the First British Dermatologist', *Mayo Clinical Proceedings*, 51 (1976), 62–6, and even the more historically grounded writing of P. J. Hare perpetuated Turner's unfavourable reputation in his *Our Credulous Countryman* (Edinburgh, 1967). One important exception is the short article by Alan Lyell, 'Daniel Turner (1667–1740) LRCP London (1711) M. D. Honorary, Yale (1723) Surgeon, Physician and Pioneer Dermatologist; The Man Seen in the Pages of His Book of the Skin', *International Journal of Dermatology*, 21 (1982), 162–70. Here (p. 168), Lyell explained Turner's reliance on authority more as a reverence for earlier works than as a blind acceptance of their word.

7. Appendix: Blondel's propositions

1 By IMAGINATIONISTS, I mean those, who believe in the Power of the Mother's Imagination over the Foetus.

2 There's no *Solutio Continui* without Force or Violence.

3 Imagination must act by some means.

4 Passion, in respect of the Mind, is a Modification of Thoughts, but Motion in Respect of the Body.

5 Passions act upon the Body by accelerating, or diminishing the velocity of Blood, and Spirits.

6 Imagination cannot act beyond the Sphere of the Soul, and of the Body.

7 There is no sensation without Nerves.

8 Nerves being once divided can never reunite.

9 A Ligature, or a Pression upon a Nerve, or a Blood Vessel, makes them useless, so long as it lasts.

10 The longer is an Artery, the slower is the Motion of Blood, at the Extremity of the Vessel.

11 The Rudiments of all Plants and Animals are from the Beginning of the world.

12 Conception is independent on the Mother's will.

13 The *ovum* is for a long Time in the Fallopian *Tube*, and in the *Uterus* without Adhesion.

14 The *Foetus* has a sensation, and a circulation of the Blood independent on the Mother.

15 Deformities ought to be less amazing than the vast Number of regular Bodies.

These propositions were listed in Blondel's *Power*, and had previously appeared in similar form in *Strength*. The earlier work also contained the proposition: 'There are not in the World, two *Atoms*, that be both alike'.

THE INFLUENCE OF MATERNAL IMPRESSIONS ON THE FETUS.

BY FORDYCE BARKER, M. D., LL. D., COLUMB. ET EDINB.

New York.

THE belief that maternal impressions may affect the nutrition and development of the fetus in utero has existed from the earliest periods of which there are any records. The oldest evidence of this belief is found in chapter xxx of the Book of Genesis, in an account of a business transaction between Jacob and his father-in-law Laban, in which this belief prompted Jacob to adopt a method which in recent times has become very common in Wall Street, that of doubling his capital " by watering the stock."

The law of Lycurgus that Spartan women when pregnant should look constantly at statues of Castor and Pollux, representing strength and beauty, so that their offspring might be similarly developed, must have been based on this belief.

Five columns of fine print in the catalogue of the Surgeon General's library at Washington demonstrate the copiousness of medical literature on this topic, and how largely it has occupied the medical mind. That maternal impressions may affect the form, development, and future character of the fetus, has been very generally accepted as true by women in all ages, and by men so far as they have any idea on the subject, without doubt.

Three of the most distinguished writers of fiction in modern times have based incidents on this belief, in a way which they would not have done if they had supposd that these incidents would be rejected by their readers as improbable.

Goethe, in his *Elective Affinities*, describes a case in which strong mental impressions at the time of conception, or soon after, affected the child. Sir Walter Scott, in the *Fortunes of Nigel,* explains the extreme horror which a drawn sword always excited in James I, owing to the brutal murder of Rizzio having been committed in the presence of his unfortunate mother before he saw the light.

The theory of "maternal impressions" is the groundwork on which is constructed *Elsie Venner,* that remarkable novel by Oliver Wendell Holmes, most original in its conception, fascinating in its dramatic development, and most suggestive in the curious speculations with which it is interspersed.[1]

Medical writers with hardly an exception, down to the beginning of the 18th century, express the belief, with more or less distinctness, that fetal marks and deformities are due to the emotions, desires, or shocks of the pregnant mother.

Writers have given quotations from supposed treatises by Hippocrates which clearly avow this doctrine, but that these are genuine treatises by him is now generally questioned by scholars. But no one doubts that they were written by some very ancient medical author of high authority. Paulus Ægineta[2] gives some interesting quotations from ancient

---

[1] An article in the *Boston Medical and Surgical Journal,* vol. xx, 1839, p. 98, quoted from the *Southern Medical and Surgical Journal,* vol. iii, 1839, p. 381, on the *Snake Man,* Robert H. Copeland, may have consciously or unconsciously suggested the character of *Elsie Venner.* The man was then twenty-nine years old. " His mother when six months pregnant was struck, but not bitten, by a rattlesnake. She was so forcibly impressed that her child when born had a face resembling that of a snake, i. e., his teeth are like fangs, his eyes and mouth like those of a snake. He has not control over his right arm and leg, the joints of which are singularly loose. At times his right arm will coil up close to his body, and then will project and strike at an object four or five times just like a snake. His right foot and leg will then execute similar movements. His face then simultaneously becomes excited, the angle of his mouth is then drawn backward, the eyes snap, the lips separate, showing the teeth, and the entire aspect becomes snaky." There are more details of a similar character for which I will refer to the original paper.

The names of six physicians are attached to the foregoing account, certifying that it is substantially true.

[2] *Sydenham Society Transl.,* 1844, Commentary on Book I.

authors, who believed strongly in the influence of maternal impressions on the fetus. Galen (ad Pisonum), Soranus, Hesiod, and Heliodorius are especially quoted.

Ambroise Paré,[1] in Book XXV, entitled *Of Monsters and Prodigies*, describes and figures many instances, and in chapter vii he very distinctly avows his belief in the influence of maternal impressions on the fetus.

In short, without referring to the many other authors who have written on this subject, I think it may be truthfully said that, down to the beginning of the 18th century, this was the accepted belief of the medical profession. Blondell, an English physician, appears to have been the first to question this theory, in 1727. He was followed by Hallé, Burdach, and Buffon.

Within the past twenty-five years, many papers have been published in which this theory has been strongly controverted.

In my judgment, the most able and the most scientific is an elaborate article of nearly sixty pages by Dr. J. G. Fisher, of Sing Sing, N. Y., entitled,[2] *Does Maternal Mental Influence have a Constructive or Destructive Power in the Production of Malformations or Monstrosities at any Stage of the Embryonic Development?* The paper concludes with twenty-three deductions, the most important of which I will quote.

1. " That traditional superstition has perpetuated the notion that malformations are the result of mental emotions."

2. " That the medical profession is in no inconsiderable degree responsible for the existence of and continuance of this popular error."

3. " That various intense emotions are common with gestating women, and apprehensions of malformation of their offspring exist in the minds of a large portion, yet abnormal births are extremely rare."

4. " That there is nothing like law in the alleged results of maternal mental influence in the production of malformations."

[1] London, 1634.   [2] *American Journal of Insanity*, January, 1870.

5. "That the occasional apparent relation of cause and effect is due, in most instances, to accidental coincidences, which would be far less frequent if the facts could be obtained *previously* instead of *subsequently* to the birth of the child."

6. "Such evidences are not sufficiently numerous and authentic to warrant a rational belief in the origin of monstrosities from the perturbed emotions of the mother's mind."

7. "Like causes produce like results, whereas we find that in a series of cases of any special variety of malformation mental emotions arising from a considerable number of dissimilar objects, even of the most diverse character, are assigned as the cause."

8. "In a large proportion of the cases of malformation, no mental or even physical explanation is offered by the parents or friends."

9. "There is no relation between the number and character of these mental emotions and apprehensions of pregnant women and the actual frequency and variety of malformations."

10. "That some of the assumed causes are alleged to have operated upon the embryo or fetus subsequently to the named period for the evolution of the part which is found to be the seat of the malformation, thereby implying a distinctive as well as a metamorphosing power."

12. "Malformations identical in kind and in degree recur again and again in the human subject, and admit of a systematic classification, definite and distinctive."

13. "Every form of malformation and monstrosity in the human subject has had its exact morphological counterpart in the lower animals."

15. "The only rational and scientific explanation is to be found in pathological histology."

16. "Monstrosities are not the result of embryological and physiological laws, they are the products of embarrassments to normal development."

17. "Vices of conformation and monstrosities are due to either retarded or excessive development."

Dr. Fisher is known as an accomplished student and authority on teratology, and his deductions on this subject will be largely accepted by most scientific men, but this is only a limited part of the question of maternal impressions.

Dugas[1] has written a strong paper in opposition to the theory of "maternal impressions," and asserts that "it originated in man's natural love of mysteries and desire to account for everything." He says that "the only rational grounds for the belief are to be found in the occasional coincidence between the alleged cause and effect, but these are so rare, when compared with the countless number of instances in which the effect fails to follow the cause, that they must lose much of their force upon the slightest investigation." He denies that there is any channel by which the mental emotion can reach the fetus, and refers every supposed result of maternal impressions to coincidence.

"If," he says, "the emotions of the mother can affect the fetus so as to induce deformity, this must be done at the precise time at which the deformed locality is undergoing evolution, for the difficulty would much increase even if we had to presume that after the evolution had been completed the emotions of the mother would destroy it and reproduce an anomalous one in its place."

I must refer to another able paper, read before the Chicago Medical Society by Dr. Norman Bridge,[2] in opposition to the doctrine of mental impressions on the fetus.

As most of the reported cases give the third month of pregnancy and after, when the limbs are already formed, he holds it to be impossible that deformities can result in such from maternal emotions.

"A thousand sufficient forms of disturbance might occur," he says, "and each might be capable of interfering with perfect development. There might be too much or too little blood supplied to the fetus—the quality of this blood might be abnormal in countless ways. Accidents may occur,

[1] *Southern Medical and Surgical Journal*, September, 1866, p. 317.
[2] *Chicago Medical Journal*, August, 1875, p. 577.

blows and falls. There may be frequent attempts at miscarriage, or the mother may be syphilitic, or may have some acute disease. The maternal organism may be abnormal; indeed it would be useless to give all the influences capable of arresting or disturbing the development of the ovum." But he admits that "mental emotions may act through the blood so as to work the failure of a perfect development of the fetus," but "mental emotion does not act through the blood to disturb in the most wonderful manner a particular part of the body of the fetus, the part varying according to the particular mental impression." "To endow the blood with such weird intelligence as this would require is too great a load for our credulity. There is no philosophy in the theory that it so acts; all the truths of anatomy, physiology, and pathology are strictly against it." "It has nothing in its favor except the fact that in an occasional case a deformity occurs as, judging from an emotion really experienced, the mother expected it would."

In a paper read by Dr. D. S. Conant before the New York Academy of Medicine[1] on "Monstrosities" he argues that anomalies are the result of arrested development. His main argument against the theory of maternal impressions is based on the statement of Virchow that there is no nervous tissue in the umbilical cord, and therefore the only communication between the mother and fetus is through the medium of the blood.

In the discussion on the paper,[2] Dr. Detmold opposed the theory of maternal impressions, and reported a case tending to show that fetal deformities are due to arrest of development. The late Dr. Peaslee agreed with Dr. Detmold that arrest of development, not maternal impressions, was the true cause of fetal deformities. But he adds, "When the pregnant woman becomes the subject of intense anxiety, fear, or other kinds of mental emotions, the offspring might be more or less impressed. The reason for this

[1] *Transactions of the New York Academy of Medicine,* vol. ii, p. 269.
[2] *Bulletin of the New York Academy of Medicine,* vol. i, p. 363.

effect on the fetus could be explained by the close sympathy between the brain and uterus.

"The blood going to an impregnated uterus may be so altered in quality as to produce fatal effects on the fetus, if after a pregnant woman is frightened, a monster is produced in a *general* instead of a *special* way by the arrest of development. For it is a well-known fact that the fetus, during its various stages of development, passes through certain conformations which in general appearance very much resemble those of the lower animals."

Many other writers might be referred to who have advocated similar views; but I do not find any arguments in support of their opinions more forcible than those which have been quoted. I may mention as prominent in this number, Velpeau,[1] Ryan,[2] Demageon,[3] and Reinvilliers.[4]

But I think the weight of authority must be conceded to be in favor of the doctrine that maternal impressions may affect the development, form, and character of the fetus.

Montgomery[5] says, "Pregnant women should not be exposed to causes likely to distress, or otherwise strongly impress their minds." Rokitansky[6] says, "The question whether mental emotions do influence the development of the embryo must be answered in the affirmative. Seeing that many malformations originate in an arrest of development, and how frequently the former bears a certain resemblance to various animals, it is just conceivable that the development of the embryo may be so arrested by maternal *emotions* as *accidentally* to occasion a likeness between the object that produced the impression and the resulting malformation." This expression of sober belief by this eminent scientific German seems entitled to great weight.

[1] *Bull. des sciences médicales*, août 1827.

[2] *London Medical and Surgical Journal*, 1883, p. 176.

[3] "L'imagination considérée dans ses effets directes sur l'homme et les animaux," Paris, 1855, p. 325.

[4] *Hygiène pratique des femmes*, Paris, 1875, p. 78.

[5] *Signs and Symptoms of Pregnancy*, Philadelphia, 1857, p. 29.

[6] *Path. Anat.*, vol. i, p. 11.

Carpenter (*Physiology*) says, "No sound physiologist of the present day is likely to fall into the popular error of supposing that marks upon the infant are to be referred to some transient though strong impression upon the imagination of the mother; but there appears to be a sufficient number of facts on record to prove that the habitual mental conditions on the part of the mother may have influence enough at an early period of pregnancy to produce bodily deformities or peculiar tendencies. But, whatever the impression transmitted, it must be of a character to modify the nutritive materials supplied by the mother to the fetus."

This is an extremely important admission on the part of an excellent and conservative physiologist. The important points to be noted are that the causes should be habitual, acting on the system of the fetus through the blood, and acting early in pregnancy.

Dalton[1] says, "There is now little room for doubt that various deformities and deficiencies of the fetus, comformably to the popular belief, really originate in certain cases from nervous impressions, such as disgust, fear, or anger, experienced by the mother."

Flint[2] says, "It is often the case that when a child is born with a deformity the mother imagines that she can explain it by some impression received during pregnancy, which she only recalls after she knows that the child is deformed. Still there are cases which can not be doubted, but which in the present state of our knowledge of development and the connection between the mother and the fetus we can not attempt to explain." MM. Grimaud de Caux et Martin St. Ange[3] say on this subject, "Pregnancy is a function of the woman, as are digestion and the acts of secretion of various kinds, and, if these latter are affected by moral impressions, why should not the former be also similarly acted upon? If the composition of the blood be altered, is it possible that the fetus which is being developed

---

[1] *Physiology*, sect. iv.   [2] *Text-book of Physiology*, p. 896.
[3] *Histoire de la génération de l'homme*, etc., Paris, 1849, p. 252.

in the mother's womb by this fluid should not undergo detrimental changes."

Devay[1] says, "Both reason and experience establish the fact that mental impressions of the mother may influence the fetus so as to give rise to an aberration of which *the form will correspond to the emotion acting upon the mother, and that there is consequently no doubt that deformed infants are thus produced.*"

I may add the names of Isidore Geoffroy Saint-Hilaire,[2] Allen Thomson,[3] and Hammond,[4] all of whom express their belief in the positive influence of maternal impressions on the fetus.

It will be observed that all who disbelieve in this doctrine base their skepticism on what they regard as physiological reasoning, and chiefly on the assertion that there is no direct nerve communication between the maternal and fetal system, and that, therefore, nerve impressions can not be transmitted to the fetus. Deformities, they urge, are due to arrest of development, but no one has brought forward any sound physiological reason why this arrest of development may not have been caused by maternal impressions, affecting fetal nutrition by their influence on the maternal blood, as well as by falls, injuries, diseases, intra-uterine amputations by ligation of the umbilical cord, and the various other causes which have been assigned. Those numerous changes in fetal development where the effect corresponds with known maternal impressions, of which hundreds perhaps have been published, are considered as simply coincidences. But if mathematical calculation could be made as to the chances for such a coincidence, I believe that the odds would be so enormous as to be almost beyond enumeration. My personal acquaintance with the profession leads me to

---

[1] *Traité spéciale d'hygiène des familles,* Paris, 1858, p. 329.

[2] *Hist. gén. et partic. des anomalies de l'organisation chez l'homme et les animaux,* Bruxelles, 1837, tome iii, p. 377.

[3] *Cycloped. of Anatomy and Physiology,* vol. ii, p. 474.

[4] *Treatise on Insanity,* p. 2.

suppose that a very large majority of obstetricians utterly disbelieve in this influence, and I ascribe this skepticism to the fact that, while they find this belief almost universal, to such an extent as to cause great anxiety in many of their patients, especially if they have been subjected to any strong emotion, yet the verification of this apprehension is so extremely rare that probably not one in a hundred of practicing obstetricians ever meets with a convincing case. How frequently after the birth are the questions asked, Is the child perfect? Has it any marks?

Extremely rare as is the occurrence of cases which prove the result of this influence, yet I think the fact is so well proved by sufficient authentic evidence as to make it as certain as any other fact which can not be explained by science, and there are many such. Indeed, in the light of all the evidence which has been accumulated on this point, it seems to me as reasonable to deny the occurrence of earthquakes because philosophy has not yet been able to give a satisfactory explanation of their cause.

I think that the subject has been obscured by the tendency to restrict the term " maternal impressions " to purely emotional causes, and that it really includes those which have a physical as well as psychical origin. Indeed, we have some reason for believing that these causes may act effectively on the ovules before fecundation, or even modify the action of the ovary in the performance of its specific function of forming and developing ovules. The idea was first suggested to me by the following case, well known to several others besides myself:

CASE I.—In February, 1859, I was requested by a well-known physician of this city to visit with him his niece, a young lady, eighteen years of age, and an only child. She had been very peculiarly insane for nine weeks, and had been visited by two prominent alienists, Dr. Benjamin Ogden and Dr. Tilden Brown, who had suggested that her mental condition might possibly be due to some uterine trouble. Previous to this illness she had been always of a bright, happy

11

temperament, fond of study and reading, and was regarded by
her teachers as unusually clever in her studies, and as possessing
quite a remarkable talent for music. The history given me was
this: During the preceding Christmas holidays she was taken
for the first time to the theatre, and witnessed the play of " Our
American Cousin," which was then on the stage at Laura Keene's
theatre, with a cast which has never since been equaled. She
was greatly excited and slept none that night, and for a day or
two talked of nothing else, until she was sharply reproved for
this by both her father and mother. From this time she entirely ceased talking, rarely answering in the briefest terms
any question, but passed her whole time, except when prevented, in writing letters to Lord Dundreary, who was to her a
real personage, and not Sothern the actor. It was said that she
must have written hundreds of these letters, which were filled
with expressions of a sentimental love, quotations from the
Songs of Solomon, Bailey's *Festus*, and such writings, but
never expressed sexual passion. Both her mother and her nurse,
who had been her wet-nurse in infancy, and had always been
with her, assured me that there never was the slightest erotic
manifestation or indelicacy of either language or conduct, and
that there was no reason to suspect self-abuse. Menstruation
had begun when she was thirteen, and had always been regular
until the previous September, when, without any known cause,
it had ceased. So far as could be learned, she never had had
leucorrhea. For some weeks it had been difficult to get her to
take sufficient food for existence, and for one period of four
days all that she did take was forced down. Her general health
improved greatly under constitutional treatment, and early in
May she menstruated for three days, and in June for five days,
her normal period. She had entirely ceased to talk about Lord
Dundreary, and would sometimes occupy herself in reading or
fancy needle-work, but was generally *distrait*, listless, and taci-
turn. I now urged an entire change by a trip to Europe, but
three years of her childhood had been passed there, and she
most strenuously objected to leaving home. She finally was
induced to consent by the argument that her father, who had
long been a sufferer from rheumatic gout, might be cured by a
course of baths at Wiesbaden. After leaving this watering-

place, they traveled in Switzerland, and then went to Italy for the winter. During this time her health, both of body and mind, was entirely restored. While in Rome she met with a young man, whose family were well known to her father and mother, and who was personally agreeable to them, and they consented to an engagement ; but, fearing a possible recurrence of her former maladies, they insisted, without giving any reason, that the marriage should be postponed for a year. The mother afterward told me that her husband and herself often seriously discussed the question whether it was not their duty to inform the young man of the previous peculiar illness of their daughter, but they could never bring themselves to do it. The second year was passed very much like the first, by a stay of six weeks in Wiesbaden, and then traveling in Rome for the winter. The civil war of this country greatly distressed the father, who had large interests in the South, and in May, 1861, the family made their arrangements to return home ; but the father was taken ill and died in Paris. Before his death, he foresaw the end, and advised immediate marriage, which took place in Paris. The family returned to New York in September. Early in February, 1863, I attended the daughter in her first confinement with a fine, healthy boy. When this child began to walk and to talk, on account of certain peculiarities his father began to call him Dundreary, greatly to the terror and distress of his grandmother and the old nurse, who feared that it would awaken painful memories in the daughter, who never once had alluded to her former illness. The boy's walk was always by a little skip, with the left foot forward. He had a very curious stammer, and his left brow was drawn down with the lids partially closed. The grandmother several times urged me to remonstrate with his father for calling him by such a name, telling me, with tears in her voice, that her daughter also was getting the habit of calling him so, and that his little playfellows called him " Dunny." I, however, persuaded her that silence on the subject was the part of wisdom. This is the only child that the lady has ever had. The child, now twenty-three, was educated abroad, and I saw him for the first time in several years last winter on the street, and then noticed that his left eyebrow had much the appearance which we see in Englishmen who are in the habit of wearing one eye-glass, and that his first two or three steps after stopping were with a little skip, his left foot forward, but he seems to have quite overcome the habit of stammering.

I have no theory to offer in regard to this case, but will simply ask if it be possible that the condition of the nervous system during insanity acted so effectively on the ovarium as to modify the development of the ovule which was fecundated several years subsequently, and thus caused the peculiarities of the child after birth. Darwin[1] says that "it is even probable that either the male or female sexual elements, or both, before their union, may be affected in such a manner as to lead to modifications in organs developed at a late period of life, in nearly the same manner as a child may inherit from his father a disease which does not appear until old age."

Case II.—A lady, a typical brunette, was first married in 1850 to a gentleman who was an equally typical blonde. She was never pregnant by him, and he died of phthisis in 1856. She married in 1861 a former partner of her first husband, and a double second cousin of herself, that is, the father of one and the mother of the other were first cousins. Her husband is as marked a brunette as herself. Her first child was born April, 1862, and has very light, almost white, hair, eyebrows and eyelashes. The extraordinary resemblance to the first husband is often spoken of by acquaintances, and I have often been asked how I accounted for it. I must say that I do not see the resemblance, except in the coloring and the habit of incessantly winking, which the daughter has in common with the first husband. But the curious point is, that all known relatives of both husband and wife are brunettes. I may add that three children which the lady has had since the birth of these first are brunettes with very dark complexions.

Many analogous cases have occurred with animals. The case of the Arabian chestnut mare of Lord Morton, which

[1] *The Variations of Animals and Plants*, etc., Appleton & Co., vol. ii, p. 257.

bore a hybrid to a quagga, and afterward produced two colts by a black Arabian horse which were striped, and had other distinctive marks of the quagga, is often quoted.[1]

Darwin[2] mentions a similar case in a horse bred by Lord Mostyn, which had previously borne a foal by a quagga. The same fact is known in regard to the influence transmitted by a first impregnation to subsequent progeny[3] of many animals.[4] Darwin says, "Similar cases have so frequently occurred that careful breeders avoid putting a choice female of any animal to an inferior male, on account of the injury to her subsequent progeny which may be expected to follow." He adds, "Some physiologists have attempted to account for these remarkable results from a previous impregnation, by the imagination of the mother having been strongly affected ; but it will hereafter be seen that there are very slight grounds for any such belief. Other physiologists attribute the result to the close attachment and freely intercommunicating blood-vessels between the modified embryo and mother. But the action of foreign pollen on the ovarium, seed-coats, and other parts of the mother-plant strongly supports the belief that

[1] *Philos. Trans.*, 1821, p. 20.

[2] *The Variation of Animals and Plants under Domestication*, Appleton & Co., New York. Vol. i, p. 435.

[3] *Idem*, note, p. 436, in which instances of this result are quoted in mares, sheep, sows, and dogs.

[4] Two years ago I was visiting a place in England whose owner had a great fondness for breeding horses, cattle, and dogs of the purest blood. From him I learned much that was most interesting and new to me, in regard to the care taken in securing the propagation of the best, and he told me a very curious story of one of his dogs. I wrote to him this summer, asking if he would kindly give me the story in writing, as I wished to be perfectly accurate in the use of the fact. The following is an extract from his reply:

"I was riding on horseback through a small village on my estate, and had with me a highly-bred greyhound bitch which was in heat. As we went by the blacksmith's shop, a number of mongrels ran out and after the bitch. My groom and myself whipped all off except a pertinacious little ugly cur, who ran along for a mile and a half, but *never touched the bitch*. He then got so tired with the race and the beating that he left. When the bitch got home, she was put with a dog of her own breed, but when she cast her puppies they were the image of the ugly little cur."

with animals the male element acts directly on the female, and not through the crossed embryo."

I will now relate three cases which have occurred in my own practice, where the evidence of the influence of maternal impressions seems to me irresistible.

CASE III.—A lady, the mother of four children, the youngest ten years of age, had, in each of her pregnancies, suffered to a severer degree than most women from nausea and vomiting up to the sixth month. At a very early period of her fifth pregnancy (it is certain that it was in the first month) her eldest daughter, aged fifteen, went into a jeweler's with some companions and they had their ears pierced for rings. Both ears became inflamed and suppurated, and they were a long time in healing. The sight of this daughter, the sound of her voice, or even the mention of her name, always brought on most violent retching and vomiting, and this was so severe and persistent as to dangerously interfere with her nutrition. The daughter was sent away to make a long visit at the house of her uncle. She was brought home fully a month after her mother's nausea had entirely ceased. The ears had become perfectly well; but when she entered the house and her mother threw her arms around her, to welcome her, the vomiting at once returned, and continued so incessant and distressing that I was extremely anxious for several days as to the result. The daughter was again sent away, and remained until after the birth of the child. I did not reach the house until two hours after the child was born, and the mother was then quietly sleeping. A very dear friend of hers was at the house, the mother of one of the Fellows of this Society, who took me into an adjoining room to see the baby, and pointed out the lobes of its ears, which had the appearance of having been bored. She then showed me that each ear had an aperture, and passed through one a twisted thread. My impression is, that it was only tried on one ear from the fear of making the child cry and awaking the mother. But it was a subject of common remark with many friends, during the childhood of this infant, that his ears looked as though they had been bored, and I well remember that his father, a graduate of West Point, and a dis-

398

tinguished officer in our army, told me that, when this son entered as a cadet, one of the officers of this institution asked him "if his son's ears had been bored on account of weak eyes."[1] I must add that the mother, a very bright, intelligent woman, was greatly amused and interested by these peculiarities in the ears of her child ; but she always assured me that the anticipation that he would be marked in this way had never once entered her mind.

CASE IV.—A lady was married at the age of twenty, when her father made her a present of a house. She was absent on her wedding-trip for two weeks, and then went to the Gramercy Park Hotel to stay while her house was being repainted and decorated, and such furniture as she wished was selected and purchased. She had not menstruated since her marriage. On her first day at this hotel she went to the *table d'hôte* and found herself seated opposite a gentleman with three daughters who all had hare-lips. (This family was well known.) The first glance at them made her so faint that she at once left the table, and always after took her meals in her private rooms until she moved to her own house. She never mentioned her reasons for this even to her husband, nor had she any suspicion that she was then pregnant. I attended her in her confinement, which was a very laborious one, and she was delivered by the forceps, profoundly under the influence of chloroform. I saw at once that the child had a double hare-lip, and sent for Dr. Carnochan, who had finished the operation before she awoke from her chloroform sleep. On becoming conscious she demanded to see her child, saying that she was certain that it had a hare-lip. I refused to allow her to see the child until the next morning, and gave her a full opiate. The operation was remarkably successful, the mother did well, and the child, now nearly thirty, would not attract attention by the appearance of his lip, but only by an indistinct articulation of a few words.[2]

---

[1] It is a popular belief in New England, and perhaps some other parts of the country, that boring of the ears and wearing rings in them is a great remedy for weak eyes.

[2] I may here say that this is the only case which has occurred in my practice in which any peculiarity of the child had been anticipated by the mother, although the apprehension has been strongly expressed by many. I may also add

CASE V.—Mrs. ——, who had been married but a few weeks, was at the theatre with her husband and other friends. Something, she knew not what, vexed him, and he placed the point of his elbow on her hand, which was resting on the arm of her seat, and held it so firmly that she could not draw it away. Not wishing to make a scene in the theatre, she bore it silently until she fainted. The fingers were much swollen and very painful for several days. She never lived with her husband afterward, and subsequently obtained a divorce on the ground of cruelty.

Thirty-five weeks and three days after the theatre incident I attended her, when she gave birth to a son. On the left hand, the first and second phalanges of all the fingers and the thumb were absent, looking as if they had been amputated. She has lived abroad most of the time since the divorce. I saw her in London, in August last, for the first time in several years, and examined the hand of the lad, now fifteen years old, and unusually bright and clever. In reply to a question from me, which she says I had repeatedly asked in the infancy of her child, she assured me that never once during her pregnancy had the thought occurred to her that her child would be born with this deficiency.

Dr. Hunter McGuire, of Richmond, Va., recently related to me the following case of which he was cognizant :

that this is the only case of hare-lip that has occurred in my private practice ; but I have seen it in three other cases in consultation, in two of which I delivered by forceps and in one by version. Not one occurred during my long service in charge of the lying-in wards of Bellevue Hospital. I may be pardoned for a few words not pertinent to the subject of this paper. In the beginning of my obstetrical practice I made a very careful study of those emergencies which may suddenly arise and demand prompt action, in order to establish in my mind the fixed principles which should govern me without doubt or hesitation. One of them was the question whether hare-lip should be operated on immediately after birth or delayed until a later period. My decision was in accordance with my action in the present case. The same course was followed in two of the cases which I saw in consultation, and with a success which caused no regret. But in the third my friend, the attending physician, held very decided convictions that the operation should be postponed until a later period. Dr. James L. Little, who was called upon afterward to operate a second time, informed me that the result of the first was very unsatisfactory.

"A slave, in order to avoid being sold to another family, cut off one of his great toes with an axe in the presence of his pregnant mistress. When her child was born one foot was without a toe, and the stump greatly resembled that of the negro. Dr. McGuire was not able to inform me as to the period of pregnancy when the self-amputation of the negro occurred, but he added that he could not learn that the lady had ever anticipated the mutilation of her child."

In closing this paper, I beg to quote the two following sentences from an editorial article on this subject in the *British Medical Journal* of June 16th, 1877, p. 748, which seems to me very sound : "When, in the early weeks, structural development is proceeding at no tardy rate, an interference of nutrition of the mother can not but impress the fetus detrimentally, and the organ interfered with would be that one in the condition of most active development, or that which could less easily bear any arrest, however transient, with impunity."

Again : "Then, too, although no nervous connection has been demonstrated to exist between the mother and fetus, yet the latter possesses nerves ; and alterations of the nutrient power of the mother can not but act on the nerves that are governing, though it may be only to a slight extent, the growth of the fetus itself."

I have not deemed it wise to occupy the time of the Society by quoting any of the very numerous cases which have been before published as supposed proofs of the influence of maternal impressions. But I have great pleasure in acknowledging my indebtedness to Dr. H. C. Coe for the trouble that he has taken in looking up for me and verifying the literature of the subject. As many may wish to read for themselves this curious collection of proofs or coincidences, as each may regard them, I have appended a reference to the most important cases published within the past quarter of a century.

APPENDIX.

The following paper is taken from a small volume[1] published forty-three years ago, and now out of print, and is the first medical paper ever published by Dr. Sayre. On account of the originality and ingenuity of the theory which it propounds, I think all will deem it well worthy of being rescued from the oblivion of a non-medical work and made known to the profession :

"NEW YORK, *May 10, 1843.*

"Agreeable to your request, I send you my *theory* explanatory of the formation of *nævi materni,* or the influence of the mind of the mother in determining the developments of the *fetus in utero.*

"It has been for a long time a disputed point whether the mother had any influence upon the *fetus in utero,* in causing it to be marked, or in any way deformed, by having any strong impression made upon her mind during gestation ; and whether there was any similarity in these marks, or deformities, and the impression under which she labored.

"It is now, however, almost incontestably proved, and generally admitted, from the number of cases that have occurred in which the mother has, previous to the birth of the child, described exactly the position and character of the deformity which has afterward been found to exist, and agree so exactly with her previous description, that it becomes our duty to inquire into the *causes* that have produced these effects, and ascertain, if possible, the intricate sympathies existing between the mother and child, and the *laws* which govern these sympathies, and see if they can not be converted to some good account.

"If, for instance, we find that from some horrid sight, or loathsome object, presented to the female during pregnancy, she becomes impressed with the idea that at birth her child will bear this or that particular deformity, and time develops her fears to have been well grounded, and her suppositions prove true, it is but reasonable to suppose, from analogy, that

[1] *Facts and Arguments on the Transmission of Intellectual and Moral Qualities from Parents to Offspring.* (Name of author not given on title-page or in the book.) New York : T. Winchester, publisher. 1844. Second edition.

could we have made an *equally strong impression* of a *different kind* we should have produced a *different* kind of growth or formation, *according to the impression under which she labored.*

"Taking, then, this principle for granted, which I hope hereafter to prove true by facts, it becomes our duty to surround the female during pregnancy with every object which would have a tendency to develop both the *physical* and *mental* frame of the fetus, in the most perfect degree, and of the highest order.

"We all admit that it is by the *nerves* we receive impressions ; that it is *through* them that the *will* is conveyed to the different parts of the system ; that the *vessels* are the *executors* of the will ; and that secretion, absorption, the different growths, developments, etc., are the *result* of this work carried on, or performed by the *vessels* and *controlled* by the *nerves ;* or, in other words, the *brain* and *nervous mass superintends*, or *orders*, the *vessels obey these orders*, and the different growths, etc., are the *result* of the work.

"If, then, the *nervous* system or *controlling* power be *disturbed*, the *orders* are given *wrong ;* the *vessels obeying* these *wrong* orders, and *acting* in *compliance with them*, an *unnatural* or *deformed product is the necessary result.*

"We all admit again that the child has *not* an *independent* existence until *extra-uterine* life ; neither has it an independent *will ;* but *it* also is dependent upon the mother, is under her control, and must, of course, *act in accordance with hers.*

"If, then, the will, thought, impressions, mind, or *controlling power*, so to speak, exists entirely in the brain and nervous masses, when endowed with life (as without them we can receive no impressions) ; and if the *vessels* act entirely under the control of these *nerves*, and the different *growths, developments*, etc., are the *result* of the *action* of *these vessels*, and if the *will* of the *child* is *dependent entirely upon that of the mother*, it follows, as a matter of course, the *developments* of the *child being the result of the action of its vessels*, which vessels are controlled by its nervous system, and it again entirely dependent on the mother, that these various developments must be in accordance with the various impressions made upon her mind.

"This, it seems to me, is the most satisfactory explanation of the various morbid developments that have occurred in children born of mothers who, during pregnancy, have labored under some strong mental impression as regards their child's deformity, and who have previous to delivery accurately described the deformity which has afterward been found to exist.

"Of the proof of this we need only refer to Dr. Elliotson's work,[1] who gives some well-described cases. I am also permitted to refer to Dr. Gilman,[2] Professor of Obstetrics in this city, who can confirm it by a number of cases;[3] and I can corroborate it by one that came under my own observation.

"If, then, this explanation be admitted, I think the immense importance of my first position clearly proved, viz., that of surrounding the female, during this most interesting period, with every influence which would have a tendency to produce the most favorable impressions for the most perfect development of the fetus, both *physically* and *mentally.*

"Again, it is generally admitted concerning any system, whether nervous, vascular, or muscular, that it is capable of performing function in an exalted or diminished degree, according to its development, as regards strength and activity.

"If, then, we admit that by the *exercise of organs* we *increase* their *power of performing function,* as is proved by comparing the arm of the blacksmith with that of the writing-master; and also that the *brain* is the seat of the intellect or mind, as proved by acephelous children, who, having no brain, are deficient in its Godlike attributes; and if the *mental* organs can be *increased* in *power as well* as the *physical,* and if the *child's* organs are developed in *harmony* with the *mother's;* with what vast importance do we find this interesting question surrounded, and what strong appeals from future generations are made upon the fondly expecting-to-be mother to exercise both her *physical* and *mental* powers to their greatest degree,

[1] Elliotson's *Physiology.*

[2] Formerly Professor of Obstetrics and Diseases of Women in the College of Physicians and Surgeons, New York.

[3] "These cases, and those referred to in Dr. Elliotson's work, are too distressing and painful in their nature for insertion in a work intended for the perusal of the most sympathetic and sensitive portion of the sex."

in order that she may be the happy bearer of an offspring gifted in these essentials for future usefulness in their highest degree of development, both as regards strength and activity.

"If these few hasty thoughts shall have a tendency to awaken in mothers an interest in this most interesting but too long neglected question, the writer will be more than amply repaid by the consciousness of having conferred a boon upon future generations.   Lewis A. Sayre."

REFERENCE TO PUBLISHED CASES.

British Medical Journal, October 5, 1878, p. 543, one case by Dr. Glyn Whittle.

British Medical Journal, July 14, 1877, p. 36, two cases by W. Whitelaw.

British Medical Journal, July 14, 1877, p. 67, one case by William Smyth.

British Medical Journal, July 28, 1877, p. 96, one case quoted from *Carter on Hysteria,* by William Sedgwick.

British Medical Journal, August 25, 1877, p. 282, one case by Dr. Augustus Hess.

British Medical Journal, November 3, 1877, p. 655, two cases by Dr. Jasper Cargill.

Medical and Surgical Reporter, January 27, 1877, six cases by Dr. J. S. Hill.

"Proceedings of Philadelphia County Medical Society," *Philadelphia Medical Times,* November 25, 1876, eight cases reported by Dr. William T. Taylor.

Cincinnati Lancet and Observer, one case reported by Dr. C. O. Wright, who also quotes two from Montgomery, *Signs and Symptoms of Pregnancy,* discussion on Dr. Wright's paper.

American Journal of Obstetrics, vol. i, 1878, p. 634, in which our President, Dr. Thad. A. Reamy, reports one case.

British Medical Journal, August 26, 1876, p. 270, one case reported by Dr. W. J. H. Wood.

British Medical Journal, March 24, 1877, p. 376, one case reported by T. D. Saunders.

The *Boston Medical and Surgical Journal,* vol. xx, 1839, p. 98, quotes from the *Southern Medical and Surgical Journal,* vol. iii, 1839, p. 381, the story of "The Snake Man."

Since the meeting of the Society, and since an abstract of the foregoing paper has appeared in several medical journals, I have received numerous letters from different parts of the country, twenty-six in number, describing cases of supposed maternal impressions on the fetus. The following three cases are the most striking. The first was related to me by my friend Dr. A. Brayton Ball, of this city, who afterward, by my request, had the kindness to give me the statement in writing.

"The facts in the case of 'maternal impression,' which I mentioned to you a few days ago, are briefly as follow : Mrs. B., a woman of highly nervous temperament, pregnant between two and three months with her first child, was much startled by seeing a child about ten years of age with an hypertrophied, prolapsed tongue.

"The child's appearance was extremely repulsive, and so shocked Mrs. B. that she nearly fainted.

"From this time on she was apprehensive that her child would be 'marked' in the same way, and this fear was shared by her aunt, who was present when the incident occurred, though the matter was never afterward referred to between them during the pregnancy. At birth, Mrs. B's. child presented exactly the same deformity. The tongue was hypertrophied, and hung down over the lower lip, but with this exception was perfectly formed. The tongue remained outside of the mouth until the child was several years old, and then gradually retreated into the cavity, but has always remained sufficiently large to interfere with the proper enunciation of words. No similar case has been known in either branch of the family, and several children have been born since then, all perfectly developed. I regret that I can not state the exact period of pregnancy when the 'maternal impression' was made, as it happened nearly thirty years ago, but the date probably fell between the limits I have mentioned. Mrs. B., though not a patient of mine at the time, became so afterward, and her account of the case agrees in every particular with that given me by her aunt, who was with her when the incident occurred, and at her confinement.

" I make no comment on the case, except to say that I regard it as in the highest degree improbable that the only relation between the two events is that of mere coincidence."

The history of the following case I received in a letter from Dr. Thomas W. Shaw, of Pittsburg, Pa.

"A singular and typical case occurred in my practice recently, that stamps the fact of such mental impressions beyond a doubt.

"A lady residing in the country, a short distance from the city, about six or eight weeks advanced in pregnancy, was horrified to find that one of her children, while playing about the stable, had the tine of a pitchfork run through the right hand where the carpal bones and forearm join. At the normal end of gestation I delivered her of a full-grown, healthy male child, who had the right hand *entirely absent.* The stump was a perfect amputation, with a very small excrescence that showed rudimentary fingers and thumbs.

"She remarked to me at once, that was just where she thought ' Jimmy's hand was cut off with the pitchfork.' "

The following is from Dr. J. A. Robison, of Chicago, Ill.

"As accumulative evidence for your paper on the 'Influence of Maternal Impressions on the Fetus,' I trust you will pardon me for relating the following : Mr. K.'s first wife was killed by the cars, both lower limbs being amputated. His second wife bore him a son with the lower extremities amputated above the knees."

This last case I regard as the most striking confirmation of the theory of Darwin, quoted in the paper, as to the direct influence of the male element on the female, that has ever been published in regard to the human race.

The question is naturally suggested, whether the impressions which led to the absence of the lower limbs in the fetus were not paternal rather than maternal.

DISCUSSION.

Dr. S. C. Busey, of Washington.—What I may have to say on this interesting question will be supplementary to the paper which you have just heard read. It is a subject difficult to discuss, because the relation of cause and effect between the single fact of the existence of a deformity and the alleged circumstance of a mental impression can not be proved. We have, however, some facts, more data, and many coincidences ; and the object I have in view is to endeavor to present these evidences in such manner as may bring you to a conclusion similar to that of Dr. Barker and myself. I do not intend to offer any dogmatic conclusion, nor have I any positive convictions to present ; but I have a belief that there is some relation of cause and effect between the mental impressions of mothers and fetal deformities. This belief is something more than mere credulity, and in support of it I will submit several propositions.

First, any prevalent concurrent belief must be based upon an element of truth. The circumstance to which Dr. Barker refers, of the exhibition at the watering-troughs of variously colored rods of poplar and chestnut to the flocks of Laban, and the creation of a race of "ring-streaked, speckled, and spotted" cattle, is, perhaps, the first recorded illustration of the effect upon the offspring of an impression made, during gestation, upon the parent. This is, perhaps, as generally and firmly believed as any other fact recorded in Genesis. It was, moreover, at that time, a common belief that animals were affected in this manner, and a commentator remarks that sheep were the most impressible of the lower order of animals. From that early date to the present, this belief has been continuously growing more prevalent. With the advances in civilization, learning, and science it has continued to increase in prevalence. Now it is a fixed and permanently accepted truth with a vast majority of intelligent women. Among men it is very generally accepted ; and as the evidences and facts accumulate, many more medical men concede the possibility of such a relation of cause and effect. If it were absolutely destitute of an element of truth, is it possible that a belief having its origin in such an apparently trivial circumstance as the trick of Jacob could have become a fixed belief in the female mind, and, notwithstanding the numerous assaults made and ridicule hurled against it by medical men, continuously acquire prevalence among all classes of people?

The second proposition is that, as in the physical world there is no effect without a cause, so it is likewise true in the world of life that there can be no effect without a cause. Nature commits no freaks. As an abstract proposition, this is probably acceded to; but it is alleged that, as deformities and blemishes occur more frequently in the vegetable kingdom, where there is neither intellect, instinct, nor brain, therefore the condition of mind and the possibility of mental impression can not enter as a factor in producing like results in the human being. To my mind this is a strong argument in favor of this relation of cause and effect. The deviations in form which occur much more frequently in the vegetable kingdom than in any other, are produced by extraneous influences not less subtle, occult, or inexplicable than the effect of mental shock and persistent mental impression upon a fetus deriving its sustenance from the mother, whose mind is indelibly impressed with a certain conviction that an injury to her offspring must follow. We are constantly witnesses of the deviations in form in vegetable life caused by conditions of the atmosphere, climate, season, heat, moisture and dryness, soil and locality. We can not have failed to observe the variations in form, in the general characteristics of growth and development, in the colors, fragrance, and beauty which the floriculturist has produced in many flowering plants, and the alterations in size, taste, and nutrient qualities of edible vegetables and fruits produced by the horticulturist. These changes, alterations, and improvements exhibit the effect of extraneous causes, either directly managed by the intellectual master-man, or by some condition of the natural elements which, as yet, we do not understand. No one can expect to find in the same field of wheat every head the same size, nor every grain in each head of the same grade and weight. No one can expect to find upon the fruit-bearing tree every blossom alike, nor every fruit of the same flavor and size. No

12

one expects to see upon the blossoming rose-bush every bud of equal size, with every petal of exact shape and shade of color. Neither does any one expect to find among any species of thorough-bred animals uniformity of size, weight, and color ; nor equal speed and power.   We see these variations ; we witness the effects, and reason from effect to cause.   In a vast majority of instances we fail to demonstrate the relation of cause and effect ; and, when in the comparatively few cases this relation is established, it is the logical or practical deduction from the multiplication of like variations under like circumstances.

The third proposition is as follows : If in a single case the relation of cause and effect can be demonstrated between the fact of fetal deformity and the circumstance of maternal impression, that one case must be accepted as proof, and the inference must be clear that if one such case does occur, others may.

Moreover, if there are any number of cases in which it can be shown that an impression was received, and that there followed a deformity of the fetus corresponding in essential particulars with the maternal impression, it must be conceded that the relationship of cause and effect is presumptively established. This latter proposition can be illustrated by a number of instances ; none more marked, perhaps, than the one related by Dr. Barker in his paper—that of pressure made upon the hand of the mother, while sitting in the theatre, and the birth of her child with absence of the first and second phalanges of the left hand.

All the cases may be divided into four classes :

1. Those classed as coincidences.   If there were no others, the theory might be discarded.

2. Those in which there was a maternal impression and fetal blemish or deformity, with absence of correspondence.   These two classes are constantly referred to in proof of the theory of chance, or mere coincidence, and, considered without reference to other evidences, they would attract but little attention.   But Nature does not uniformly present results in a definite form and manner.   The ultimate fact can not always be established without consideration of the trivial evidences which, when

grouped in orderly arrangement, constitute a continuous chain
of evidence, leading in the direction of a definite conclusion.
These two classes should be regarded as the initial stage in the
process of inductive reasoning by which I am attempting to
establish a conclusion, and must, at least, be accepted as proof
of the presence of an effect, even though the cause of the
blemish or abnormality may not be so manifest.

3. This class includes those cases in which there is no previous mental impression or conviction, but correspondence between an observation and fetal deformity. The mother did
not receive a shock, was not disturbed concerning the probable deformity of her child, but had observed a certain thing,
and when the child was born the deformity was present, corresponding with the observation. In such cases there is
neither maternal shock, fright, nor conviction, nevertheless
there is correspondence between the observation and fetal deformity. These circumstances remove such cases from the possibilities of freak, coincidence, or chance, and point directly to
some change in the complex economy of the pregnant woman,
produced by an extraneous influence, and transmitted to the
dependent fetus. Every one admits that virtues and vices,
whether hereditary or acquired, may be transmitted. If this
be true, why may not a vice of the animal economy, even
though originating during the progress of utero-gestation, influence the physical development of the fetus? In fact, such
an effect is not an uncommon occurrence. If the general development and formative energy of the fetus can be influenced
by the physical condition of the mother, why may not the development of some special part be influenced by some sudden
and unusual change or disturbance of the reproductive activities? If a father with a cleft palate or supernumerary digits
can beget a child with a cleft palate or supernumerary digits,
why may not a pregnant woman, whose impressible nature may
be greatly changed by trivial circumstances, transmit to the
formless embryo an impression, or the influence of a disgusting
observation upon her physical economy? If a child begotten
during the inebriation of the father may, and usually does,
suffer some evil effect, why may not the maternal economy,
changed by extraneous conditions, be equally effective in modi-

fying fetal development? It is not the alcohol, but its effect upon the man, that is transmitted. If a father with supernumerary digits may beget a child with like deformity, it does not follow that a pregnant woman who may have observed such a deformity in another person will give birth to a child with like deformity ; but may not the observation in each case be the element of causation ? The greater probability of such fetal deformity in cases where the father is thus afflicted may be the result of the more constant observation of the mother. These speculations might be multiplied *ad infinitum.* They do not demonstrate the relation of cause and effect, but they do establish a basis for a rational belief.

4. This class refers to the cases of correspondence between the maternal impression and the fetal deformity. I have not examined the literature of this subject very carefully, but will cite a few cases.[1] The first to which I will refer is the case reported by Dr. Goodell in the *American Journal of Obstetrics*, May, 1871, p. 131.

Dr. Goodell stated, that while he scouted the extravagant statements made by the laity with regard to the influence of maternal impressions upon the fetus, yet he was inclined to the belief that there is more in them than physiologists are willing to concede. In support of this he would narrate a remarkable case. It occurred in the family of a Fellow of the Obstetrical Society of Philadelphia, to which Dr. Goodell, with the permission of the father, had narrated the circumstances. They were published, but somewhat imperfectly, in the *American Journal of Obstetrics*, May, 1871, p. 131.

The lady menstruated for the last time May 6, 1870 ; and on July 7th her husband was invited to assist at the rite of circumcision in the family of a Hebrew friend, living directly opposite. The lady was intensely interested in the description of the operation, of which she demanded the minutest details, and which she deemed a very "cruel" one. It, indeed, made so great an impression upon her that for several days it was the constant burden of her thoughts and conversation. She would even wake up her husband at night to talk with him about the

[1] The illustrations cited comprise only those to be found in my private library I have not had time to refer to the library of the Surgeon-General's office.

cruelty of the rite and the sufferings of the child. As the result will show, her husband at that time took alarm lest this morbidness on his wife's part should affect the future child. She was delivered on February 6th, Dr. Goodell being in attendance. The child, a boy, was born during the momentary absence of the father, who was called out of the room to see an office-patient ; but he returned before the cord was cut, and immediately asked what the sex was, and whether the child was perfectly formed. Being on the further side of the bed, he could not see the child. Dr. Goodell replied that it seemed to be sound. " Examine the penis," anxiously demanded the father, "and see whether it is all right." The room being dark, Dr. Goodell could not see very well, but thought that he detected a hypospadias, and so informed the father. Without looking at the child, he at once said, " You don't mean hypospadias, but circumcision." Sure enough, upon a closer inspection, the glans penis was found exposed, while the retracted prepuce, adherent to the corona glandis, actually showed the yet granulating sore of what seemed to be a recent circumcision. Dr. Goodell stated that this case had converted him to the belief that there sometimes exists in the early months of gestation a relation of cause and effect between a maternal emotion, especially if of a powerful nature, and a birthmark.

Dr. Busey, continuing.—It does not seem possible that such precise correspondence between the maternal impression and the condition of the prepuce could have been a coincidence.

Case 2.—Ashburton Thompson (*Trans. Obstet. Soc. Lond.*, vol. xix, p. 94). A mother received at her door a visitor, who had in the median line of his neck an aperture where a tracheal tube could be worn ; in fact, it was a cleft left by such a tube. The mother was impressed with the conviction that her child would be deformed, and it was born with a cleft in the median line of its neck, almost identical in appearance with the observation.

Case 3.—The same author reports another case, in which the mother received during the same pregnancy two impressions at different times, and differing entirely in their nature.

Her child was born with two distinct deformities, corresponding with the separate impressions received. It is more logical to conclude that these effects were the results of the maternal impressions, than that two such remarkable coincidences should have occurred during the same pregnancy independently of the nervous perturbation and mental anguish which were known to be present.

Case 4.—A fetus,[1] at the fifth month, was born marked with a compact mass of hair continuous with the eyebrows, and extending evenly and uniformly over the whole forehead, which "gave the head a very singular expression, very closely resembling a squirrel." The mother stated that when "only a few weeks gone in pregnancy she had been greatly startled by a pet squirrel that had attempted to bite her."

This child also exhibited two well developed lower incisor teeth, which were ascribed to her "frequent repugnance at the sight of some poorly-constructed false teeth worn by her aunt."

Case 5.—The child of Mrs. T.[2] was born with a red mark on its back, and also a mark in the center of its forehead. The mother had, during the fourth month of her pregnancy, received a blow on her lumbar region, and a month later was struck on her forehead by something falling.

Coincidences may repeat themselves, but the chance of coincidence in such cases where there is direct correspondence between the maternal impression and the effect is infinitesimally small. If the facts as stated are correct, the relation between the phenomena is direct.

Case 6.—Fearn[3] reports the case of absence of the same metacarpal bone of the same hand of the child of a mother who witnessed the removal of the corresponding bone from the hand of her husband. She was much shocked and alarmed at the sight.

Case 7.—Dr. G.[4] sustained a fracture of "his leg, midway between the ankle and knee. His wife was about five months

[1] Stevens, *Obstet. Gaz.*, vol. iii, p. 465.
[2] Wilson, *Obstet. Jour.*, G. B. & I., vol. viii, p. 333.
[3] *Report Med. Ass. Ala.*, 1850.
[4] Dossey, *Trans. Med. Ass. Ala.*, 1850.

advanced in pregnancy. When the child of which she was pregnant was born, it had on the leg corresponding with the injured limb of the father, and at precisely the same spot, the appearance of a fracture of a limb, and there was also a decided shattering of the leg."

CASE 8.—A woman,[1] when three months pregnant, was frightened by the sight of a "dog's foot sticking through the crack of a door in her room." Her son was born with a deformed hand, bearing some resemblance to a dog's foot."

CASE 9.—"A lady,[2] three months advanced in pregnancy, saw a pig, driven furiously out of an inclosure, have its bowels torn out by the stake of a fence." She was greatly shocked, and fainted. "Her child, when born, had the entire front of the abdomen covered only by a thin film, and the intestines were visible through it."

CASE 10.—A pregnant woman[3] suddenly saw one of her children covered with blood by some accident. "The child she was carrying was born with a large red stain upon its face. This woman had not thought of or brooded over the occurrence, nor had she any apprehension that her infant would be marked."

CASE 11.—A pregnant mother[4] had one of her ears torn through by the forcible dragging away of one of her ear-rings. Her child was born with a fissure in the ear corresponding to the laceration in its mother's.

CASE 12.—Adams[5] delivered a child with a forearm terminating in a conical stump just above the wrist. The mother, during her pregnancy, had nursed a brother who had had his hand torn off by machinery, and the forearm afterward amputated. The malformation of the child was upon the same arm.

CASE 13.—A girl,[6] thirteen years old, very small and delicate for her age, had a middle finger upon one hand equal in size to that of a man. The corresponding metacarpal bone was also enlarged. The mother, during her pregnancy, had

[1] Baker, *Obstet. Gaz.*, vol. i, p. 347.
[2] Parker, *Amer. Jour. Med. Sci.*, vol. xxv, p. 360.
[3] Hayward, *Amer. Jour. Med. Sci.*, vol. xxv, p. 359.
[4] Doane, *Amer. Jour. Med. Sci.*, vol. xxv, p. 358.
[5] *Amer. Jour. Med. Sci.*, vol. xxv, 358.   [6] Jackson, *Ibid.*

for a long time dressed a felon or whitlow for an old uncle. "The affected finger corresponded to the one malformed in the case of the daughter. The operation was always disagreeable to her, as she was a woman of a nervous temperament."

CASE 14.—A lady,[1] when two months and a half pregnant, though not at the time aware of it, suddenly saw a man, recently killed, lying with one upper extremity exposed, bloody, and so twisted that the hand lay upon the upper part of the neck. At this sight she nearly fainted, was ill for a month, and during the remainder of her pregnancy could not banish the sight from her mind. She also feared danger to the child *in utero*. The infant exhibited an extensive blood-mark covering the back of the corresponding hand, and extending along the extremity to the shoulder, and somewhat upon the neck.

CASE 15.—A lady,[2] "four weeks after her marriage, saw a hen injured, by the breaking of one of its legs and the removal of the lower portion. She was exceedingly troubled at this, continually dwelt upon the subject, and insisted that her child would be deformed. The child, perfectly formed in other respects, exhibited upon one of its lower extremities simply a heel, and the rudiments of five toes with microscopic nails."

CASE 16.—Haldeman[3] was present at the birth of a child with absence of both parietal and upper three fourths of the frontal and occipital bones. The eyes were large, full, and bright. The superciliary ridges were very prominent, and densely covered with brown hair. When this child was shown to the mother, she exclaimed, "Oh! those are the eyes and brows of my brother John." John had been killed on a railroad, and the body was brought home for interment. Her second month of pregnancy had just passed when she saw the disfigured body, and the "ghastly face and eyebrows."

CASE 17.—A lady,[4] in the third month of her pregnancy, was so horrified at the appearance of her husband with a severe wound of his face, from which the blood was streaming,

---

[1] Jackson, *Amer. Jour. Med. Sci.*, vol. xxv, 358.
[2] Storer, *Amer. Jour. Med. Sci.*, vol. xxv, p. 356.
[3] *Obstet. Gaz.*, vol. v, p. 233.
[4] Hammond, *Psychological Journal*, vol. ii, 1868.

that she fainted, and subsequently had an hysterical attack. She "could not get rid of the impression the sight of her husband's bloody face made on her," and was afraid the child would be affected. It was born "with a dark red mark upon the face, corresponding in situation and extent with that which had been upon the father's face."

Case 18.—The wife[1] of a janitor of the College of Physicians and Surgeons, during her pregnancy, dreamed that she saw a man who had lost a part of the external ear. This dream made a great impression, and she mentioned it to her husband. The child was born with one ear "exactly like the defective ear she had seen in her dream." Dr. H. says it looked "as if a portion had been cut off with a sharp knife."

Case 19.—Stewart[2] was asked by a mother, immediately after the birth of her child, if the hands were well formed. Each hand had a supernumerary finger. The mother had been impressed by seeing a man with supernumerary fingers.

Case 20.—Taylor[3] has seen a child whose right hand was without fingers. The mother, early in her gestation, had been approached by a beggar, at the same time thrusting out a mutilated hand.

Case 21.—Miller[4] narrates the case of a man who, by an accident, had lost a part of his scalp. The ghastly sight so frightened his pregnant wife that she fainted, and the child was born with a bald spot on the top of his head, which is permanent.

Case 22.—A lady[5] whose mother had a cancerous tumor between her eyes, which she had seen frequently during the early months of her pregnancy, and about which she was much worried, gave birth to a child marked with a nævus "projecting out between the eyes, the size of a cherry."

Kerr reports a case, cited farther on, of a subsequent pregnancy without any maternal impression, but with the birth of a child with a blemish corresponding to an impression received during the previous pregnancy, and to the blemish on the child of that pregnancy.

[1] Hammond, *Psychological Journal*, vol. ii, 1868.
[2] *Amer. Jour. Obstet.*, vol. vi, p. 641.   [3] *Ibid.*
[4] *Obstet. Gaz.*, vol. iv, p. 67.
[5] Taylor, *Phila. Med. Times*, vol. vi, p. 307.

My credulity will not permit me to accept the doctrine of chance or coincidence in explanation of the correspondence between the maternal impressions and the fetal deformities in this group of cases. Upon the common doctrine of chance, the coincidence is too remarkable to be explained so readily, and, if one is suggestive, a second adds great weight, and a third is almost conclusive. The element of chance is eliminated by the great variety of causes with corresponding effects ; that is, in each of the foregoing cases the circumstance producing the impression is different ; yet in each case the effect is, to a greater or less degree, in correspondence with the causal circumstance. In a few of the cases the maternal impression was absent or forgotten. It is not improbable, in such cases, that the impression was effaced while the effect remained. The susceptibility and impressibility of pregnant women differ ; and the degree of mental anguish which different women may suffer from a similar disgusting and shocking observation will vary very greatly. The frequency of deformities of children after some shocking sight is the test of the truth of such cause of deformity. I can not trace the connection between the two phenomena in each case, but the effect succeeds the impression with more definiteness and precision than logical sequences usually do. I can not dismiss as mere chance the fact, that a mother who had received two separate and different impressions gave birth to a child marked by two distinct and corresponding deformities or blemishes ; nor the other fact, that a woman in two consecutive pregnancies gave birth to a child marked alike and corresponding to an impression received during the first pregnancy. In this connection it may be stated, that a mare once folded by a quagga will ever afterward, when folded by a stallion, bear striped colts ; and that the peculiarities of the first husband may be transmitted to the children of the widow by a second husband.

The effect of maternal impression may be more fully illustrated by the two following cases :

CASE 23.—Miller cites the case of Mrs. Wilkins,[1] who was suddenly seized with an uncontrollable longing for oysters, which could not be gratified, and, fearing that her intense

---

[1] *Obstet. Gaz.*, vol. iv, p. 67.

longing and disappointment would result in marking her child, she clapped her hand upon her buttocks, with the wish that it should be there, if it occurred. "The youngster was graced with a large and well-formed oyster upon his buttock." This case seems to prove too much, and would not have been referred to but that it is corroborated by the second case, which has been reported by a physician whose accuracy and fairness no one will doubt.

CASE 24.—Mrs. P.,[1] during the fourth month of her pregnancy, received a visitor whose face was disfigured by a mark of bright scarlet color, covering one half of her nose and extending on the cheek. The vivid account of her mortification and troubles, and of the failure of her efforts to have it removed, made a profound impression upon Mrs. P. When the visitor discovered that her friend was *enceinte,* she was horrified, and expressed fears that the baby would be marked as she was. Mrs. P. had the same fears, and remarked, " Well, if my baby is to be marked, I will mark it here," slapping herself on the right buttock. The child was born in November following, at full term, with a bright red mark on the right buttock, irregular in shape, and measuring two and a half inches. This case is reported by Dr. Prentiss, to whom the interview was related at the time of its occurrence, and who was present at the birth of the child.

These two cases are as closely allied as two earthquakes, occurring at different times and in widely separated localities, can be. The phenomena in both are so alike, that a like cause must have been common to both. Chance does not offer such precision. Freaks of Nature can not be so exact in concomitant detail. Similar coincidences vary sufficiently to dismiss the suggestion of like causes. After-thought is eliminated. There is no circumstance in the history of either case which attaches to heredity. If the first, by itself, should appear as an event proceeding from an unknown cause, the second is surrounded by all the conditions of intelligent deliberation.

These considerations may properly be followed by the citation of cases, which show that in the matter of maternal impressions, as in other physical conditions, like causes will produce like results.

[1] Prentiss, *Phila. Med. Times,* vol. xii, p. 385.

CASE 25.—A lady,[1] of a highly nervous and impressible temperament, with a cultivated mind, during the third or fourth month of her pregnancy was greatly disturbed and made sick and faint at the observation of her maid, who had been very badly burned about the eyes, causing considerable ecchymosis around the eyes, and active congestion of the conjunctiva. Her child was born marked upon the conjunctiva of both eyes.

CASE 26.—A pregnant woman,[2] whose little daughter fell against a hot cooking-stove and was badly burned on the face, hands, and arms, was greatly shocked and frightened. She frequently referred to the accident. Three months afterward her child was born marked with blisters on the lips, in the mouth, on the right ear, right elbow, both hands, each knee, and both ankles, resembling those caused by burns.

CASE 27.—Thirteen months after the birth[3] above referred to Mrs. H. gave birth to another child "marked precisely on the same parts and in the same manner as the above described one. The mother had for some years enjoyed good health, and was altogether free from disease at the time."

CASE 28.—The child of Mrs. M.[4] was born with two distinct vesicles on the left hand, one over the metacarpal bone, and the other on the phalanx of the index finger. Previous to the birth the mother had burned her hand, and the vesicles on her hand corresponded exactly with those on the hand of the child.

CASE 29.—A lady[5] who resided next door to a woman with a double hare-lip, and who had seen this person daily during her pregnancy, was firmly convinced that her child would be marked. It was born with a single hare-lip and cleft palate.

CASE 30.—A lady,[6] when two months pregnant, was impressed with the belief, by the sudden observation of a woman with a double hare-lip, that her child would be born with a similar deformity. It had a double hare-lip, and double cleft palate.

[1] Heddens, *Amer. Jour. Med. Sci.*, vol. xxiii, p. 558.

[2] Kerr, *Amer. Jour. Med. Sci.*, vol. xxxiv, p. 285.   [3] *Ibid.*

[4] Wilson, *Obstet. Jour.*, Great Britain and Ireland, vol. viii, p. 333.

[5] Baker, *Obstet. Gaz.*, vol. i, p. 347.   [6] *Ibid.*

CASE 31.—A woman,[1] between four and five months pregnant, was much impressed by the narration of the details of an operation for hare-lip. Her child was born with a hare-lip.

CASE 32.—A woman,[2] during her first pregnancy, having constantly before her a mental picture of a former fellow factory workman who had a hare-lip and cleft palate, was haunted with the idea that her child would have a deformed mouth. The child was born with a hare-lip and cleft palate.

CASE 33.—A woman[3] had been, during the early months of her pregnancy, disturbed by visits from a beggar-woman with a hare-lip, and had had a "horrible picture in her mind" ever since, and was distressed with the fear that her baby would "have a mouth like the old beggar-woman." Her fears were realized.

CASES 34 and 35.—Carnochan[4] gives an account of two cases of hare-lip. One, he states, was caused by a dentist, who roughly lifted the mother's lip at the sixth month of pregnancy ; the other, by the mother, at the eighth week of her pregnancy, seeing two girls suddenly enter her room who had been imperfectly relieved of the deformity.

It is claimed that maternal impressions can not exercise any agency in the production of fetal blemishes and deformities, because, in many cases, the time of their occurrence is either not coincident with the evolution of the part of the fetus affected, or is prior to the period when the ovum acquires an intimate attachment to the womb ; and because it has been proved that like deformities have been caused by injuries to the mother's abdomen, diseases of the uterus, secundines, and ovum, heredity, diathesis, the formation of fibrous bands, placental adhesions, pressure of a loop of the umbilical cord, and fracture.[5] To make this argument conclusive, it is furthermore maintained that malformations, for the most part, have their origin during the period of embryonic life in which the ovum is formless *blastema.*

[1] Channing, *Amer. Jour. Med. Sci.*, vol. xxv, p. 360.
[2] Jameson, *Amer. Pract.*, vol. xviii, p. 76.
[3] *Ibid.*
[4] *Richmond and Louisville Jour.*, vol. xxv, p. 424.
[5] Waddell, *Richmond and Louisville Med. Jour.*, vol. xxv, p. 420.

No one has claimed, nor even expressed a belief in the doctrine, that every case of fetal deformity is attributable to a maternal impression. Neither has any one who has assailed this belief or doctrine satisfactorily explained the cases in which the correspondence between the impression and the malformation has been demonstrated. It would be stretching one's credulity beyond the capacity of human intellect to assume that any one of the pathological conditions before enumerated could adapt a vice of conformation with such precision to either a previous or coincident maternal impression. Admitting, then, to its fullest extent, the argument of exclusion from lack of coincidence between the time of mental excitement or depression of the pregnant woman and the period of evolution of the part affected, and that like malformations may be caused by a variety of morbid conditions, there remain many cases, some of which have been cited, where prolonged mental emotion, protracted grief, distress, or shock, occasioned by some thrilling recital, disgusting observation, or sudden terror, offers the only explanation of the two corresponding phenomena.

If the etiology is incomplete without the factor of hereditary or acquired diathesis, the concession carries with it an element of causation even more occult and inexplicable than the theory of maternal impressions, because it implies that in those cases presenting the phenomenon of correspondence between the mental disturbance and fetal deformity, the diathetic vices must oftentimes, in some incomprehensible manner, verify the fears and predictions of the mother. If a diathesis is an admitted and recognized cause, why may not a shock, grief, sudden terror, mental distress, and anguish, which may affect a pregnant woman's health, deprive her of sleep, destroy her appetite, interfere with the assimilation of her food, disturb the secretions and produce emaciation, interrupt the progress of fetal growth and development? The proper nutrition of the fetus is certainly influenced by conditions of the mother's health, and it does not seem irrational to conclude that some delay, arrest, or misdirection[1] of fetal growth might result from such temporary interference with the developmental pro-

[1] Miller, *Trans. Obstet. Soc. Lond.*, vol. xxvi.

cesses as a deep and protracted mental impression might produce.

Dr. Arthur Mitchel, Commissioner in Lunacy for Scotland, seems to have demonstrated that such perturbations of a mother's mind may cause imperfections in the child. From four hundred and forty-three cases of idiocy or imbecility, examined with special reference to the effect of "strong mental emotion affecting pregnant women as a cause of idiocy in the offspring," he has selected the following six cases, which did not in the history of the children present any other circumstance which "had a preferential claim to be considered the cause of the imperfection."

CASE 36.—"A woman,[1] while pregnant, witnessed from the shore the drowning of her husband, a fisherman, during a storm. She was in a deplorable state of terror while watching his danger, and fainted when the catastrophe came. Long afterward she remained in feeble health. Her child, when born, was small and weakly, and turned out an idiot."

CASE 37.—"A woman, while pregnant, lost three of her children in one week of epidemic fever. Her grief and agitation at the time were excessive, overwhelming, and she continued in a state of deep depression, never quitting her bedroom till she was delivered, several months after the bereavement, being then in a wretched state of bodily health. Her child was an idiot when born, and her next and last child was stillborn."

CASE 38.—"A woman was in the sixth month of pregnancy when a great flood occurred, which threatened such danger to her and her family, that a boat was made fast to the door of her house, by which they were to escape if necessary. She and her children were for a short time left alone in the house ; and while thus situated, a tall man, unknown to her, dripping wet, and in apparent agitation, walked into her cottage, sat down by the fireside, and, after a few minutes, rose abruptly and left, never having spoken. She became most alarmingly terrified, and for several days could not be tranquilized. She sat watching the door for the re-appearance of what she regarded as a mysterious visitor, and screamed violently if

[1] *Trans. Obstet. Soc. Lond.*, vol. xxvi, p. 127.

any movement or sound could be interpreted by her fancy into an indication of his approach. The child's movements *in utero* were observed to be quick and violent, and she complained of the pain they gave her. It was not, however, born before the full term, and soon after birth was seen to be idiotic."

CASE 39.—"When in a state of pregnancy, a young woman was plunged into deep and protracted grief by the sudden and distressing death of her husband—a loaded cart having passed over him. She was left in extreme poverty, and to her grief was added anxiety about the maintenance of her children. Her bodily health suffered greatly. Her child, born at full term some months after the accident, was small at birth, and was soon recognized to be defective in mind."

CASE 40.—"A pregnant woman saw one of her children gored to death by a cow. Her mental disturbance and agitation were excessive, and could not be subdued or controlled. The motions of the fetus in this case are described as having been so intense as to give the woman and her friends alarm. Abortion was threatened, but did not occur. Her child is now a chronic idiot."

CASE 41.—"A woman was driving a dog-cart when the horse ran away. The vehicle was upset, and the accident caused the immediate death of the horse. The woman is said to have been physically uninjured, but she continued for a day or two in a state of abject terror, from which she could not be aroused. She was pregnant at the time, and her child, which was born about the full period, was partially paralyzed at birth, and is now a complete idiot. It is possible, of course, that in this case bodily injury may have been inflicted on the mother, though it was not perceived. The mental emotion, however, was certainly of a very unusual character, and it was the belief of the woman herself, and of her friends, that this accounted for the condition of her child."

These cases Mitchell cites as proof that "protracted violent mental excitement or deep mental impression may cause defects of the offspring." He has given the subject the most careful study, and "can see no reason why it should not be regarded as sufficient."

The effects and influences of heredity furnish very many

corroborative circumstances and conditions. Peculiarities of physical conformation, temperament, disposition, mental defects, and special characteristics, virtues, vices, and habits, are transmissible to the offspring. We recognize types that distinguish races, nations, communities, and families, and yet the inequalities and dissimilarities in the offspring of common parents are numerous and multiform, and everywhere, among all civilized nations, in all countries and climates, in every sphere of life and grade of society, in all trades, occupations, and professions, individuality is a characteristic of the human race. The special peculiarities which differentiate individuals may be inherited from either or both parents. We also know that mental and physical conditions acquired by the mother during the period of pregnancy may be inherited by the child. If a virtue or a vice, an idiosyncrasy, a mental defect or a habit, a disease, either inherited or acquired by the mother during pregnancy, can be transmitted to a fetus *in utero,* it does not seem any less possible that a shocking circumstance or observation occurring during the earlier months of utero-gestation, and continuously during the remaining months operating through its perturbating influences on her mind and constitution, should impress the fetus with its analogue. It is a well known fact that fright, anger, grief, or any sudden and violent mental shock, may so change and deteriorate the quality of the milk, especially during the earlier months of lactation, as not only to render it unfit for use, but quickly and fatally poisonous to the nursling.

In view of this classification of the cases, and the grouping of a few of the most striking, does it not appear manifest that I have established a basis for a reasonable belief in the relation of cause and effect between maternal impressions and fetal deformity ?

There are two theories in regard to the *modus operandi* of maternal impressions : One, and the more popular, is that they operate through the blood ; the other, through the nervous system. If there is any truth in the doctrine, it is more than probable that the detrimental influences are exercised in both ways. Food, medicines, poisons, and diseases are conveyed to the fetus *in utero.* Children have been born with measles, scarlet fever, small-pox, and other communicable diseases. Con-

13

genital chorea, hysteria, and epilepsy have been observed. There have been entire families of choreic persons, in which the disease has been propagated through several generations. Mothers, who had suffered a severe fright when advanced in pregnancy, have given birth to choreic children. The transmission of these nervous diseases is very rare ; but the transmission of a tendency to hysteria, chorea, and epilepsy, and of a special susceptibility of the nervous system, is very often demonstrable.

The most remarkable demonstration of the transmissibility of disease, and of the continuous duration of the predisposition through remote generations, has been made by Dr. Billings, in his recent address at Brighton, before the British Medical Association. He has shown that the prevalence of certain diseases, in certain localities in this country, is due to the fact that the population of these regions of country consists mainly of the descendants of emigrants of European races among which the diseases had been for an unlimited period very prevalent.

Thus, Mr. President, I have endeavored to present to you the evidences, some slight, some more positive, and others leading directly up to the conclusion which we desire to establish. I do not claim to have demonstrated the relation of cause and effect, but I hope I have presented the doctrine which Dr. Barker and myself maintain is tenable, in such manner as to command your favorable consideration.

DR. JOHN S. BILLINGS, of Washington, Honorary Member. —With regard to the question as to the influence of a pregnancy on the sex and other characteristics of the product of a subsequent pregnancy, we have almost no scientific information, for only scattered cases are reported. In order to establish a scientific basis, we must take into account not only exceptional cases, but the whole mass of cases, and get at the average results. If we could have statistics as to the sex, and the physical and mental peculiarities of the children, of women who have made two marriages and had children by each husband, we might have some scientific data. Such data can be obtained only by co-operative effort.

In the field of physiological experiment I need not point to the possibilities of control in this matter.

I do not consider it disadvantageous to bring up such a subject in a society of this kind, for it is occasionally well to get upon the outer boundaries of our knowledge, and obtain some conception of our ignorance on certain subjects. It is impossible to conceive of any explanation, according to the ordinary laws of physiology, of the influence which shall be exerted through connections with the mother upon an ovum, which has been fecundated and has been growing for two or three months, so as to produce some of the results reported this morning, such as the loss of fingers from the hand from pressure on the fingers of the mother, or the production of hare-lip from the sight of an individual having a hare-lip. If there is a direct causal connection, we must assume the existence of forces of which, as we have no scientific knowledge, the best thing is to recognize our ignorance on the subject, to make experiments where experimentation is feasible, to collect such facts as we can, and be content to admit that, on this subject as on many others, " we do not know."

Dr. Goodell, of Philadelphia.—I simply wish to say, that the case which I narrated this morning certainly staggered me. Before this I was a skeptic on the question of maternal impressions. Of course, I believed that strong maternal impressions, prior to conception, can mold the ovum both mentally and physically. Hence, the case reported this morning, of characteristics of the first husband transmitted to the offspring of the second husband, I can understand. It is merely a modified heredity. But the question of conveying maternal impressions to the body of a fetus which has already been conceived, and is in the process of development, that is a point on which I was skeptical, until my case of prenatal circumcision had to a certain extent converted me. There is one check upon that, however, and it is, that since then I have delivered a woman, who had no maternal impressions whatever, of a child that presented a very analogous condition. There had been apparently an amputation of the foreskin, and a red line indicated the cicatrix. But there was not, as in the first instance, the actual granulating surface of a raw sore.

Dr. Barker.—I have only a few remarks to make in closing the discussion. One point is, to correct an impression which

Dr. Billings seems to have had with regard to two cases.   In the case of the child who was born with the absence of fingers on the left hand, the mother had passed but a single menstrual period when the injury was received.   The other was the case in which there were marks in the ears.   The incident of the impression of the daughter's ears was in the first month of pregnancy, and so with all the cases, there was no evidence that the period since conception had been more than six or seven weeks.

For my own part, I reject as unscientific evidence all cases where pregnancy existed for three or four months before the mental impression was made.   The one with the hare-lip was the only one who had a strong anticipation of it ; in the others the deformity was not anticipated.

One other point, which was incidentally mentioned but not discussed, is with reference to the influence which may have been produced upon the ovary, and hence upon the ovum, months or years before fecundation.   In the Dundreary case, it was three or four years before impregnation occurred that the impression was made.

Dr. Chadwick moved that a committee of three be appointed to investigate this subject, and report at some subsequent meeting of the Society.   Carried.

ACKNOWLEDGMENTS

Rucker, M. Pierce. "An Eighteenth Century Method of Pain Relief in Obstetrics." *Journal of the History of Medicine and Allied Sciences* 5 (1950): 101–05. Reprinted with the permission of the *Journal of the History of Medicine and Allied Sciences*.

Simpson, J.Y. "Notes on the Employment of the Inhalation of Sulfuric Ether in the Practice of Midwifery." *Monthly Journal of Medical Science* 7, No.2 (1847): 721–28.

Playfair, W.S. "Anæsthesia in Labor." In *A Treatise on Science and Practice of Midwifery*. (Philadelphia: Lea Brothers & Co., 1885): 295–98.

Channing, Walter. "Introduction." *A Treatise on Etherization in Childbirth* (Boston: William D. Ticknor and Co., 1848): 1–25.

Duffy, John. "Anglo-American Reaction to Obstetrical Anesthesia." *Bulletin of the History of Medicine* 38 (1964): 32–44. Reprinted with the permission of Johns Hopkins University Press.

Farr, A.D. "Religious Opposition to Obstetric Anaesthesia: A Myth?" *Annals of Science* 40 (1983): 159–77. Reprinted with the permission of Taylor and Francis, Ltd.

Leavitt, Judith Walzer. "Birthing and Anesthesia: The Debate over Twilight Sleep." *Signs* 6, No.1 (1980): 147–64. Reprinted with the permission of the University of Chicago Press, publisher. Copyright 1980 University of Chicago Press.

Melzack, Ronald. "The Myth of Painless Childbirth." *Pain* 19 (1984): 321–37. Reprinted with the permission of Elsevier Science B.V.

Stewart, Duncan. "The Cæsarean Operation Done with Success by a Midwife." *Medical Essays and Observations* 5 (1752): 360–62.

Richmond, John L. "History of a Successful Case of Casarean Operation." *Western Journal of Medical and Physical Science* 3 (1830): 485–89.

Eastman, Nicholson J. "The Role of Frontier America in the Development of Cesarean Section." *American Journal of Obstetrics and Gynecology* 24 (1932): 919–29. Reprinted with the permission of Mosby Year Book, Inc.

Francome, Colin and Peter J. Huntingford. "Births by Caesarean Section in the United States of America and in Britain." *Journal of Biosocial Science* 12 (1980): 353–62. Reprinted with the permission of the Biosocial Society.

Enkin, Murray W. "Having a Section Is Having a Baby." *Birth and the Family Journal* 4, No.3 (1977): 99–102. Reprinted with the permission of Blackwell Scientific Publications, Inc.

Mandy, Arthur J., et al. "Is Natural Childbirth Natural?" *Psychosomatic Medicine* 14, No.6 (1952): 431–38. Reprinted with the permission of Williams & Wilkins.

Dick-Read, Grantly. "The Relief of Pain in Labour." *Western Journal of Surgery, Obstetrics and Gynecology* 62, No.12 (1954): 591–97. Reprinted with the permission of the California Medical Association.

Cosslett, Tess. "Grantley Dick Read and Sheila Kitzinger: Towards a Woman-Centred Story of Childbirth." *Journal of Gender Studies* 1, No.1 (1991): 29–43. Reprinted with the permission of the Carfax Publishing Company.

Felton, Gary S., and Florrie B. Segelman. "Lamaze Childbirth Training and Changes in Belief about Personal Control." *Birth and the Family Journal* 5, No.3 (1978): 141–50. Reprinted with the permission of Blackwell Scientific Publications, Inc.

Devitt, Neal. "The Transition from Home to Hospital Birth in the United States, 1930–1960." *Birth and the Family Journal* 4, No.2 (1977): 45–58. Reprinted with the permission of Blackwell Scientific Publications, Inc.

Silberman, Sara Lee. "Pioneering in Family-Centered Maternity and Infant Care: Edith B. Jackson and the Yale Rooming-In Research Project." *Bulletin of the History of Medicine* 64 (1990): 262–87. Reprinted with the permission of Johns Hopkins University Press.

Eakins, Pamela S. "The Rise of the Free Standing Birth Center: Principles and Practice." *Women and Health* 9, No.4 (1984): 49–64. Reprinted with the permission of Haworth Press, Inc. Copyright 1984.

Stewart, Mary, and Pat Erickson. "The Sociology of Birth: A

Critical Assessment of Theory and Research." *Social Science Journal* 14 (April 1977): 33–47. Reprinted with the permission of JAI Press, Inc.

Doering, Susan G., Doris R. Entwisle, and Daniel Quinlan. "Modeling the Quality of Women's Birth Experience." *Journal of Health and Social Behavior* 21 (1980): 12–21. Reprinted with the permission of the American Sociological Association.

O'Connor, Bonnie B. "The Home Birth Movement in the United States." *Journal of Medicine and Philosophy* 18 (1993): 147–74. Reprinted with the permission of Kluwer Academic Publishers.

Engelmann, George J. "Pregnancy, Parturition, and Childbed among Primitive People." *American Journal of Obstetrics* 14 (1881): 602–18; 828–47.

Blakely, Stuart B. "Superstitions in Obstetrics." *New York State Journal of Medicine* 22, No.3 (1922): 117–21. Reprinted with the permission of the Medical Society of the State of New York.

Snow, Loudell F., Shirley M. Johnson, and Harry E. Mayhew. "The Behavioral Implications of Some Old Wives' Tales." *Obstetrics and Gynecology* 51, No.6 (1978): 727–32. Reprinted with the permission of Elsevier Science Inc.

Wilson, Philip K. "'Out of Sight, Out of Mind?': The Daniel Turner–James Blondel Dispute over the Power of the Maternal Imagination." *Annals of Science* 49 (1992): 63–85. Reprinted with the permission of Taylor and Francis, Ltd.

Barker, Fordyce. "The Influence of Maternal Impressions on the Fetus." *Transactions of the American Gynecological Society* 11 (1887): 152–96.

EDITORS

Series Editor

Philip K. Wilson, MA, Ph.D., is an assistant professor of the history of science at Truman State University (formerly Northeast Missouri State University) in Kirksville, Missouri. After receiving his undergraduate degree in human biology from the University of Kansas, he pursued work towards an MA in medical history at the William H. Welch Institute for the History of Medicine at The Johns Hopkins School of Medicine and received his Ph.D. in the history of medicine from the University of London. He has held postdoctoral positions at the University of Hawaii-Manoa and Yale University School of Medicine before settling in Missouri.

Wilson has received scholarly support including a Logan Clendening Summer Fellowship, an Owsei Temkin Scholarship, a Folger Shakespeare Library Fellowship, a Wellcome Trust Research Scholarship, and grants from the Hawaii and Missouri Committees for the Humanities for medical and science history projects. He was a founding member of the Hawaii Society for the History of Medicine and Public Health. Wilson has contributed chapters to volumes including *The Popularization of Medicine 1650–1850* (Routledge), *Medicine in the Enlightenment* (Rodopi), and *The Secret Malady: Venereal Disease in Eighteenth-Century Britain and France* (University Press of Kentucky), articles in the *Annals of Science,* the *London Journal,* and the *Journal of the Royal Society of Medicine,* and is a regular contributor of medical and science history entries to many dictionaries and encyclopedias. Currently, Wilson is pursuing research on women's diseases, osteopathy, and eugenics in Kirksville, Missouri, where he lives with his wife, Janice, and son, James.

Assistant Editors

Ann Dally, MA, MD, received her Master's degree from Oxford University, having been an exhibitioner in modern history at Somerville College. She then studied medicine at St. Thomas' Hospital, London, qualifying in 1953. After some years of general medical practice, she specialized in psychiatry, a specialty she practiced until her retirement in 1994. Meanwhile she pursued her interests in the history of medicine, receiving her doctorate in that subject in 1993. The book based on her doctoral thesis, *Fantasy Surgery, 1880–1930,* will shortly be published as part of the Wellcome Institute for the History of Medicine (London) series. Her most recent book, *Women Under the Knife. A History of Surgery* (Routledge), follows a long publishing history of books including *The Morbid Streak, Why Women Fail, Mothers: Their Power and Influence, Inventing Motherhood: The Consequences of an Ideal,* and a book of memoirs, *A Doctor's Story.* Currently a Research Fellow at the Wellcome Institute for the History of Medicine (London), she lives with her husband Philip Egerton in West Sussex, England and has four children and seven grandchildren.

Charles R. King, MD, MA, is a professor of obstetrics and gynecology at the Medical College of Ohio. He received his BA from Kansas State University, an MD from the University of Kansas, and has completed post graduate medical training at the University of Kansas and the University of Oregon. He has since received an MA in medical history from the University of Kansas. King has been the recipient of Rockefeller Foundation, National Endowment for the Humanities, American College of Obstetricians and Gynecologists-Ortho, and Newberry Library Fellowships for projects in medical history. He is the author of numerous publications regarding women's health, including articles in the *Bulletin of the History of Medicine, Kansas History,* and the *Great Plains Quarterly,* and has recently completed *Child Health in America* (Twain). He currently lives with his wife, Lynn, in Temperance, Michigan.

DATE DUE

GAYLORD			PRINTED IN U.S.A.